Frontiers in Neurosurgery
(Volume 1)

NeuroEndovascular Challenges

Editor

Simone Peschillo M.D., Ph.D.

Department of Neurology and Psychiatry
Endovascular Neurosurgery/Interventional Neuroradiology
"Sapienza" University of Rome
Rome
Italy

CONTENTS

FOREWORD

This well written book shows the fascinating evolution and rapid growth of the discipline of endovascular neurosurgery from the early pioneering days until today. In a Pindaric flight, it comes to my mind that the early pioneering days of endovascular therapy resemble the work carried out in a garage by Wozniak and Jobs at the beginning of the Apple era, as the worked to create a revolutionary computer. In our discipline I was part, together with a few fellow enthusiasts, of the "garage work" of our discipline and, although now retired, I cannot resist in keeping myself au courant on the progeniture that came from that early work. I am happy that the young generation of interventionalists, leveraging from the work of pioneers, is so active and inclined to improvement. This book clearly depicts how our discipline inexorably evolved step by step to form a marvellous, revolutionary, and exciting era. The vast majority of aneurysms, for example, are nowadays treated by the endovascular approach, worldwide. Cooperation between physicians and industry is a key factor leading to advancement. Enthusiasm and academic work also play a pivotal role.

This book is enlightening in that it spans from the history (outstandingly presented by the Editor) to the most recent technical advancements (superbly portrayed by the authors of chapter VII). Given the fast pace and creativity of the young generation of physicians and engineers, one may rightly think that the best is still to come! In my days I used to say: "largo ai giovani!" (give way to the young people!).

This book teaches and confirms that, differently from the past, the current evaluation of novel techniques and devices (and the consequent clinical impact) is no longer based on personal, often irrational, opinions or, worse, "gut feelings". On the contrary, nowadays multicenter studies and clinical trials allow for a more rational, scientifically sound, empirically accurate and fact-based way of evaluation, influencing the decision making process in a positive and logical manner.

Undeniably, treatment of brain arteriovenous malformations constitutes, by tradition, a setback in our discipline, that often, but not always, leads to dissatisfaction and to the impossibility to cure, even with the more recent embolic agents. It is my opinion that in any kind of neuroendovascular disease, the use of liquid agents (namely glue) implies a significant degree of uncontrollability, and carries a not negligeable risk of incurring in "problems". This is not a good thing.

On a similar topic, this book provides in the appendix, with good reason, an always welcomed description of the "dangerous anastomosis", tacitly reiterating the importance of not injecting glue in particular areas of the vascular tree.

This book offers a well documented, extensive, and up to date panorama of the revascularization techniques utilized in acute ischemic insults. This is a field in continuous evolution that already allows tremendous results in brain salvaging endeavors.

The in depth, analytic, and accurate description of the complex issue of double antiplatetet therapy in neuroendovascular procedures provides highly valuable information and practical guidelines.

On a personal note, I would like to reiterate that our procedures should not be called "minimally invasive", specially when interacting with patients and their families. It may give a false sense of an innocuous, easy procedure. Instead, our procedures, although less invasive than surgery, are indeed invasive: in fact the reality is that they may become very complex, treacherous, and potentially life-threatening.

I would like to congratulate the Editor, Simone Peschillo, M.D., Ph.D, and all the other authors for giving our community a precious instrument of knowledge.

Guido Guglielmi, M.D.
Department of Interventional Neuroradiology
University of California at Los Angeles
Los Angeles, California
USA

PREFACE

An appreciation of the history of vascular and endovascular neurosurgery requires a journey that starts far from the modern age, in the ancient past. Undeniable traces can be uncovered more than 2700 years before Christ, when the first description of an arterial aneurysm was made. From that moment on, neurosurgery matured through the millennia toward a discipline which, during the last century, has seen tremendous advancements.

This particular history is scattered with both anecdotal and fascinating events, which led the first neurosurgeons to develop increasingly complex techniques, and also to take risks and, not uncommonly, to make hazardous choices. Passing through the era of pure extravascular extracranial approaches, vascular neurosurgery evolved toward ever less invasive procedures making its way through the intracranial and finally into the endovascular space.

We symbolically fixed the year in which modern endovascular neurosurgery was born as 1927: this was the year in which a Portuguese professor of neurology, Egas Moniz, performed the first cerebral angiography marking the beginning of the endovascular era.

As the product of different disciplines, endovascular neurosurgery matured thanks to the efforts of pioneers from different domains in medical sciences. Initially, endovascular intracranial navigation was exclusively guided by blood flow; subsequently, magnetically guided devices, among others, made their appearance and were followed by the modern micro-catheters equipped with guide-wires which finally allowed arterial bifurcations to be negotiated. An undeniable contribution was provided by Serbinenko, the father of the detachable balloon embolization technique. Nevertheless, when an Italian neurosurgeon, Guido Guglielmi, presented his endovascular detachable coil embolization system in 1991, everything changed and endovascular neurosurgery was endowed with new perspectives.

None of this would have been possible without those ground-breakers whose effort, dedication and passion made massive contributions to vascular and endovascular neurosurgery as we know it. During the past 10 years, the most remarkable advances have been made in embolization of cerebral aneurysms, arteriovenous malformations and stroke treatment.

Endovascular techniques are less invasive than other forms of neurosurgery; however, endovascular neurosurgery is becoming more complicated as the technology is becoming more sophisticated. In the early stage, a single microcatheter was required to deliver a coil into an aneurysm. Nowadays, the artery is usually congested with multiple catheters, balloons or stents for the treatment of challenging aneurysms.

The current situation presents the neurosurgical community with the dualism of "open surgery versus endovascular treatment" for the management of intracranial cerebrovascular disease. Endovascular neurosurgery is, however, rapidly delineating an exclusive domain in neurosurgery and most contemporary authors already no longer consider the dualism in terms of opposition but rather in terms of synergy.

The history of endovascular neurosurgery has gifted the authors of this book, and we hope the readers too, with the inspiration required for the pro-active creation of a better future. This very particular history encourages us to pursue innovation regardless of currently shared convictions and dogmas. It teaches us that scientists must broaden their horizons, crossing the boundaries existing between different disciplines, seeking innovation by treading as yet unbeaten paths. Modern medical science is moving toward an increasingly hyper-specialized universe, in which the galaxies cross each other very rarely. And yet, an intersection between the galaxies is essential for further development. For the very same reason, young neurosurgeons should make efforts to broaden their range of feasible therapeutic options grasping, for instance, both the art of the catheter as well as the art of the knife.

The target audience of this e-book includes endovascular neurosurgeons, vascular neurosurgeons, neuroradiologists and neurologists. The detailed and comprehensive nature of the book makes it most suitable for practicing endovascular and vascular neurosurgeons who have a solid knowledge of neuroangiography. This is not an introductory level text on the neurosciences: the Editor's and authors' intent is to share information they feel is useful for the performance of endovascular neurosurgery. The rapid growth in the number of those performing endovascular neurosurgery is evidence of the need for such a book.

The main idea of this work is to trigger discussion on the principal issues that are still debated in this field, and not to reiterate the same topics that are easily found in other texts.

ACKNOWLEDGEMENTS

The editor would like to thank all the authors for the excellent work done. Furthermore, special thanks goes to Guido Guglielmi, M.D., Alessandro Caporlingua. M.D. and Antonio Santodirocco M.D.

Simone Peschillo, M.D., Ph.D.
Department of Neurology and Psychiatry
Endovascular Neurosurgery/Interventional Neuroradiology
"Sapienza" University of Rome
Rome
Italy
E-mail: simone.peschillo@gmail.com

List of Contributors

Alain Bonafé	Centre Hospitalier Universitaire Gui de Chauliac, Montpellier, France
Alberto Debernardi	Department of Neurorsurgery, Niguarda Ca' Granda Hospital, Milan, Italy
Alessandro Caporlingua	Department of Neurology and Psychiatry, Neurosurgery, "Sapienza" University of Rome, Rome, Italy
Antonio Santodirocco	Department of Neurology and Psychiatry, Interventional Neuroradiology, "Sapienza" University of Rome, Rome, Italy
Antonio Santoro	Department of Neurology and Psychiatry, Neurosurgery, "Sapienza" University of Rome, Rome, Italy
Arani Bose	Interventional Neuroradiologist, New York, USA and Penumbra Inc., Alameda, California, USA
Claudio Colonnese	Department of Neurology and Psychiatry, Neuroradiology, "Sapienza" University of Rome, Rome, Italy
Dave Barry	Penumbra Inc., Alameda, California, USA
Delia Cannizzaro	Department of Neurology and Psychiatry, Neurosurgery, "Sapienza" University of Rome, Rome, Italy
Emanuele Orrù	Neuroradiology Service, University Hospital of Padua, Padua, Italy
Fabio M. Pulcinelli	Department of Experimental Medicine, "Sapienza" University of Rome, Rome, Italy
Federico Caporlingua	Department of Neurology and Psychiatry, Neurosurgery, "Sapienza" University of Rome, Rome, Italy
Filippo Pecorari	Department of Cardiovascular, Respiratory, Nephrologic, Anesthesiology and Geriatric Sciences, "Sapienza" University, Rome, Italy
Flavia Temperilli	Department of Experimental Medicine, "Sapienza" University of Rome, Rome, Italy
Francesco Causin	Neuroradiology Service, University Hospital of Padua, Padua, Italy
Gianluigi Guarnieri	Neuroradiology Service, AO Cardarelli Hospital, Naples, Italy
Giorgio Re	Department of Cardiovascular, Respiratory, Nephrologic, Anesthesiology and Geriatric Sciences, "Sapienza" University, Rome, Italy
Giovanni Rosa	Department of Cardiovascular, Respiratory, Nephrologic, Anesthesiology and Geriatric Sciences, "Sapienza" University, Rome, Italy

Guglielmo Pero   Department of Neuroradiology, Niguarda Ca' Granda Hospital, Milan, Italy

Italia La Rosa   Department of Cardiovascular, Respiratory, Nephrologic, Anesthesiology and Geriatric Sciences, "Sapienza" University, Rome, Italy

John Lockhart   Penumbra Inc., Alameda, California, USA

Joseph Gabrieli   Neuroradiology Service, University Hospital of Padua, Padua, Italy

Kiriakos Lobotesis   Imperial College Healthcare NHS, London, United Kingdom

Marco Cenzato   Department of Neurorsurgery, Niguarda Ca' Granda Hospital, Milan, Italy

Mario Muto   Neuroradiology Service, AO Cardarelli Hospital, Naples, Italy

Paolo Machì   Centre Hospitalier Universitaire Gui de Chauliac, Montpellier, France

Roberto Delfini   Department of Neurology and Psychiatry, Neurosurgery, "Sapienza" University of Rome, Rome, Italy

Simone Peschillo   Department of Neurology and Psychiatry, Endovascular Neurosurgery/Interventional Neuroradiology, "Sapienza" University of Rome, Rome, Italy

Sophia S. Kuo   Penumbra Inc., Alameda, California, USA

2

Frontiers in Neurosurgery, Vol. 1, 2015, 3-32

CHAPTER 1

Introduction: The New Era of Endovascular Treatment

A. Caporlingua[1], C. Colonnese[2] and S. Peschillo[3,*]

[1]Department of Neurology and Psychiatry, Neurosurgery, "Sapienza" University of Rome, Rome, Italy; [2]Department of Neurology and Psychiatry, Neuroradiology, "Sapienza" University of Rome, Rome, Italy; [3]Department of Neurology and Psychiatry, Endovascular Neurosurgery/Interventional Neuroradiology, "Sapienza" University of Rome, Rome, Italy

Abstract: This introductory chapter provides the readers with an insight into the history of neuroendovascular surgery. Acknowledging the past is of the utmost importance to understanding and interpreting present dynamics and future directions in such a young, yet quickly evolving medical field. Starting from ancient history with the first descriptions of cerebral aneurysms, we describe the era of the extravascular approach to cerebrovascular disease with a focus on the main techniques conceived such as arterial ligation, aneurysm wrapping, trapping and packing. With the invention of the aneurysmal clip, the direct surgical approach to cerebral aneurysms gained a privileged place in the management of intracranial vascular disease which it retained throughout most of the second half of the 20th century. Nevertheless, marked by the invention of cerebral angiography, the endovascular era symbolically began in 1927. Ingenious, sometimes bizarre and hazardous, endovascular approaches to cerebrovascular disease are recounted, touching the history of the evolution of endovascular techniques, embolic materials and navigation devices. Modern neuroendovascular surgery is described with a focus on the development of coil technology which represents an essential milestone as it gave a massive impulse toward the birth of a new subspecialty in neurosurgery. At the end of the chapter we discuss how the training of young neurosurgeons is changing and should cope with these new acquisitions. The role of neuroendovascular surgery in neurosurgical residency programs is summarized for the United States, Japan and Europe. Should this be part of the neurosurgeon's armamentarium? Could it be delegated completely to the neurointerventional radiologist or might it be best part of a completely new specialty?

Keywords: Cerebrovascular disease, history, interventional, neuroradiology, stroke, subarachnoid hemorrhage.

The concept of endovascular therapy emerged at the beginning of the 20th century thanks to the sparkling ideas of pioneers who conceived innovative approaches to

***Corresponding author S. Peschillo:** Department of Neurology and Psychiatry, Endovascular Neurosurgery/ Interventional Neuroradiology, "Sapienza" University of Rome, Rome, Italy; Tel/Fax: +390649979185; E-mail: simone.peschillo@gmail.com*

yet unsolved medical problems. The ability to cross boundaries between different disciplines, to make innovations and, ultimately, to create a new field of medical interest is what led to the birth of neuroendovascular surgery. In this introductory chapter we would like to take the readers on a journey through history to acknowledge the efforts of these pioneers and to describe how different disciplines such as neurosurgery and neuroradiology, among others, have actively influenced the evolution of the treatment of cerebrovascular disease [1]. What makes this historical journey so important is that it shows unequivocally that the training of the people carrying out such treatment must necessarily be part of a multidisciplinary curriculum embracing neurosurgery as well as neuro-endovascular surgery, "mastering the knife as well as the catheter" [2].

The first known description of an arterial aneurysm, contained in the Ebers Papyrus, dates back to 2725 BC. According to this archeological document, Egyptian physicians performed surgical explorations with instruments previously cauterized with fire [3]. A physician from Ephesus, Flaenius Rufus, wrote about the risk of post-traumatic arterial dilatation in 117 BC [4, 5]. Galen himself (AD 129-210), a Roman physician born in Pergamum, whose principles based on the then-current humorism influenced Western medicine for thirteen centuries until the work of Vesalio, described the entity of aneurysm [6]. Although during ancient history numerous descriptions and documented observations clarified the nature and features of arterial aneurysms, the correlation between cerebral aneurysms and subarachnoid hemorrhage is relatively recent. During the 1600s and 1700s forensic studies conducted on patients, often socially highly placed or even political figures whose death was sudden and inexplicable, led to the proposal that cerebral aneurysms could be a possible cause of subarachnoid hemorrhage. In 1680 Dionis described the cases of the Duke of Aurelia and the Prince of Espinoy, both of whom died suddenly. Autopsies revealed that the cerebral ventricles were distended with a "sanguineous extravasation of blood" in both cases [7]. Later, in 1818, Blackall described the anatomical features of ruptured cerebral aneurysms ruling out any suspicion of poisoning in the case of the sudden death of the Crown Prince Charles August which led to a new royal dynasty in Sweden in the early 19th century [8]. In 1761, the Italian researcher Morgagni of Padua described dilatations of both posterior branches of the carotid arteries which may very well have been aneurysms [9] and Biumi, another Italian, described a ruptured intracavernous carotid aneurysm found at an autopsy in Milan in 1765 [10].

Decades passed until a therapeutic approach was offered for the management of such a delicate condition. As sometimes happens, the first step toward innovation was taken by someone who would see the potential benefit of an already existing surgical technique to approach a then untreatable condition. Nowadays the term "Hunterian ligation", born at the end of the 18th century and consecrated in 1835 [11], refers to a surgical technique of arterial ligation but it is also used to designate the period of its major success for the management of peripheral vascular lesions. The surgeon and scientist, John Hunter (1728-1793), described a case of false symptomatic popliteal aneurysm whose rupture on the fifth day after a first attempt of classical proximal ligation at its neck was the motive for an ipsilateral femoral artery ligation. After his first procedure, in December 1785, Hunter carried out four more documented procedures. Three were successful with one patient surviving for 50 years thereafter [12]. Despite that, the first reports of peripheral vascular ligation are even older. Ambroise Paré in 1552 is credited with the first documented operative carotid artery and internal jugular vein ligation [12, 13]. Later available reports date from two centuries after that of Paré's, such as the case treated by Abernathy, a pupil of John Hunter, who ligated the carotid artery of a man whose neck was gored by the horns of a cow in 1798; this case, published not before 1804, is considered the first ever reported in English literature [14-18]. Jean Louis Petit, according to Cutter, was the first to state that the brain could survive even without the contribution of one carotid artery, pointing the way toward elective carotid artery ligation for conditions other than injury. He made his observations in a patient with an aneurysm of the common carotid artery who he had followed for 7 years. When the patient died, at autopsy Petit found complete thrombotic occlusion of the affected common carotid artery without any reason to believe this was the cause of death [17]. In 1793 the first elective carotid artery ligation with survival was performed and reported by Hebenstreit [16, 17]. Only a few years later, when its potential was finally grasped, this procedure was used in the management of aneurysms of the cervical carotid artery. In 1803 Cogswell was the first to apply a ligature to the carotid artery in order to treat a carotid aneurysm [19]; others were to follow. Cooper (1768-1841) reported detailed accounts of two of his patients afflicted by cervical carotid artery aneurysms treated at Guy's Hospital between 1805 and 1809. The first, published in 1806, was that of a 44-year old woman whose aneurysm was so voluminous that she presented with dysphagia, a violent cough and an evident, swollen formation occupying two-thirds of her neck. After surgical ligation of the common carotid artery the patient developed hemiplegia on the 8th post-operative day and then eventually died on the 21st day of respiratory failure [20]. The following patient, a 50-year old porter, came to Cooper's attention in July 1808;

this patient's aneurysm of the left internal carotid artery (ICA) was considerably less advanced than the one in the previous patient. Presenting with the size of a walnut it was successfully treated by proximal ligation of the common carotid artery; the patient was able to return to his former occupation and was seen in a healthy condition 8 months after the procedure. Interestingly, Cooper already noted how, despite its evolution being arrested, the aneurysm continued to be filled with blood by retrograde flow [21]. In 1811, Cooper's colleague at Guy's Hospital, Travers (1783-1858) first reported the successful treatment of a carotid-cavernous fistula by ligature of the common carotid artery in a 34-year old pregnant woman, carried out in 1809. Portraits of the patient, before and 2 years after the procedure, clearly show the outcome in this particular case [22]. It was an accidental finding that led Horsley (1857-1916) to attempt the first carotid artery ligation for the management of a giant intracranial middle fossa aneurysm initially mistaken for a tumor [23]. A later report by Keen confirmed that the patient operated upon by Horsley was in "extremely good condition" 5 years after surgery [24].

Considerable efforts were made during the early 20th century to perfect ligation techniques to minimize complications such as infections, neurological morbidity in patients with a malformed or incomplete circle of Willis and above all thromboembolic accidents, often due to intimal damage caused by the ligature itself. In 1905, Halstead tested aluminum strips which would slowly tighten around a band embracing the ligated artery enabling gradual occlusion of the vessel [25]; in a seemingly similar way Matas used aluminum bands with a slowly tightening mechanism to test the efficiency of collateral circulation prior to permanent occlusion [26]. Perthes and Nasette proposed autologous fascia as the material for the bands used to prevent intimal damage induced by sutures on the arterial wall [27]; occlusion by application of particular clamps was introduced [28]. In 1950 Poppen's sequential placation technique of the carotid artery, which considerably reduced arterial intimal damage, was described and used on 50 patients who survived for more than 3 years after the procedure [29, 30].

Carotid ligation remained the most reliable and consistently used technique in the management of intracranial aneurysms at the beginning of the 20th century and reports describing it continued to be published even during the second half of the 1900s [31-35]. In 1966 Tonnis and Walter published a review based on a series of cases of carotid artery ligation for intracranial aneurysms collected between 1933-1960; they reported a mortality rate of 3-41% and significant morbidity mainly associated with high rates of post-operative infection and thrombosis [36].

Although later reports described mortality rates below 20% [30, 37] it was clear that a transition toward an intracranial approach was inevitable.

A mere accident prevented Zeller in 1911 from being the first person to successfully perform intracranial carotid artery occlusion for the treatment of a cavernous carotid fistula. Unfortunately his assistant accidentally pulled the ligature applied to the ICA with subsequent massive and regrettably fatal hemorrhage [38]. Twenty-two years had to pass to see the first carotid-cavernous fistula treated with success by Hamby and Gardner [39]. Intracranial surgery opened new horizons for the management of aneurysms, providing the possibility of directly manipulating the aneurysm itself and its parent vessel by trapping, wrapping and, ultimately, clipping techniques. Although Dr. Harvey W. Cushing's had a pessimistic attitude toward the surgical management of aneurysms of the circle of Willis and completely disagreed about Hunterian carotid ligation techniques, not unreasonably considered as "futile" or even "foolish", a review of Cushing's personal, meticulously organized, patients' records uncovered a few cases of intracranial aneurysms among those of brain tumors, these latter being Cushing's predilection [40]. In his "Little Black Book" describing personally performed operations, in the section dedicated to patients suspected of harboring a brain tumor, nine were discovered to have intracranial aneurysms during surgery. His notorious "exploratory craniotomies" in these patients revealed pulsating tumors, then correctly identified as aneurysms, which he used to puncture arbitrarily, not without apprehension, with a lumbar needle after ipsilateral cervical carotid artery ligation. He would then pack the aneurysm immediately and wrap it with strands of muscle, which he commonly used for general hemostatic purposes, to block the inevitable massive hemorrhage following clot removal from the aneurysmal sac. Norman McComish Dott (1897-1973), one of Cushing's residents, is considered to be the first to plan and perform a craniotomy for a ruptured intracranial aneurysm. His patient, a 54-year old man suffering from recurrent spontaneous subarachnoid hemorrhage, underwent surgery after the third hemorrhage on the 22nd of April, 1931: he was in a coma and chances of success were poor. A bleeding 3-mm aneurysm of the ICA bifurcation was isolated and steadily wrapped in muscle for twelve minutes and a subtemporal decompression was performed. The following day the patient was awake and able to speak. Until his death, which occurred eleven years after, no others hemorrhagic events were reported [41]. Building on the success of wrapping techniques, Tonnis and Jefferson added their contribution on the subject in the literature [42, 43].

Six years after Dott's famous operation, Walter E. Dandy (1886-1946) gave a further impulse to cerebrovascular surgery. Although better known for the introduction of pneumoventriculography and his studies on hydrocephalus, Dandy's contribution to vascular surgery is undeniable [44-46]. In 1935 he published his results on the treatment of carotid cavernous sinus fistula, at that time commonly referred to as pulsating exophthalmos, using a trapping technique consisting of the isolation of the fistulous communication by ligation of the cervical carotid artery and clipping of the intracranial ICA just before its bifurcation. The purpose was to induce thrombosis somewhere in the vascular apparatus participating in the fistula, thus interrupting it. Further publications about trapping techniques followed, with reports from Poppen [30], Logue [47] and Tindall [48]. However what made Dandy stand out as the father of modern vascular neurosurgery was the first planned direct clipping procedure for intracranial aneurysm performed on the 23rd March, 1937. For the purpose he used a Cushing silver clip, originally introduced by the aforementioned in 1911 for hemostatic purposes during surgery for brain tumors [49] and subsequently modified by McKenzie to satisfy Dandy's particular requirements. The patient, a 43-year old alcoholic, presented with third oculomotor nerve palsy, right frontal headache, right eye pain, diplopia and right ptosis. Suspecting an aneurysm of the circle of Willis, Dandy decided to perform a right "hypophyseal approach" (frontotemporal craniotomy) hoping to find a right ICA or a posterior communicating artery aneurysm. His supposition, based solely on clinical observation, was correct: a "pea-sized" ICA aneurysm with a narrow neck, developing right next to the posterior communicating artery, was exposed and successfully clipped [27, 46].

Although clip technology has improved greatly throughout history until the present day, the basic principles of Dandy's technique remained unchanged. In 1949 Duane changed Cushing's V-shape clip to a new U-shape clip, improving clipping efficiency [50]; Norlèn and Olivecrona made the clip adjustable and above all repositionable [51]. A temporary clip for arterial occlusion was developed by Schwartz in 1950; this clip, called a cross-action alpha clip, was later modified by Mayfield in 1971 to achieve better ergonomics and handling of the applicator while preserving the possibility of removing the clip if needed, thus allowing trial and error in clip placement [52]. Fenestrated clips were introduced starting from the original Mayfield-Kees clip by Drake, giving birth to the Drake-Kees clip [53, 54]. Among the numerous variants of aneurysmal clips, Sundt designed the so-called encircling clip-graft [55] which enables the repair of diseased major intracranial arterial branches. The Housepian clip, safer and controllable during deployment, was introduced during 1976 [53]. In the same year a major contribution to vascular neurosurgery was given by Sugita with the development of a bayoneted clip which provided better visualization and maneuverability during clip application [56]. Sugita is also credited with the introduction of many neurosurgical instruments such as the surgical microscope and the operative chair and table [57]. Microsurgical techniques evolved rapidly not only due to such technological assets but also thanks to a better understanding and awareness of microsurgical anatomy provided by gifted neurosurgeons such as Yasargil, who meticulously refined microsurgical approaches and techniques thus undeniably improving outcomes of these extremely difficult operations [58].

Concomitantly with the evolution of extravascular therapeutic approaches to cerebral aneurysms and vascular malformations, pioneering and, one may say, hazardous attempts were made to take the endovascular route to deliver innovative therapeutic solutions. Experimental results on intra-arterial thrombosis induced by metallic devices such as needles date back to 1831 with Velpeau [59] and Phillips, the latter suggesting an even faster thrombotic reaction if an electric current was applied to the needle [60]. Following these early generic results, subsequent reports on the use of endovascular techniques can be traced to the beginning of the 20th century. In 1904, Dawbarn, with his so-called "starvation operation" was the first to use an embolic agent, liquid paraffin in the specific instance, to embolize a malignant tumor in the region of the external carotid artery [61]. Although seemingly a reasonable strategy, "starving" a tumor growing in an anatomical area fed by so many anastomotic arterial branches was soon found to be futile, as Dawbarn himself was to point out [62].

The dawn of the endovascular era is historically rooted in 1927. In the early 1920s no-one really considered that it would be possible to undertake radiographic imaging of the brain in a living human subject. The only approach available was Dandy's method of introducing air into the ventricular system [46]. Pneumoventriculography provided distorted, faint images of the cerebral ventricles: the brain itself could not be seen. Unfortunately this procedure did not come without cost. The patient, strapped to a chair, put in awkward positions and even turned upside down, endured agony and pain; vomiting and headache were common side effects. Egas Moniz, professor of neurology in Lisbon, Portugal, supposed that a radiopaque material, introduced and accumulated in the brain would opacify its structure making it visible on X-ray films [63]. Affected by gout since the age of 24 he could not perform any neurosurgical procedures, even the ones he had personally developed, because of the deformities caused by his illness. In his book entitled "Confidências de um Investigador Científico" (Confidences of a scientific researcher), he describes, in a detailed and personal style, the several steps leading to the discovery of cerebral angiography. He performed numerous experiments in dogs and then cadavers prior to his first *in vivo* attempt. The procedure was technically difficult given the technology available at that time: after the injection of the contrast agent directly into the carotid artery, it was possible to take only three films in sequence, hand pulled [64]. Building on the inspiration drawn from the work of Sicard on iodized oil myelography for the study of spinal cord compression [65], Moniz initially used angiography for the diagnosis of intracranial tumors [66]. In 1933 he published an article demonstrating how this new method could be used for the diagnosis of cerebral aneurysms. Interestingly, Moniz was awarded with the Nobel Prize in 1949 not for the invention of cerebral angiography, but for the development of a surgical procedure known as "pre-frontal lobe leucotomy" used for the treatment of mental disorders and subsequently discarded. Quickly understanding the dramatic advances afforded by cerebral angiography as a diagnostic tool, the first to capitalize on Moniz's revolutionizing invention was Dott, who established a laboratory in Edinburgh equipped to perform such procedures and on 24th March, 1933 produced the first angiogram demonstrating a cerebral aneurysm [41]. More than a decade later Radner performed the first vertebral angiography through catheterization of a surgically exposed and ligated radial artery [67].

Barney Brooks from Nashville is widely reported to be the first person to attempt an endovascular treatment for a carotid cavernous sinus fistula (CCSF) with a strip of free muscle released in the ICA in 1930. It was hoped that the blood flow would propel the embolus to the fistulous opening, leading to embolization [68]. Although universally considered as the father of the thereafter so-called "Brooks method", discrepancies have been recently highlighted discrediting Brooks contribution to the treatment of CCSF [69, 70]. According to Vitek and Smith the first to describe embolization of CCSF were Hamby and Gardner in 1933. Following what they considered the Brooks method they reported on the use of a pea-sized piece of muscle clamped with a silver clip to provide radio-traceability in the ICA after temporarily occluding the common carotid artery. Following the operation the typical "bruit" initially disappeared, but recurred faintly only three days later. Two months after they had to ligate the ICA and only at this point did the bruit disappear completely and permanently. They cured the CCSF, but the patency of the ICA could not be preserved [39].

The first report on the use of a catheter to treat a CCSF dates back to 1964, even though the procedure was materially performed in 1962 by Speakman. The patient, a 27-year old woman suffering from a post-traumatic CCSF, was treated with an extravascular approach by staged trapping procedures consisting of an initial gradual occlusion of the affected left cervical common carotid artery with a Selverstone clamp then replaced by ligatures to minimize the risk of neurological complications such as hemiparesis and aphasia; subsequently a left frontal craniotomy allowed the left ICA and ophthalmic arteries to be clipped. Two months later, the patient's symptoms recurred. A catheter was then pushed inside the ICA (catheter technology at that time prevented Speakman from reaching the point of the fistula endovascularly) and marked pieces of Gelfoam were released in the blood flow under radiographic control. The dimensions of these pieces of Gelfoam, designed specifically for the purpose, allowed them to stick to the point of the fistula, definitively curing it [71]. A few years later a Japanese author, Ishimori, described a similar technique in two successfully cured cases but he used Gelfoam marked with a gold film [72]. In 1970, Isamat is credited with the first successfully performed embolization of a post-traumatic CCSF with reported ICA patency in an 86-year old woman. Given the patient's age, frailty and numerous comorbidities the intervention had to be as simple as possible: all classical aggressive treatment options were immediately rejected and artificial embolization by marked autologous muscle was adopted. The embolus was released through a modest arteriotomy performed on a clamped segment of the external carotid artery. When the proximal clamp was removed, the small piece of omohyoid muscle with a clip attached to it was immediately propelled in the ICA. In this case systemic hypertension worked in science's favor because an enormous pressure gradient between the ICA and the cavernous sinus led the muscle right to the point of the fistula. The patency of the ICA was demonstrated by angiography after the procedure. Unfortunately the patient, free of any neurological deficits or ocular complaints, eventually died from heart failure a few weeks after the procedure [73].

At this point of our history it was rather common to see neurosurgeons treat cerebrovascular disease with combined extravascular and intravascular approaches. The aforementioned Harvey W. Cushing, after surgical ligation of the common carotid artery, used to open the sac of surgically exposed cerebral aneurysms packing them with muscle strands and wrapping then with autologous muscle, thereby using extravascular and transfundal approaches [40]. Packing techniques were often used as an emergency measure when dealing with accidental intraoperative aneurysm rupture. Performed through the transfundal route, this clearly required an open surgical approach. Gardner used cotton sponges to pack a giant ICA aneurysm initially thought to be a brain tumor [74]. Differently from Gardner, in 1942 Walter E. Dandy, faced with an unclippable giant cavernous ICA aneurysm, decided to introduce silk sutures inside its sac; persistent filling observed during re-intervention 5 days later necessitated the use of the canonical trapping technique [75].

Although the basic principles of packing evolved during the following decades, the idea of filling the aneurysmal sac with an embolic material needed to be further refined and ultimately the route taken to deliver the embolus changed from the transfundal route to the endovascular route thanks to the development of new and reliable endovascular navigation techniques. Following Phillips' experiments [60], Werner attempted electrothrombosis, or rather electrothermic coagulation, by the transfundal approach for a giant ICA aneurysm so voluminous that it was eroding the orbital roof of a 15-year old girl who had not responded to any canonical trapping or extravascular approach attempted thus far. He introduced 9 m of silver enameled wire after a transorbital puncture of the aneurysmal sac passing laterally from the retracted ocular globe. Heat was applied for 40 seconds at 80 °C. The young patient recovered from the intervention with no further reported recurrence [76]. Further steps toward modern endovascular embolization were taken by Luessenhop and Spence in 1960. They performed intraoperative catheterization of the cervical ICA through a ligated branch of the external carotid artery and then deliberately released hand-made spheres of methacrylate, a polymerizing plastic, in the blood flow to embolize a brain arteriovenous malformation (bAVM). The rationale behind this seemingly hazardous procedure was to take advantage of pathological hemodynamics. In other words it was supposed that the spheres would more likely be sucked into the bAVM nidus than into the normal brain circulation. The problem was that it could not be known at which point during embolization the spheres would be propelled in normal arterial branches giving the progressive nidus embolization and reduced "sump effect"; disastrous effects were to be feared. Luckily the patient tolerated the procedure and after ligature of the exposed ICA he awakened without any neurological morbidity [77, 78]. A few years later Sano [79] and Boulos [80] described a similar technique to treat arteriovenous malformations, but they used different materials such as polymerizing silicone known also as "liquid plastic", silicon spheres, pieces of dura or polyvinyl alcohol foam particles.

Finding the right embolic agent was not an easy task and extravagant solutions were not uncommonly taken into consideration. For instance Kerber described as primitive embolic materials other than autologous muscle or fat, ground up sponges or even pellets retrieved from disassembled shot gun shells [78]. In 1963 Gallagher reported the first case of cerebral aneurysm treated with "pilojection" [81]. Using a transfundal approach, thrombosis of an anterior cerebral artery aneurysm was achieved using shafts of hog hair literally shot at high velocity with a pneumatic "pilojector gun" into the aneurysm sac. Although this particular patient died from a thrombotic accident following carotid arteriography, Gallagher treated another 16 patients using this method in 1963 including a case of arteriovenous malformation of the spinal cord. In 1965 Mullan conceived a method which avoided open surgery by craniotomy to achieve aneurysm thrombosis, thus improving outcomes in patients during the early period following a subarachnoid hemorrhage. After successful experiments conducted on artificially induced aneurysms of the femoral artery in dogs [82], he proposed a technique which consisted of the insertion of a special steel electrode with an exquisitely sharp end through a burr hole, guided under biplanar radiographic control, into the aneurysm sac. Once the aneurysm had been punctured, an electric current applied for a variable period depending on each particular case (from 62 to 390 minutes!) would not only trigger electrothrombosis, but also erode the tip of the electrode by electrolysis after a certain amount of time (usually 15 minutes) allowing safe retraction of the needle at the end of the process. However Mullan did not consider his technique as a stand-alone procedure; its primary objective was the prevention of early recurrent hemorrhage making it a bridging intervention to a subsequent clipping procedure. It was clear that without an embolic material permanently deployed in the aneurysmal sac the thrombi induced would be only temporary and the aneurysm would undoubtedly refill [83]. Acknowledging this limitation, Mullan worked on the materials used during the following years. He described a mild fibrotic reaction induced by electrothrombosis with copper-plated electrodes which made the thrombosis permanent instead of that achieved with an "inactive" steel needle. Results of his work on berry aneurysms, giant aneurysms and CCSF were published in 1974 [84, 85].

Between 1965 and 1966 Alksne and Rosomoff independently developed another technique which could prevent the need for craniotomy to treat cerebral aneurysms. To overcome one of the problems of the past experiences – the inability to "guide" the embolic agent inside the aneurysm in a safe and reliable way – they thought of using iron microspheres magnetically guided with a magnet positioned on the dome of the aneurysm using a stereotactic technique [86-88]. The magnetic probe, 6 mm in diameter, was introduced through a standard 1-cm burr hole and directed at 1 mm from the aneurysmal sac under biplanar radiographic control. Initially Alksne used to release a carbonyl iron powder suspended in human serum albumin in the previously cannulated cervical ICA but further experience with this technique encouraged him to shift toward a transfundal approach. The embolic agent was injected directly inside the aneurysm after puncturing it with a needle equipped with a transducer that could record arterial blood pressure thus confirming successful entry into the aneurysmal sac. In 1977 Alksne further modified his "recipe" for the embolic material with dramatic improvements, including shorter solidification times and a decreased risk of distal embolic dissemination [89]. In 1980 he finally published the results in a series of 22 patients treated with this method, of whom 16 did well [90]. Nevertheless, the procedure was eventually abandoned, mainly because of one insurmountable limit: the impossibility of always achieving complete aneurysm occlusion without taking a non-negligible risk of distal embolic dissemination.

During the second half of the 20th century the development of endovascular navigation techniques was at the right stage to allow tremendous widening of horizons in neuroendovascular surgery. The first experiments on the tolerance of brain arteries to catheterization using flexible tubes were conducted by Luessenhop and Velasquez in 1964. Well aware of the risk of vasospasm, these authors first investigated intraluminal trauma induced by catheters and emboli as a possible trigger for segmental or diffuse narrowing of cerebral arteries just as external mechanical stimulation or stretching of arterial walls would do. Furthermore tortuosity of the cerebral circulation hampered any means of navigation and the constant risk of occlusion or thrombosis by the catheter itself could not be neglected. Tests on glass reproduction models of the ICA, cadavers and animals were performed prior to choosing silastic tubing for the purpose of intracranial endovascular navigation. It was not possible to direct or deflect the silastic microcatheter in order to deal with arterial bifurcations, so the only means of guidance was blood flow [91]. Finally they used their equipment in three patients, two with a bAVM and one with a bleeding berry aneurysm.

Luessenhop merely imported catheterization methods which were already well-known in others fields of surgery. Indeed the bases of endovascular navigation were laid back in the beginning of the 20th century. In his book entitled "Experiments on myself", Forssmann described, maybe not only for the sake of scientific progress, how he could catheterize his own heart in 1929 [92]. A critical and undeniable advance was made by Seldinger in 1953 when he described the now universally used percutaneous arterial entry technique: a procedure as simple as it was ingenious which changed the philosophy of endovascular navigation at its very roots [93]. However, as already pointed out by Luessenhop and Velasquez, once inside the endovascular space, few means were then available to negotiate arterial bifurcations and to guide catheters at will. A possible solution came with the invention of the POD or "para-operational device", first described in 1966 by Frei [94]. This device consisted of a microcatheter with a magnetic tip which could be guided thanks to a magnetic field created by a powerful external magnet. A slight variation of the POD was presented in 1967 by Yodh who introduced a detachable platinum-cobalt magnet tip which could be released in berry aneurysms thus improving the safety of the original procedure described by Alksne and Rosomoff [95]. Further variations of the original POD made the system work remarkably well and, building on this, in 1974 Hilal *et al.* published data on a series of 120 patients treated with this device, including patients with bAVM, cerebral aneurysms and, last but not least, a case of basilar artery aneurysm which is credited in the literature with being the first to be treated by endovascular embolization [96].

The 1960s were flourishing and very productive years for endovascular surgery. Guglielmi, an Italian neuroendovascular surgeon and neuroradiologist, who we will discuss later in this chapter, would consider those years as part of the "pre-balloon era" which ended exactly in 1974 when Serbinenko published results from an outstanding series of 300 patients in whom a balloon-based, microcatheter system had been used. Although officially baptized in neuroendovascular procedures by Serbinenko, the use of endovascular balloons was certainly not a novelty. As a young resident just graduated in medicine in 1960, Fogarty invented and later patented a soft plastic catheter with an inflatable balloon at its end which was initially used to perform embolectomy procedures in thrombosed peripheral arteries. The catheter could pass through a clotted arterial lumen, after which the balloon could be inflated and then the catheter withdrawn to remove the clot [97]. Starting from the original Fogarty catheter, presented in 1963, several variants and different applications were subsequently developed. In 1962 Rothenberg described a rather creative device, which was literally called an "angiotactic instrument" [98], composed of a polyester sleeve double folded around a neoprene bladder both contained in a carrier made of two metal hemispheres. The whole device was attached to a 4-French catheter delivery system. The sleeve could be deployed *in situ* by disengaging the metal hemispheres and by inflating the neoprene balloon. Preliminary tests on animals allowed Rothenberg to suggest that the device could be applied for cerebral aneurysms, the purposeful occlusion of vessels afferent to bAVM or neoplasms, and to perform endovascular angioplasty for stenosed vessels. Later in 1970 Kessler and Wholey reported on the use of a non-detachable balloon deployed in the carotid artery to treat ICA aneurysms in two patients [99]. Based on these robust foundations and having meticulously conducted several preliminary studies as a young neurosurgeon working at the N. N. Burdenko Institute [100-103], Serbinenko finally published his results on endovascular diagnostic and therapeutic procedures using an inflatable balloon-tipped microcatheter on a series a 300 patients collected between 1969 and 1972 [104]. The technique described enabled temporary or permanent occlusion of cerebral arterial vessels. Temporary occlusion could be used to testing the efficiency of collateral blood supply and even perform angiographic, clinical and electrophysiological investigations (local anesthesia was commonly used to carry out such procedures). If, instead of normal contrast medium filler for the balloon, which was essential to enable radiographic control of the system, an opaque, rapidly solidifying filler were to be used, permanent occlusion would be achieved. Particular balloons equipped with an internal lumen would permit angiographic studies distal or proximal to an occluded vessel, injection of embolic agents such as fluid-hardening plastics for cerebral aneurysm and radiopaque materials for tumor staining, and the delivery of chemotherapeutic drugs to brain tumors. Most importantly, Serbinenko introduced detachable balloons which represented a cornerstone in the management of cerebrovascular pathologies, allowing treatment options for lesions such as cerebral aneurysms by "blowing" a balloon in their cavity or in the parent vessel, bAVM and CCSF.

Endovascular detachable balloons rapidly became notorious and improvements or variants were promptly proposed [105, 106] such as the addition of latex strings to the base of the catheter to prevent contrast agent leakage and the use of iodine solution as a filler for the balloon as suggested by Debrun who applied the newly modified equipment to the treatment of cavernous and vertebral fistulas and cerebral aneurysms [107, 108]. Despite the growing interest in inflatable balloons in neuroendovascular procedures, it was not always possible to reproduce Serbinenko's technique in the "Western hemisphere" during the years of the cold war because of technical difficulties in obtaining reliable and functional inflatable equipment. Di Tullio tried to overcome these problems by designing his own detachable balloon microcatheter after encountering consistent problems when trying to reproduce Debrun's technique in his own laboratories. In his experimental study on dogs with artificially induced carotid-jugular fistula he used silastic microcatheters attached to balloons of various sizes. Contrast leakage from the balloons was prevented by a unique micro one-way flap valve available only for balloons with a diameter greater than 1 mm. Once the balloon had been filled, it was separated from the apparatus by means of friction detachment [109, 110].

Balloon-based procedures flourished until the end of the 1980s and results of large series of patients treated with these techniques began to be published. In 1982 a series of 119 patients treated with detachable, silicon-filled latex balloons was published by Romodanov and Scheglov. They reported a 73% rate of preservation of the parent vessel and described contraindications to the embolization procedure, such as small aneurysms, wide-necked aneurysms, the acute phase of subarachnoid hemorrhage or in the presence of vasospasm (in such conditions the mortality rate could reach 22%) [111]. Higashida reported 18% mortality and 11% morbidity rates in a series of 84 patients with aneurysms not suitable for a classical surgical approach treated with balloon embolization. Furthermore he described the use of 2-hydroxyethylmetacrylate (HEMA) as a filling solution for balloons [112, 113]. It was finally possible to evaluate the impact of balloon-based endovascular techniques on the management of cerebrovascular disease and given the first encouraging results several authors designed studies focusing on comparisons with the classic surgical approach even though surgical experience was vastly greater than endovascular experience at this point in history. During the XIIth International Congress of Head and Neck Radiology in 1991 Moret presented his experience with berry aneurysms treated with endovascular balloon embolization and showed how 71% of his series of 124 patients had been successfully treated with selective aneurysmal sac occlusion, with the success rate increasing to 79% if the patients treated with aneurysm and parent vessel occlusion were added. Complication rates (6.5% mortality and 7% morbidity) were lower than those in previous studies, as could be expected from longer experience and superior mastery of the technique [114]. Although apparently flawless, the idea behind the use of inflated detachable balloons does have inherent limitations especially when it comes to the management of cerebral berry aneurysms. At the end of the 20th century neurosurgeons and neuroradiologists were endowed with a thorough understanding of pathological cerebrovascular anatomy and both direct and indirect investigations made clear that only very uncommonly would cerebral berry aneurysms have a perfect spheroid or oblate shape. So it soon became evident that an inflated balloon inside the aneurysm sac, given its intrinsic characteristics, would never provide reliable anatomical results and that embolization of the aneurysm often came at the cost of loss of patency of the parent vessel. Moret himself reported a 20% recurrence rate by recanalization for aneurysms treated with selective occlusion of their sac and described how a neck remnant could be noted on the immediate control angiogram in most cases. Furthermore, the risk of intraoperative aneurysm rupture due to the balloon inflation was not negligible [114].

Where detachable balloons failed, new technologies were put to test and new brilliant minds played their role in neuroendovascular history. In 1991, during the very same congress in which Moret showed his results with detachable balloons, the aforementioned Guglielmi and Viuela presented their work entitled "Endovascular Electrothrombosis of Intracranial Aneurysms: Experimental Research and Initial Clinical Applications". It was the beginning of the era of coil technology [114-116].

But let us take a few steps back in history to acknowledge what made it possible for this new turn of events to take place at the beginning of the 1990s. Guglielmi himself considered his work as the sum of three different disciplines: neurosurgery, electronics and interventional radiology. To achieve success he took advantage of the latest acquisitions of each discipline, especially interventional radiology as new catheter designs were to widen horizons in intracranial endovascular navigation in terms of accessibility, control and safety. During those years the POD was still quite popular and building on Serbinenko's success the device was even equipped with a detachable balloon first described by Cares, who tested it in mongrel dogs [117]. The filling solution for the balloon was serum albumin which allowed inflation and, if necessary, deflation of the device. This constituted a great improvement as detachable balloons had previously been commonly inflated with hardening solution which prevented any attempt at deflation. The detachment system was developed using a technique already introduced by Walker and Burton [118]: the catheter tip was equipped with a magnetic guidance system and the balloon was attached to a carbon steel tip. Using a radiofrequency induction coil the carbon steel tip would be heated remotely. When the temperature reached approximately 55 °C the serum albumin coagulated sealing the orifice of the balloon. Further injection of serum albumin into the catheter would finally blow off the inflated balloon. Eventually, however, the POD was abandoned, mainly due to the appearance on the market of newly designed microcatheters with superior guidance systems. Concomitantly, catheterization techniques evolved dramatically. Working mostly on arteriovenous malformations and tumors in the external carotid and medullary territories during the 1970s, Djindjian described how to achieve super-selective catheterization of arterial branches using a tapered tip catheter passed through the transfemoral route which was considered both less traumatic and more profitable than the classic puncture and cannulation of the cervical common carotid artery, as it avoided carotid spasm or thrombosis and made it possible to perform vertebral artery investigations [104, 119]. Interestingly, Djindjian, a Frenchman who was a highly esteemed expert in super-selective catheterization, considered that it was hazardous to perform such a technique in the intracranial circulation given the risk of arterial wall stress and damage. In the mid-1980s, restraints and doubts about the safety and reliability of intracranial endovascular navigation were resolved thanks to the introduction of a new microcatheter, the "Tracker", patented by Egelson in 1986 [120, 121] and presented by Daniels, owner of Target Therapeutics, in 1985 [122]. Specifically intended for intracranial navigation, this microcatheter could be pushed over a steerable microguide wire allowing arterial bifurcations to be negotiated. Its tip was steam-shapeable, making navigation through tortuous vascular anatomy possible. Before the introduction of the Tracker, intracranial endovascular navigation relied mostly on blood flow, the effect of abrupt saline injection through the soft microcatheter and the flexibility and shape of the catheter making the whole procedure difficult and, most of the time, unreliable. Tracker microcatheters changed all this, revolutionizing endovascular navigation.

Traveling through neuroendovascular history we have already witnessed how innovation very rarely started from scratch. Usually, already existing devices or techniques just needed to be perfected, revisited, or simply readapted to fit into different therapeutic contexts to bring novelty. This is exactly what happened with neuroendovascular coil technology, successfully introduced by Guglielmi at the beginning of the 1990s (Figs. **1-5**). Gianturco, way back in 1975, described his experience using new mechanical embolic devices including a very particular and primitive coil model. During those years embolization was commonly achieved by using autologous matter, for instance clots, clots augmented with thrombin, or platelets, or synthetic materials such as Gelfoam, metallic or silastic spheres, silicone preparations or radioactive particles. Starting from experimental investigations Gianturco attempted to use "cotton tails" and "wool coils". Wool coils consisted of woolen strands attached to a tightly coiled segment of steel microguide wire deprived of its core and were successfully used to treat hypernephromas in two patients [123]. Ten years later, Braun reported the first documented embolization of a giant ICA aneurysm treated with endovascular coil embolization after failure of detachable balloon occlusion methods [124]. At the end of the 1980s, in order to improve thrombosis, Dacron fibers were implemented with the coil, as described by Hilal [125]. Nonetheless the materials used were still inadequate as dense aneurysm packing was not possible because of the coil's stiffness and, above all, retrieving the embolus once deployed was not an option given that the coils were pushed freely inside the catheter and a detachment mechanism did not exist: the risk of incorrect positioning was, therefore, high and the parent vessel patency was often jeopardized [126].

Motivated by all these factors, Guglielmi conducted years of experimentation prior to the conception of detachable coils [128, 129]. In his laboratories in the "Sapienza" University in Rome, artificially created aneurysms in rabbits were treated through electrothrombosis, a technique originally adopted by Mullan in 1965. Unfortunately occlusion of the aneurysm was minimal; nevertheless, Guglielmi noticed a rather interesting phenomenon which he described as a "rat tail" erosion of the intra-aneurysmal stainless steel electrode. Electrolysis was taking place, a natural process triggered by the electric current which was previously exploited to minimize damage to the aneurysm when withdrawing needles employed during aneurysmal electrothrombosis by the transfundal approach.

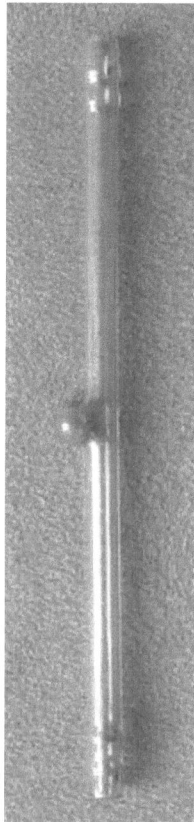

Figure 1: The first glass model were the GDC coils were tested. (Courtesy Prof. G. Guglielmi).

3 mm diameter tip

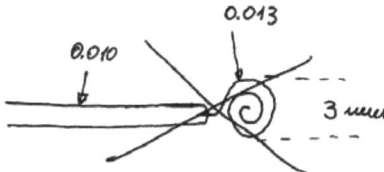

0.010　　　0.013

PROTOTYPE
n° 4 5

3 mm

instead of

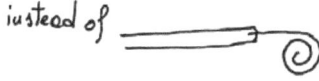

7 mm diameter tip

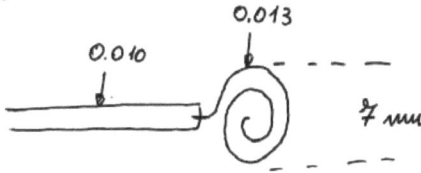

0.010　　0.013

PROTOTYPE
n° 6

7 mm

instead of

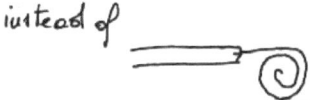

A different question:
is it possible to have one or
two prototypes n° 3
with a diameter of
0,009 ?

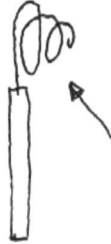

BOTH PROTOTYPES
HAVE TO BE
THREE-DIMENSIONAL

Thank-you

Figure 2: Exclusive drawings from the private archive of Prof Guglielmi, that show the first prototype of the GDC coils.

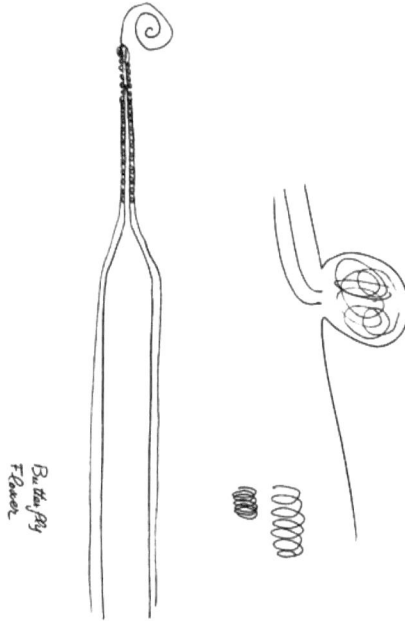

Figure 3: Exclusive drawings from the private archive of Prof Guglielmi, that show the first prototype of the GDC coils.

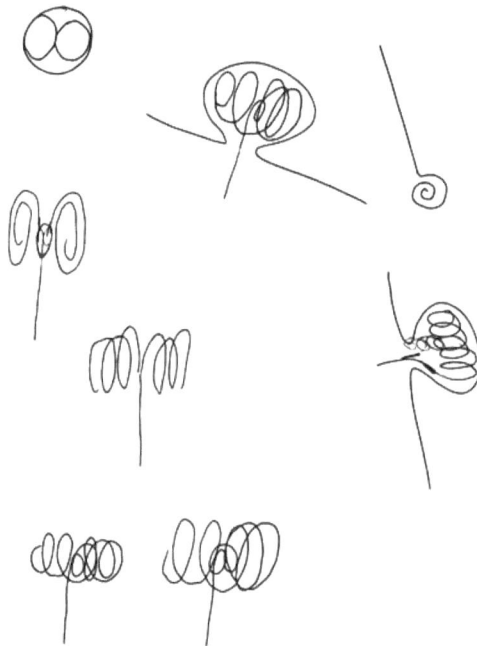

Figure 4: Exclusive drawings from the private archive of Prof Guglielmi, that show the first prototype of the GDC coils.

TO   IVAN SEPETKA

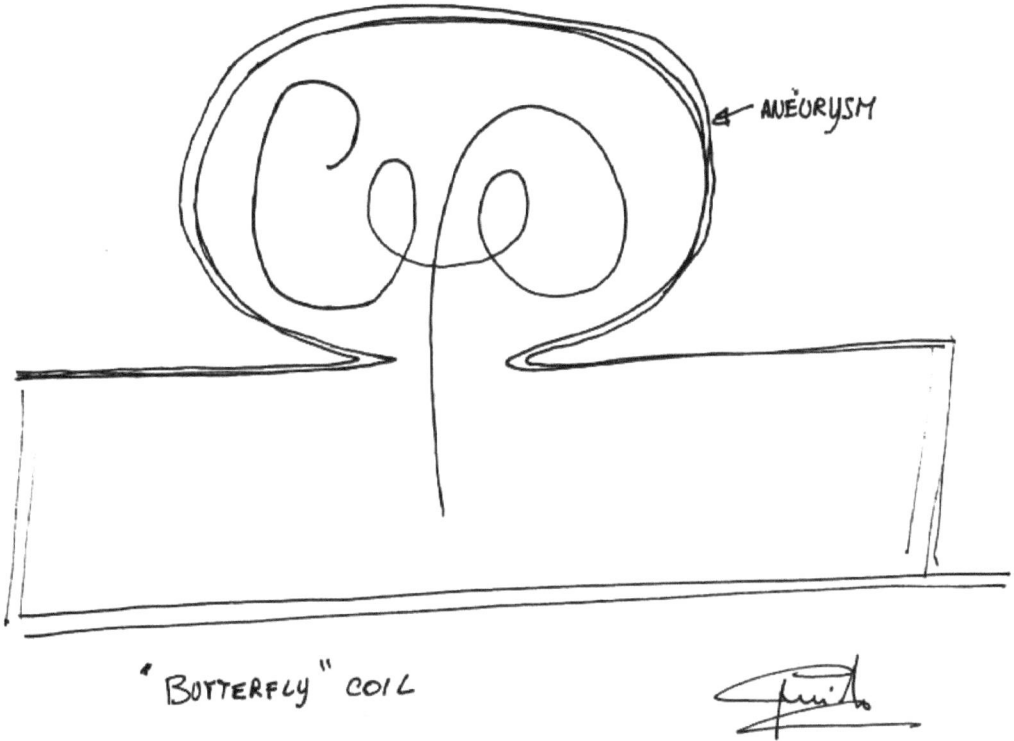

←— ANEURYSM

"BUTTERFLY" COIL

Figure 5: Exclusive drawings from the private archive of Prof Guglielmi, that show the first prototype of the GDC coils.
These images have never been published before.

Subsequently he tested embolization of artificial glass aneurysms with magnetically guided iron microspheres. A micro-magnet was attached to the tip of a stainless steel wire introduced into the glass aneurysm; microspheres released in the circulation were attracted by the magnet and enlarged it causing partial occlusion of the artificial aneurysm. When tested on animals with artificially created common carotid artery aneurysms, an electric current was applied to the magnet to boost the thrombotic reaction but occlusion was still unsatisfactory. Nonetheless, Guglielmi and colleagues noted an erosion of the wire next to the magnet caused by the electric current. This observation led to the discovery of a reliable and innovative detachment mechanism based on electrolysis!

Further efforts were made to determine the embolic agent which could best benefit from the newly discovered detachment mechanism. An existing stainless steel, platinum-tipped microguide wire was modified for the purpose. Platinum had the essential properties: biocompatibility, radiopacity and, above all, as a noble metal, resistance to electrolysis. The platinum coil, initially only 1 cm long, was soldered to the stainless steel microguidewire. The detachable coil was born. It was finally possible to navigate the cerebral circulation, enter an aneurysmal sac and fill it with a platinum coil which was then detached from the microguidewire simply by applying a 4 mA positive current which dissolved the stainless steel next to the platinum coil by electrolysis (migration of the ferrous ions from the anode to the cathode). The detachable coils were first named Guglielmi electrolytic microcoils (GEMs) and then later renamed Guglielmi detachable coils (GDCs, Boston Scientific). Finally, on the 6th March, 1990, the first patient was treated with the new device [128, 129].

Modifications of the original coil design and delivery system were numerous and involved coil and wire softness, length and shape. One of the most important was applied in order to decrease the coil detachment time, which initially could be as long as 45 minutes, and to add markers to the platinum coil to improve its radiopacity thus allowing more precise deployment. Most of these modifications were made thanks to collaboration with an engineer at Target Therapeutics, Ivan Sepetka [127, 130-132]. Furthermore the original two-dimensional design of the coil, which did not consistently ensure good neck coverage, was changed when Target Therapeutics introduced a three-dimensional coil, well known as the "framing coil", with an intrinsic shape that would seek to retain an overall spherical configuration when fully deployed.

In 1997 Vinuela reported on the use of GDCs for the treatment of aneurysmal subarachnoid hemorrhage within 48 hours of onset in an extensive series of 403 patients. Complete occlusion rates ranged from 70.8% for small-necked aneurysms to 35% for large-necked aneurysms and 50% for giant aneurysms. A neck remnant was observed more often for giant and large-necked aneurysms (50% and 57.1%, respectively) than for small-necked aneurysms (21.4%). The procedure-related mortality rate was 1.74% and the incidence of immediate morbidity was below 10%: these immediate complications were primarily intraoperative aneurysm rupture, unintentional parent artery occlusion and untoward cerebral embolization [133]. These outstanding results gave impulse to a dramatically fast spread of the technique introduced by Guglielmi. Nevertheless, further experience led to the acknowledgment of the limits of the GDC already outlined by Vinuela's work. One not negligible issue regarding the management of wide-necked aneurysms emerged. The presence of a large neck is correlated with a high probability of post-embolization neck remnant which in turn is a risk factor for recanalization. Furthermore the risk of unintentional cerebral embolization from distal coil detachment could not to be ignored [134]. To overcome these problems, several attempts were made to improve the original technique, including the "balloon remodeling technique" described by Moret in 1997. With the aid of a balloon temporarily inflated across the aneurysm neck, coils were packed more densely, which resulted in a lower rate of recanalization and parent vessel coil protrusion [135]. A few years later Murayama proposed using bioadsorbable polymers as a coat to the GDC to produce better healing of the interface between the parent vessel and aneurysm neck thus improving the anatomical outcome of endovascular embolization procedures [136]. Others pursued completely different strategies using liquid embolic agents, as Taki did. In 1991, Taki used a liquid, ethylene vinyl alcohol copolymer also known as EVAL, to embolize an intracranial aneurysm. Subsequent improvements applied to EVAL eventually led to the development of the currently employed copolymer Onyx (Microtherapeutics, Inc., Irvine, CA, USA), mostly used in spinal cord arteriovenous malformations. Nevertheless, according to the Cerebral Aneurysm Multicenter European Onyx (CAMEO) trial [137], the use of Onyx can represent a viable alternative to coil embolization when the latter is unsuitable. A recent retrospective analysis studied trends in endovascular coiling procedures. Using the "National inpatient sample", the largest inpatient health care database in the United States, Andaluz found that, in the period 1992-2003, endovascular techniques for aneurysm occlusion doubled with steady numbers of clipping procedures. Overall outcomes were better toward the end of the study period, probably because of progressively greater expertise in endovascular neurosurgery and further technological improvements in the field [138]. A similar study by Brinjikji for the period 2001 – 2008 concluded that the proportion of unruptured aneurysms treated with endovascular techniques had risen to 63% with lower rates of long-term hospitalization and mortality [139,140].

Although numerous refinements and technological innovations ameliorated endovascular coil embolization techniques, the overall treatment results were not consistently improved. The anatomical outcome and the long-term results in wide-necked or terminal-type aneurysms remained challenging issues.

At the beginning of the 21st century, in attempts to solve the problem of wide-necked and terminal aneurysms, stent technology was introduced into neuroendovascular surgery. Stents, broadly used in coronary angioplasty procedures and originally conceived during the 1960s for the endovascular management of atherosclerotic disease [141, 142], were not planned for intracranial use because of the naturally tortuous intracranial circulation anatomy. However, as soon as new, adequate models became available, stents, both alone [143] and in support of coil embolization [144, 145], were put to the test. Delivered and positioned in the parent artery across the aneurysm neck, they act as a scaffold providing a physical matrix for endothelial growth, they promote thrombosis within the aneurysm by flow diversion from the sac and, when coupled with coiling through the stent struts inside the aneurysm, they ensure the best filling possible [146]. The "Y" stent type was used in terminal-type aneurysms and "covered" stents were used to obliterate the orifice of the aneurysm while maintaining patency of the parent vessel. Toward the end of the first decade of the new century, the introduction of "flow diverter stents" further changed the philosophy of intracerebral aneurysm embolization; these stents can cure aneurysms without the need for coils. They are braided, tubular, tiny-holed, microcell-like and less porous so that once deployed across the neck of the aneurysm they divert the blood flow away from the aneurysm. This kind of device introduced a new concept: endovascular reconstruction. During endosaccular aneurysm coiling, the operator is obliged to fill the aneurysm as densely as possible with embolic material with the goal of achieving complete aneurysm occlusion at the time of the initial procedure; the technique of reconstruction with flow diverter stents differs fundamentally from the operator's perspective. The curative reconstruction that is induced by flow diverter stents occurs over a period of weeks to months and three potential mechanisms of action have been suggested: improved anatomical reconstruction of the parent artery, functional modification of flow across the orifice of the aneurysm, and biological repair of the aneurysm neck by neointimal overgrowth. Further laboratory experiments demonstrated that, depending on their mesh attenuation, stents alter and reduce the velocities of vortical flow within the aneurysm, increasing the intra-aneurysmal circulation time and affecting momentum exchange between the sac and the parent vessel. A new endovascular era has begun.

Our journey through history has finally reached its end in the present day. Although we have described it trying to respect chronological order, as if referring to a straight timeline, neuroendovascular history would be more realistically depicted as a tree with numerous branches, each branch representing different sub-fields such as coil, stent or liquid embolization technologies and each represented by different timelines, sometimes crossing one another.

Being such a relatively young discipline compared to neurosurgery, the issue of training junior neuroendovascular residents has recently emerged. Standards and requirements for neuroendovascular surgery certification have been quite clearly established in the United States and Japan. Debate on the subject is still open in Europe where neuroendovascular procedures are not uncommonly delegated completely to interventional neuroradiologists [147]. Japanese neurosurgeons currently carry out both the surgical and the endovascular treatments. Starting from the first year of residency, junior neurosurgeons are expected to be able to manage acute neurological illnesses such as a subarachnoid hemorrhage from the emergency room through to the operating room and the skills required to perform a cerebral angiography are, therefore, acquired early [2, 148].

ACKNOWLEDGEMENTS

Declared none.

CONFLICT OF INTEREST

The authors confirm that this chapter contents have no conflict of interest.

REFERENCES

[1]   Prestigiacomo CJ. Historical perspectives: the microsurgical and endovascular treatment of aneurysms. Neurosurgery 2006; 59: S39-47; discussion S3-13.
[2]   Sauvageau E, Hopkins LN. Training in cerebrovascular disease: do we need to change the way we train residents? Neurosurgery 2006; 59: S282-6; discussion S3-13.
[3]   Lippi D. An aneurysm in the Papyrus of Ebers (108, 3-9). Med Secoli 1990; 2: 1- 4.
[4]   De Moullin D. Aneurysms in antiquity. Arch Chir Neerl 1961; 13: 49-63.
[5]   von Ephesus R. De sanguinis eruptione. Latin Aetios edition by J. Cornarius, Lyons 1549, lib. XIV, Chapt. 51: 778-81.
[6]   Magnus V. Aneurysm of the internal carotid artery. JAMA 1927; 88: 1712-3.
[7]   Dionis P. Disseration sur la mort subite et sur la catalepsie; avec la relation de plusieurs personnes qui en ont ete attaques. Ld'Houry, Paris. [Quoted by Walton, 1956].
[8]   Blackall J. Observations on the nature and cure of dropsies. 2nd ed. London: Longman, Hurst, Rees, Orme & Brown 1813; 132-5.
[9]   Morgagni JB. De Sedibus et Causis Morborum per Anatomen Indagatis. Venetis, ex typog. Remodiniana. Vol. 1. New York: Hafner, 1960.
[10]   Biumi F. Observatio V. Carotis ad receptaculum vieussenii aneurysmatica etc. Eduard Sandifort: Thesaurus disseratationum. Milano: S & C Luctmans, 1765(new print 1778); 3: 373
[11]   Hunter J. Works. London, Jas F. Palmer, 1835.
[12]   Robicsek F, Roush TS, Cook JW, Reames MK. From Hippocrates to Palmaz-Schatz, the history of carotid surgery. Eur J Vasc Endovasc Surg 2004; 27: 389-97.
[13]   Paré A. The works of that famous chirurgion Ambrose Parey, translated out of Latin and compared with the French by Thomas Johnson: From the first English edition, London, 1634. New York: Milford House, 1968.
[14]   Abernathy J. Surgical observations. Surgical works. London. 1804.
[15]   Abernathy J. Surgical observations on injuries of the head. Philadelphia: Dobson, 1811.

[16]   Hamby WB. Intracranial aneurysms. Springfield, Charles C. Thomas, 1952.
[17]   Cutter I. Ligation of the common carotid artery: Amos Twitchell. Surg Gynecol Obstet (Internat Obstet Surg) 1920; 48: 1-3.
[18]   Garrison FH. An introduction to the history of medicine. Philadelphia, Saunders, 1924.
[19]   Cogswell M. Account of an operation for the extirpation of a tumour, in which a ligature was applied to the carotid artery. N Eng J Med 1824; 13: 357-360.
[20]   Cooper A. A case of aneurism of the carotid artery. Med Chir Trans 1806.
[21]   Cooper A. Second case of carotid aneurism. Med Chir Trans 1809.
[22]   Travers B. A case of aneurism by anastomosis in the orbit, cured by the ligature of the common carotid artery. Med Chir Trans 1811; II
[23]   Drake CG. Earlier times in aneurysm surgery. Clin Neurosurg 1985; 32: 41-50.
[24]   Keen WW. Intracranial lesions. M News New York 1890; 57: 443.
[25]   Halstead WS: The partial occlusion of blood vessels, especially of the abdominal aorta. Bull Johns Hopkins Hosp 1905; 14: 346.
[26]   Matas R. Occlusion of large surgical arteries with removable metallic bands to test the efficiency of the collateral circulation. JAMA 1911; 56: 233-9.
[27]   Dandy WE. Intracranial aneurysm of the internal carotid artery cured by operation. Ann Surg 1938; 107: 654-9.
[28]   Neff JM. A method for gradual automatic occlusion of larger blood vessels. JAMA 1911; 57: 700-8.
[29]   Poppen JL. Ligation of the internal carotid artery in the neck; prevention of certain complications. J Neurosurg 1950; 7: 532-8.
[30]   Poppen J. Specific treatment of intracranial aneurysms: experiences with 143 surgically treated patients. J Neurosurg 1951; 8: 75-102.
[31]   Giannotta S, McGillicuddy J, Kindt G. Gradual carotid artery occlusion in the treatment of inaccessible internal carotid artery aneurysms. Neurosurgery 1979; 5: 417-21.
[32]   Cunningham AT. Gradual occlusion of common carotid artery in treatment of pulsating exophthalmos. JAMA 1904; 62: 373-4.
[33]   Dott NM. Intracranial aneurysm formation. Clin Neurosurg 1969; 16: 1-16.
[34]   Selverstone B, White JC. A new technique for gradual occlusion of the carotid artery. Arch Neurol Psychiatry 1951; 66: 246.
[35]   Selverstone B, White JC. A method for the gradual occlusion of the internal carotid artery in the treatment of aneurysm. Proc N Engl Cardiovasc Soc 1952; 9: 24-5.
[36]   Tonnis W, Walter W. Die behandlung der sackformigen intracraniellen aneurysmen. In: Olivecrona H, Tonnis W (eds): Klinik und Behandlung der raumbeengenden intrakraniellen prozesse. Handbuch der neurochirurgie [in German]. Berlin, Springer-Verlag 1966, pp 212-363.
[37]   Schorstein J. Carotid ligation in saccular intracranial aneurysms. Br J Surg 1940; 28: 50-70.
[38]   Zeller O. Die chirurgische behanding der durch aneurysma arterio-venosum der carotis int. im sin. Cavernous hervorgerufenen pulsierenden. Exophtalmos: ein neues verfahren [in German]. Dtsch Z Chir 1911; 111: 1-39.
[39]   Hamby WB, Gardner WJ: Treatment of pulsating exophthalmos with report of 2 cases. Arch Surg 1933; 27: 676-85.
[40]   Cohen-Gadol A, Spencer D. Harvey W. Cushing and cerebrovascular surgery: Part I, aneurysms. J Neurosurg 2004; 101: 547-52.
[41]   Todd NV, Howie JE, Miller JD. Norman Dott's contribution to aneurysm surgery. J Neurol Neurosurg Psychiatry 1990: 53: 455-8.
[42]   Tonnis W. Zur behandlung intrakranieller aneurysmen [in German]. Arch F Klin Chir 1936: 189: 474-6.
[43]   Jefferson G. Compression of the chiasm, optic nerves, and optic tracts by intracranial aneurysms. Brain 1937; 60: 444-97.
[44]   Dandy WE. The treatment of carotid cavernous arteriovenous aneurysms. Ann Surg 1935; 102: 916-26.
[45]   Dandy WE. Intracranial Aneurysms. Ithaca, Comstock, 1944.
[46]   Kretzer RM, Coon AL, Tamargo RJ. Walter E. Dandy's contributions to vascular neurosurgery. J Neurosurg 2010; 112: 1182-91.

[47] Logue V. Surgery in spontaneous subarachnoid haemorrhage: operative treatment of aneurysms on the anterior cerebral and anterior communicating artery. Br Med J 1956; 1: 473-9.

[48] Tindall GT, Kapp J, Odom G, Robinson S. A combined technique for treating certain aneurysms of the anterior communicating artery. J Neurosurg 1970; 33: 41-7.

[49] Cushing H. Original memoirs: the control of bleeding in operations for brain tumors: with the description of silver "clips" for the occlusion of vessels inaccessible to the ligature. 1911. Yale J Biol Med 2002; 74: 399-412.

[50] Duane W. A modification of the McKenzie silver clip. J Neurosurg 1950; 7: 92-3.

[51] Norlen G, Olivecrona H. The treatment of aneurysms of the circle of Willis. J Neurosurg 1953; 10: 404-15.

[52] Mayfield FH, Kees G. A brief history of the development of the Mayfield clip. Technical note. J Neurosurg 1971; 35: 97-100.

[53] Fox JL. Vascular clips for the microsurgical treatment of stroke. Stroke 1976; 7: 489-500.

[54] Del Maestro RF. Origin of the Drake fenestrated aneurysm clip. J Neurosurg 2000; 92: 1056-64.

[55] Sundt TM. Clip-grafts for aneurysm and small vessel surgery. J Neurosurg 1969; 31: 59-71.

[56] Sugita K, Hirota T, Iguchi I, Mizutani T. Comparative study of the pressure of various aneurysm clips. J Neurosurg 1976; 44: 723-7.

[57] Al-Shatoury HA, Raja AI, Ausman JI. Timeline: pioneers in cerebral aneurysms. Surg Neurol 2000; 54: 465-70.

[58] Yasargil GM, Fox JL. The microsurgical approach to intracranial aneurysms. Surg Neurol 1975; 3: 7-14.

[59] Velpeau A. Memoire sur la Piqureou l'acupuncturedes arteres dans les traitement des aneurismes [in French]. Gaz Med Paris 1831; 2: 1-4.

[60] Phillips B. A series of experiments performed for the purpose of showing that arteries may be obliterated without ligature compression or knife. London, Longman, 1834.

[61] Berenstein A, Song JK, Niimi Y. Personal accounts of the evolution of endovascular neurosurgery. Neurosurgery 2006; 59: S15-21; discussion S3-13.

[62] Dawbarn RH. The starvation operation for malignancy in the external carotid area. JAMA 1904; 17: 792-5.

[63] Doby T. Cerebral angiography and Egas Moniz. Am J Radiol 1992; 159: 364.

[64] Ferro JM. Egas Moniz (1874-1955). J Neurol 2003; 250: 376-7.

[65] Sicard JA, Forestier J. Methode generale d'exploration radiologique par l'huite iodee (lipiodol) [in French]. Bull Mem Soc Med Hop Paris 1922; 46: 463.

[66] Moniz E. L'encephalographie arterielle, son importance dans la localization des tumeurs cerebrales [in French]. Rev Neurol 1927; 2: 72-90.

[67] Radner S. Intracranial angiography *via* the vertebral artery. Preliminary report on a new technique. Acta Radiologica 1947; 28: 838-42.

[68] Brooks B. The treatment of traumatic arteriovenous fistula. South Med J 1930; 23: 100-6.

[69] Vitek JJ, Smith MJ. The myth of the Brooks method of embolization: a brief history of the endovascular treatment of carotid-cavernous sinus fistula. J Neurointerv Surg 2009; 1: 108-11.

[70] Tarr RW. Yes Virginia there is a Santa Claus. J Neurointerv Surg 2009; 1: 99.

[71] Speakman TJ. Internal occlusion of a carotid-cavernous fistula. J Neurosurg 1964; 21: 303-5.

[72] Ishimori S, Hattori M, Shibata Y, Shizawa H, Fujinaga R. Treatment of carotid-cavernous fistula by gelfoam embolization. J Neurosurg 1967; 27: 315-9.

[73] Isamat F, Salleras V, Miranda AM. Artificial embolization of carotid-cavernous fistula with post-operative patency of internal carotid artery. J Neurol Neurosurg Psychiatry 1970; 33: 674-8.

[74] Gardner WJ. Cerebral angiomas and aneurysms. Surg Clin North Am 1936; 16: 1019-30.

[75] Dandy WE. Intracranial arterial aneurysms in the carotid canal. Diagnosis and treatment. Arch Surg 1942; 45: 335-50.

[76] Werner SC, Blakemore AH, King BG. Aneurysm of the internal carotid artery within the skull: wiring and electrothermic coagulation. JAMA 1941; 116: 578-82.

[77] Luessenhop AJ, Spence W. Artificial embolization of cerebral arteries. Report of use in a case of arteriovenous malformation. JAMA 1960; 172: 1153-5.

[78] Kerber C. History of endovascular neurosurgery: a personal view. Neurosurgery 2006; 59: 22-9.

[79]   Sano K, Jimbo M, Saito I, Basugi N: Artificial embolization of inoperable angioma with polymerizing substance. In Pia HW *et al.* (eds): Cerebral Angioma. Berlin-Heidelberg-New York, Springer, 1975, pp 222-9.

[80]   Boulos R, Kricheff II, Chase NE. Value of cerebral angiography in the embolization treatment of cerebral arteriovenous malformations. Radiology 1970; 97: 65-70.

[81]   Gallagher JP. Pilojection for intracranial aneurysms. J Neurosurg 1968; 21: 129-34.

[82]   Mullan S, Beckman F, Vailati G, Karasick J, Dobben G. An experimental approach to the problem of cerebral aneurysm. J Neurosurg 1964; 21: 838-45.

[83]   Mullan S, Raimondi AJ, Dobben G, Vailati G, Hekmatpanah J. Electrically induced thrombosis in intracranial aneurysms. J Neurosurg 1965; 22: 539-47.

[84]   Mullan S, Reyes C, Dawley J. Stereotactic copper electric thrombosis of intracranial aneurysms. Prog Neurol Surg 1969; 3: 193-211.

[85]   Mullan S. Experiences with surgical thrombosis of intracranial berry aneurysms and carotid cavernous fistulas. J Neurosurg 1974; 41: 657-70.

[86]   Alksne JF, Fingerhut AG, Rand RW. Magnetically controlled metallic thrombosis of intracranial aneurysms. Surgery 1966; 60: 212-8.

[87]   Alksne JF, Fingerhut AG, Rand RW. Magnetic probe for the stereotactic thrombosis of intracranial aneurysms. J Neuro Neurosurg Psychiatry 1967; 30: 159-62.

[88]   Rosomoff HL. Stereomagnetic occlusion of intracranial aneurysm: principles and application. Trans Am Neurol Assoc 1966; 91: 330-1.

[89]   Alksne JF, Smith RW. Iron-acrylic compound for steriotaxic aneurysm thrombosis. J Neurosurg 1977; 47: 137-41.

[90]   Alksne JF, Smith RW. Stereotaxic occlusion of 22 consecutive anterior communicating artery aneurysms. J Neurosurg 1980; 52: 790-3.

[91]   Luessenhop AJ, Velasquez AC. Observations on the tolerance of the intracranial arteries to catheterization. J Neurosurg 1964; 21: 85-91.

[92]   Forssmann W. Experiments on Myself: Memoirs of a Surgeon in Germany. New York, St. Martin's Press, 1974.

[93]   Seldinger SI. Catheter replacement of the needle in percutaneous arteriography. A new technique. Acta Radiol Suppl (Stockholm) 2008; 434: 47-52.

[94]   Frei EH, Driller J, Neufeld HN, Barr I, Bleiden L, Askenzay HN. The POD and its applications. Med Res Eng 1966; 8: 11-8.

[95]   Yodh S, Pierce N. A new magnet system for "intravascular navigation." Med Biol Eng 1968; 6: 143-7.

[96]   Hilal SK, Michelsen WJ, Driller J, Leonard E. Magnetically guided devices for vascular exploration and treatment: Laboratory and clinical investigation. Radiology 1974; 113: 529-40.

[97]   Fogarty TJ, Cranley JJ, Krause RJ, *et al.* A method for extraction of arterial emboli and thrombi. Surg Gynecol Obstet 1963; 116: 241-4.

[98]   Rothenberg SF, Penka EJ, Conway LW. Angiotactic surgery: preliminary studies. J Neurol Neurosurg Psychiatry 1962; 19: 877-83.

[99]   Kessler LA, Wholey MH. Internal carotid occlusion for the treatment of intracranial aneurysms: a new percutaneous technique. Radiology 1970; 95: 581-3.

[100]   Serbinenko FA. Catheterization and occlusion of major cerebral vessels and prospects for the development of vascular neurosurgery [in Russian]. Vopr Neirokhir 1971; 35: 17-27.

[101]   Serbinenko FA. Balloon occlusion of cavernous portion of the carotid artery as a method of treating carotid-cavernous fistulae [in Russian]. Vopr Neirokhir 1971; 6: 3-9.

[102]   Serbinenko FA. Catheterisation and occlusion of major vessels of the brain [in Russian]), in Perviy vsesouzniy s'ezd neuroshirurgov, Tom I. Moscva, 1971; 114-9.

[103]   Serbinenko FA. Reconstruction of cavernous part of carotid artery in case of carotid- cavernous fistulae [in Russian]. Vopr Neirokhir 1972; 36: 3-9.

[104]   Serbinenko F. Balloon catheterization and occlusion of major cerebral vessels. J Neurosurg 1974; 107: 684-705.

[105]   Pevsner PH. Micro-balloon catheter for superselective angiography and therapeutic occlusion. Am J Roentgenol 1977; 128: 225-30.

[106]   Kerber C. Calibrated leak balloon microcatheter: a device for arterial exploration and occlusive therapy. Am J Roentgenol 1979; 132: 207-12.
[107]   Debrun G, Lacour P, Caron J, Hurth M. Experimental approach to the treatment of carotid cavernous fistulas with an inflatable and isolated balloon. Neuroradiology 1975; 112: 9-12.
[108]   Debrun G, Lacour P, Caron J, Hurth M. Inflatable and released balloon technique experimentation in dog — application in man. Neuroradiology 1975; 9: 267-71.
[109]   DiTullio MV Jr, Rand RW, Frisch E. Development of a detachable vascular balloon catheter: a preliminary report. Bull Los Angeles Neurol Soc 1976; 41: 2-5.
[110]   DiTullio M, Rand RW, Frisch E. Detachable balloon catheter. Its application in experimental arteriovenous fistulae. J Neurosurg 1978; 48: 717-23.
[111]   Romodanov AP, Shcheglov IV. Intravascular occlusion of saccular aneurysms of the cerebral arteries by means of a detachable balloon catheter. In: Krayenbu¨hl H (ed): Advances in Technical Standards in Neurosurgery. New York, Springer-Verlag 1982, pp 25-48.
[112]   Higashida RT, Halbach VV, Barnwell SL, *et al*. Treatment of intracranial aneurysms with preservation of the parent vessel: result of percutaneous balloon embolization in 84 patients. AJNR Am J Neuroradiol 1990; 11: 633-40.
[113]   Higashida T, Halbach VV, Hieshima B, Weinstein PR, Hoyt F. Treatment of a giant carotid ophthalmic balloon embolization artery aneurysm by intravascular therapy. Surg Neurol 1988; 30: 382-6.
[114]   Fisch U, Valavanis A. Xllth International Congress of Head and Neck Radiology 1991.
[115]   Guglielmi G. The beginning and the evolution of the endovascular treatment of intracranial aneurysms: from the first catheterization of brain arteries to the new stents. J Neurointerv Surg 2009; 1: 53-5.
[116]   Guglielmi G. History of the genesis of detachable coils. A review. J Neurosurg 2009; 111: 1-8.
[117]   Cares HL, Hale JR, Montgomery DB, Richter HA, Sweet WH. Laboratory experience with a magnetically guided intravascular catheter system. J Neurosurg 1973; 38: 145-54.
[118]   Walker AE, Burton CV. Radiofrequency telethermocoagulation. JAMA 1966; 197: 700-4.
[119]   Djindjian R, Cophignon J, Theron J. Embolization by superselective arteriography from the femoral route in neuroradiology: review of 60 cases. Neuroradiology 1973; 26: 20-6.
[120]   Engelson E. Catheter for guide-wire tracking. US Patent No. 4739768, 1986.
[121]   Kikuchi Y, Strother CM, Boyer M. New catheter for endovascular interventional procedures. Radiology 1987; 165: 870-1.
[122]   Richling B. History of endovascular surgery: personal accounts of the evolution. Neurosurgery 2006; 59: S30-8; discussion S3-13.
[123]   Gianturco C. Mechanical devices for arterial occlusion. Am J Rad 1975; 124: 428-35.
[124]   Braun IF, Hoffman JC Jr, Casarella WJ, Davis PC. Use of coils for transcatheter carotid occlusion. AJNR Am J Neuroradiol 1985; 6: 953-6.
[125]   Hilal SK, Khandji AG, Chi TL. Synthetic fiber-coated platinum coils successfully used for the endovascular treatment of arteriovenous malformations, aneurysms and direct arteriovenous fistulas of the CNS. Presented at the American Society of Neuroradiology, Chicago, May 16, 1988.
[126]   Hilal SK, Khandji A, Solomon RW. Obliteration of intracranial aneurysms with pre-shaped highly thrombogenic coils. Radiology 1989; 173: 250-7.
[127]   Guglielmi G, Vinuela F, Sepetka I. Electrothrombosis of saccular aneurysms *via* endovascular approach part I. J Neurosurg 1991; 75: 1-7.
[128]   Guglielmi G, Vinuela F, Dion J, Duckwiler G. Electrothrombosis of saccular aneurysms *via* endovascular approach. Part II. J Neurosurg 1991; 75: 8-14.
[129]   Guglielmi G, Viñuela F, Briganti F, Duckwiler G. Carotid-cavernous fistula caused by a ruptured intracavernous aneurysm: endovascular treatment by electrothrombosis with detachable coils. Neurosurgery 1992; 31: 591-7.
[130]   Guglielmi G, Viñuela F, Duckwiler G, *et al*. Endovascular treatment of posterior circulation aneurysms by electrothrombosis using electrically detachable coils. J Neurosurg 1992; 77: 515-24.
[131]   Guglielmi G, Viñuela F, Duckwiler G, Dion J, Stocker A. Highflow, small-hole arteriovenous fistulas: treatment with electrodetachable coils. AJNR Am J Neuroradiol 1995; 16: 325-8.
[132]   Guglielmi G, Vinuela F, Dazzi M. The Guglielmi detachable coil "crescent" in the endovascular treatment of peripheral brain aneurysms: technical case report 2007; 61.

[133]   Viñuela F, Duckwiler G, Mawad M. Guglielmi detachable coil embolization of acute intracranial aneurysm: perioperative anatomical and clinical outcome in 403 patients. 1997. J Neurosurg 2008; 108: 832-9.

[134]   Hayakawa M, Murayama Y, Duckwiler GR, Gobin YP, Guglielmi G, Viñuela F. Natural history of the neck remnant of a cerebral aneurysm treated with the Guglielmi detachable coil system. J Neurosurg 2000; 93: 561-8.

[135]   Moret J, Cognard C, Weill A. The "remodeling technique" in the treatment of wide neck intracranial aneurysms: angiographic results and clinical follow-up in 56 cases. Intervent Neuroradiol 1997; 3: 21-35.

[136]   Murayama Y, Viñuela F, Tateshima S, Song JK, Gonzalez NR, Wallace MP. Bioabsorbable polymeric material coils for embolization of intracranial aneurysms: a preliminary experimental study. J Neurosurg 2001; 94: 454-63.

[137]   Molyneux AJ, Cekirge S, Saatci I, Gal G. Cerebral Aneurysm Multicenter European Onyx (CAMEO) trial: results of a prospective observational study in 20 European centers. AJNR Am J Neuroradiol 2004; 25: 39-51.

[138]   Andaluz N, Zuccarello M. Recent trends in the treatment of cerebral aneurysms: analysis of a nationwide inpatient database. J Neurosurg 2008; 108: 1163-9.

[139]   Brinjikji W, Rabinstein AA, Nasr DM, *et al.* Better outcomes with treatment by coiling relative to clipping of unruptured intracranial aneurysms in the United States, 2001-2008. AJNR Am J Neuroradiol 2011; 32: 1071-5.

[140]   Hui FK, Fiorella D, Masaryk TJ, Rasmussen PA, Dion JE. A history of detachable coils: 1987-2012. J Neurointerv Surg 2014; 6: 134-8.

[141]   Dotter CT, Judkins MP. Transluminal treatment of arteriosclerotic obstruction: Description of a new technique and preliminary report of its application. Circulation 1964; 30: 654-70.

[142]   Dotter CT. Transluminally-placed coilspring endarterial tube grafts: Long-term patency in canine popliteal artery. Invest Radiol 1969; 4: 329-32.

[143]   Wakhloo AK, Schellhammer F, de Vries J, Haberstroh J, Schumacher M. Self-expanding and balloon-expandable stents in the treatment of carotid aneurysms: an experimental study in a canine model. AJNR Am J Neuroradiol 1994; 15: 493-502.

[144]   Szikora I, Guterman LR, Wells KM, Hopkins LN. Combined use of stents and coils to treat experimental wide-necked carotid aneurysms: preliminary results. AJNR Am J Neuroradiol 1994; 15: 1091-102.

[145]   Turjman F, Massoud TF, Ji C, Guglielmi G, Viñuela F, Robert J. Combined stent implantation and endosaccular coil placement for treatment of experimental wide-necked aneurysms: A feasibility study in swine. AJNR Am J Neuroradiol 1994; 15: 1087-90.

[146]   Fiorella D, Albuquerque FC, Han P, McDougall CG. Preliminary experience using the neuroform stent for the treatment of cerebral aneurysms. Neurosurgery 2004; 54: 6-17.

[147]   Peschillo S, Delfini R. Endovascular neurosurgery in Europe and in Italy: what is in the future? World Neurosurg 2012; 77: 248-51.

[148]   Ecker RD, Levy EI, Hopkins LN. Workforce needs for endovascular neurosurgery. Neurosurgery 2006; 59: S271-6; discussion S3-13.

CHAPTER 2

Challenging Cranial Arteriovenous Fistulas

Guglielmo Pero[*]

Department of Neuroradiology, Niguarda Ca' Granda Hospital, Milan, Italy

Abstract: Arteriovenous fistulas, both pial and dural, are neurovascular malformations which frequently have a poor natural history. Their treatment can be either endovascular or neurosurgical. The evolution of neurointerventional materials and techniques extended the indication for endovascular treatment to most of the arteriovenous fistulas.

A clear understanding of the vascular anatomy of arteriovenous fistulas is essential in order to be able to treat them. Familiarity with neurovascular techniques and devices is also important for choosing the proper treatment strategy in each case.

In this chapter the different types of fistulas are discussed with the most appropriate treatment strategies in each situation, also taking into consideration the neurovascular materials now available.

Keywords: Dural arteriovenous fistula, endovascular treatment, pial arteriovenous fistula.

INTRODUCTION

Arteriovenous fistulas are abnormal connections between arteries and veins without intervening vessels. They can be cranial and spinal and can involve both dural vessels and pial vessels. Moreover arteriovenous fistulas can be "direct" shunts between one artery and one vein (direct arteriovenous fistulas) or composed of multiple arteriovenous shunts between arterioles of the wall of a dural sinus and the sinus itself.

A clear understanding of the angioarchitecture of an arteriovenous fistula is essential for the endovascular treatment of the fistula. The aim of the treatment is the obliteration, *via* either the arterial or venous route, of the shunting point, which is not always easy to identify. Proximal occlusions will result in recanalization of the fistulas, whereas too distal occlusions risk transforming the fistulas into more aggressive lesions, recruiting cortical veins proximal to the occlusion point.

---

*Corresponding author Guglielmo Pero: Department of Neuroradiology, Niguarda Ca' Granda Hospital, Milano, Italy; Tel:/Fax: +39 02 6444.2773; E-mail: guglielmo.pero@ospedaleniguarda.it

Simone Peschillo (Ed.)

CRANIAL DURAL ARTERIOVENOUS FISTULAS

Dural arteriovenous fistulas (DAVFs) are composed of multiple arteriovenous shunts between the arterioles of the dural wall of the sinus and its venous compartment. They can occur at any point of the dura but the transverse-sigmoid sinus and cavernous sinus are the most frequent locations.

Generally the arterial supply comes from meningeal branches of the external or internal carotid arteries, or of the vertebral arteries but a supply from the pial arteries is frequent in larger and high-flow fistulas [1].

The venous outflow is the main feature of a DAVF that influences the prognosis and, therefore, the decision to treat the fistula.

Various classifications of DAVFs have been proposed; almost all are designed to distinguish between benign and aggressive DAVFs. Benign DAVFs drain into dural sinuses not involving the cortical veins; they are associated with headache, bruit and orbital signs [2].

Drainage into cerebral veins makes the prognosis significantly worse, increasing the annual mortality risk up to 10.4% and the risk of any neurological event to 15% [3]; the involvement of cerebral veins can cause hemorrhage or neurological symptoms related to venous hypertension (*i.e.* seizures, focal neurological deficits, cognitive impairment and myelopathy).

Of the various classifications of DAVFs, in our clinical practice we most frequently use the Borden classification (Table **1**) [4] because it is based on a simple subdivision of three types of fistulas. Type I fistulas drain into the dural venous sinus or meningeal veins; they are often asymptomatic or present with a bruit and the risk that they bleed is very low. Type II fistulas drain into the dural sinus and then into leptomeningeal veins. Type III fistulas drain directly into a cerebral vein without the interposition of the dural sinuses. This classification is used in this chapter unless otherwise specified.

The classification of Djindjian and Merland, published in 1973, formerly clarified the role of venous drainage in assessing the prognosis of DAVFs (Table **2**) [5]. This classification comprises four types of DAVFs; the first three types are similar to the three types of the Borden classification. Djindjian and Merland type IV fistulas have cerebral venous drainage with large venous dilatations (lakes) that may behave with a mass effect.

Table 1. Classification of dural arteriovenous fistulas according to Borden *et al.*

Type	Venous Drainage
I	Anterograde or retrograde drainage into dural venous sinuses only
II	Anterograde or retrograde drainage into dural venous sinuses and then into cortical veins
III	Retrograde cortical venous drainage only

Table 2. Classification of dural arteriovenous fistulas according to Djindjian and Merland.

Type	Venous Drainage
I	Located in the sinus with anterograde or retrograde flow
II	Located in the sinus with reflux into cortical veins
III	Direct cortical venous drainage
IV	Cortical venous drainage into large venous lakes

In 1995 Cognard *et al.* proposed a revision of this classification emphasizing the role of the venous drainage in predicting the risk of each DAVF (Table **3**) [3]. They expanded the classification of Djindjian and Merland and included five types of DAVFs with three subtypes of type II fistulas. Type V DAVFs drain into spinal perimedullary veins and all these fistulas, in their series, had an aggressive presentation (progressive myelopathy, subarachnoid hemorrhage or focal neurological deficit).

Table 3. Classification of dural arteriovenous fistulas according to Cognard *et al.*

Type	Venous Drainage
I	Located in the sinus with anterograde flow
II a	Located in the sinus with reflux into the sinus
II b	Located in the sinus with reflux into cortical veins
II a+b	Located in the sinus with reflux into both the sinus and cortical veins
III	Direct cortical venous drainage
IV	Direct cortical venous drainage with venous ectasia
V	Direct cortical venous drainage with spinal venous drainage

Most of DAVFs are located in the transverse-sigmoid sinus or in the cavernous sinus. Other frequent locations are the superior sagittal sinus, the *confluens sinuum* (torcular Herophili), the tentorium (the straight sinus and the superior petrosal sinus) and the anterior cranial fossa (in the region of the olfactory fossa).

It should be noted that the location of DAVFs is related to the clinical symptoms, either because of the structures located near the fistula or because of the different venous structures that can be involved [1]. The anatomic location of the fistula also influences the endovascular approach and the chances of treatment being successful.

The treatment of DAVFs can be palliative or curative. The former type of treatment has the aim of reducing the symptoms related to the fistula and can be proposed for type I fistulas with unbearable symptoms (typically the bruit related to DAVFs of the transverse-sigmoid sinus). This type of treatment is carried out mainly by transarterial embolization with polyvinyl alcohol particles. Nevertheless a progression from benign to aggressive fistulas has been rarely reported as a consequence of palliative treatments [6]. Spontaneous occlusions of the fistula occur in up to 10% of DAVFs of the cavernous sinus and less frequently in fistulas of the transverse-sigmoid sinus [7]. Multiple daily manual compression of the carotid artery and the jugular vein at the neck has been used in the past as a conservative treatment of DAVFs of the cavernous sinus or the transverse-sigmoid sinus, with some reports of complete occlusion of the fistulas [8].

The curative treatment of DAVFs consists of occluding the fistulous arteriovenous connection and the first segment of the venous outflow. It can be achieved either by surgical disconnection of the vein or by endovascular occlusion of the fistula and its abnormal venous outlet. The current endovascular techniques consist mainly of Onyx (Covidien, EV3, Irvine, CA, USA) injection (transarterial or transvenous) and transvenous coiling of the dural sinus or of the vein. In complex cases both approaches can be used in the same procedure.

Dural Arteriovenous Fistulas of the Transverse-Sigmoid Sinus

DAVFs of the transverse-sigmoid sinus are most often type I fistulas with non-aggressive symptoms [1, 3]. They frequently cause a bruit and pulsatile tinnitus because there is an increased blood flow near the middle ear, both in the arterial branches of the external carotid artery supplying the fistula and in the venous sinus. Nevertheless, in some series, DAVFs of the transverse-sigmoid sinus were mainly type II and III fistulas [9]. The progression of a type I fistula to a type II one is related to progressive venous hypertension that causes stenosis and occlusion of the draining sinus [6]. The symptoms of type II and III fistulas of the transverse-sigmoid sinus are headache, focal neurological signs and cognitive impairment.

In our clinical practice, we do not treat type I fistulas of the transverse-sigmoid sinus unless an extreme bruit becomes unbearable and prevents daily routine. In such cases, endovascular embolization with polyvinyl alcohol particles was the usual treatment until the advent of Onyx for the occlusion of DAVFs [10]. Embolization of DAVFs with polyvinal alcohol particles is only a palliative treatment that reduces the flow temporarily, occluding the feeding arteries; nowadays we reserve this treatment to patients who cannot undergo more aggressive but curative treatments. The advantage of this kind of procedure is that it can be done under local anesthesia.

The advent of Onyx and the availability of large remodeling balloons changed the treatment of DAVFs of the transverse-sigmoid sinus. Onyx injection always requires general anesthesia because of the intense pain caused by the irritant action of the dimethylsulfoxide (DMSO) [11]. It also requires that the patient remains still for very long time.

Onyx can be used to occlude a fistula either *via* a transarterial or transvenous approach. Factors that need to be evaluated when choosing the treatment strategy in transverse-sigmoid sinus fistulas (both types I and II) are the complete patency of the sinus, the presence of normal cortical veins that drain into the sinus (especially the vein of Labbé) and the navigability of arterial feeders and the sinus. Generally a transarterial injection has the advantage that Onyx starts to occlude the vein from the point of the fistula making the injection more easily understandable; furthermore, a smaller amount of Onyx is required.

When the transverse sinus is patent we prefer to proceed with transarterial injection of Onyx, protecting the patency of the sinus with a balloon. The Copernic 8 x 80 mm (Balt Extrusion, Montmorency, France) is a large low-pressure, compliant remodeling balloon [12]. It protects the patency of the sinus during the injection of Onyx from the arterial feeders of the DAVF and steers the Onyx directly into the arteries, reducing the amount of Onyx that needs to be injected and the time of treatment (Fig. **1**). The balloon can be positioned in the dural sinus through a venous femoral access with a 6 French guiding catheter in the jugular vein; it supports 0.014 inch microguidewires and can also reach the superior sagittal sinus or the straight sinus.

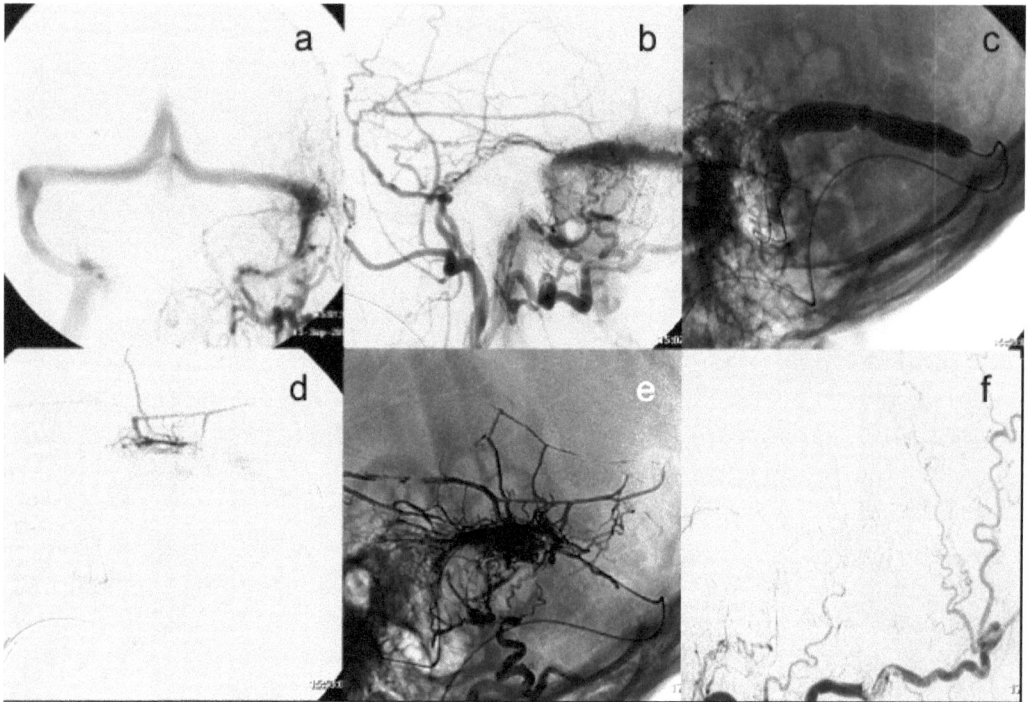

Figure 1: (a) and (b) DAVF of the left transverse-sigmoid sinus that drains into the right transverse-sinus with simultaneous occlusion of the left jugular vein. (c) A Copernic 8 x 80 mm remodeling balloon is inflated in the left transverse-sigmoid sinus approaching from the right side; the microcatheter is in the left middle meningeal artery. (d) The contrast injection from the microcatheter during inflation of the balloon. (e) and (f) The final Onyx cast with complete occlusion of the fistula. (Courtesy of Dr. E. Boccardi).

It is recommended that, before starting the Onyx injection, a test angiographic series is performed from the arterial side while inflating the venous balloon in order to identify collateral venous drainage of the fistula and also to understand the arterial feeders better. Test angiography will also demonstrate the junction of the cerebral veins with the sinus, which is important because occluding them with Onyx could cause hemorrhagic complications due to the impairment of the cerebral venous drainage.

Strategies that can be used in the case of very large sinuses, with diameters greater than the 8 mm Copernic balloon, are the introduction of two 8 mm Copernic balloons in parallel or folding one balloon or more in the sinus if it is occluded [13]; otherwise, one larger non-compliant balloon for peripheral vascular angioplasty can be used. Peripheral vascular angioplasty balloons are stiffer and their navigation through the jugular gulf and the sigmoid sinus is more difficult than that of the Copernic balloon, so they require an 8 French direct internal jugular vein access and, frequently, an 8 French guiding catheter in the transverse sinus.

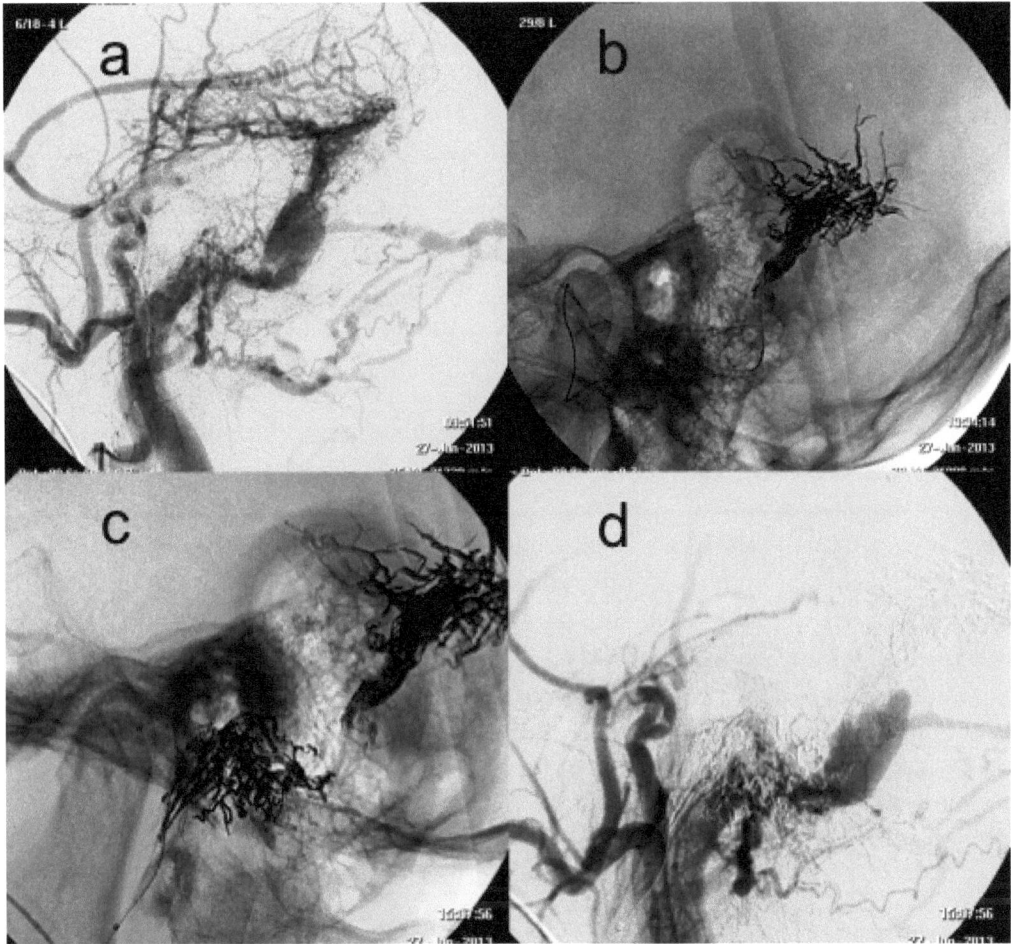

Figure 2: DAVF of the transverse-sigmoid sinus causing an unbearable bruit. (a) There are two different fistula sites: the transverse-sigmoid sinus and the jugular gulf; the sinus is occluded behind the fistula. (b) The distal fistula was closed with coils and Onyx, occluding the sinus. (c) Onyx injection from the neuromeningeal branch of the ascending pharyngeal artery to occlude the jugular gulf fistula. (d) This fistula was partially occluded because during the injection an anastomosis with the intrapetrous internal carotid artery appeared. Nevertheless, the symptoms were resolved completely.

Partially occluded transverse-sigmoid sinuses that do not drain normal cerebral veins can be sacrificed. In such situations there is no need for patency to be protected with a balloon; frequently an easier treatment consists of occluding the fistula and the sinus transvenously with coils and Onyx (Fig. **2**). In such situations, extreme care is necessary to seal the fistula completely because occlusion of the sinus without complete occlusion of the fistula can result in the evolution of the fistula into a more aggressive type: the venous outflow of the fistula can be redirected to cortical veins converting a type I fistula in a type II or III fistula.

Sometimes in type II DAVFs of the transverse-sigmoid sinus the sinus is patent only in the fistulous segment and it is occluded both distally and proximally. The easiest way to occlude these fistulas is injection of Onyx from the arterial feeders. Unfortunately this strategy is not always practicable because the feeding arteries are extremely tortuous or thin or because the route is occluded by previous unsuccessful treatments.

If the microcatheter cannot reach a position adequately proximal to the fistula, the penetration of the Onyx can be improved by occluding the artery just proximal to the tip of the microcatheter. This can be achieved either by using coils and glue and injecting the Onyx through a detachable tip microcatheter [13] or by injecting Onyx from a dual lumen balloon microcatheter [14]. These techniques allow a more comprehensive, forceful and controlled Onyx embolization, avoiding too prolonged reflux of Onyx particularly in large arteries (Fig. **3**).

When the fistula cannot be reached endovascularly, the options remaining are direct surgical occlusion or endovascular occlusion of the isolated sinus previously surgically exposed (Fig. **4**).

Type III DAVFs of the transverse-sigmoid sinus are located at the junction of a cortical vein with the transverse sinus; the sinus is often, but not necessarily, occluded. The management of this type of fistula is commonly occlusion by transarterial Onyx embolization.

DAVFs of the transverse-sigmoid sinus frequently extend to the jugular gulf or to the torcular herophili. Extension to the jugular gulf is generally associated with type I fistulas and increases the bruit because of its position near the middle ear (Fig. **2**).

Torcular involvement, on the other hand, is associated with more aggressive types of fistula, with greater flow and more symptoms related to cerebral venous outflow impairment. Distal catheterization of the posterior meningeal artery or occipital artery is frequently required to treat torcular DAVFs.

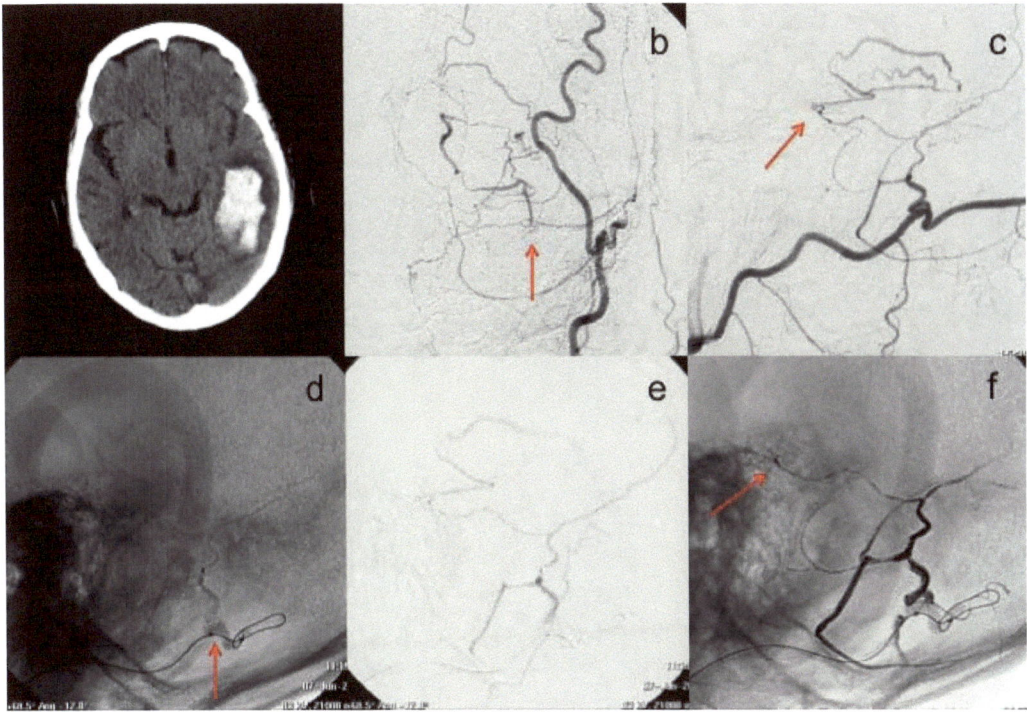

Figure 3: Left temporal basal hemorrhage (a) caused by a small DAVF of the superior petrous sinus, filled by the petrous branch of the occipital artery (arrows in b and c). (d) A remodeling balloon (arrow) was inflated in the occipital artery to allow easier catheterization of the branch and to improve the progression of the Onyx toward the fistula; nevertheless the microcatheter did not pass the intradiploic tract of the artery (e). (f) The Onyx just reached the point of the fistula (arrow), not passing entirely into the vein; however, the fistula was completely occluded at the angiographic control after 6 months.

Dural Arteriovenous Fistulas of the Cavernous Sinus

The cavernous sinus is the second more frequent site of DAVFs. A premise is essential before discussing their endovascular treatment.

DAVFs of the cavernous sinus need to be distinguished from carotid-cavernous fistulas (CCFs); they have different pathophysiology, different vascular architecture and, therefore, different endovascular treatments.

CCFs are direct connections of the cavernous segment of the internal carotid artery (ICA) with the cavernous sinus; they can be post-traumatic due to laceration of the ICA caused by a fracture of the base of the skull, or spontaneous due to the rupture of an intracavernous aneurysm. So frequently there is a single fistulous hole in the arterial wall that can be passed through with different systems (microcatheters or detachable balloons). CCFs are analyzed in depth in a separate section of this chapter.

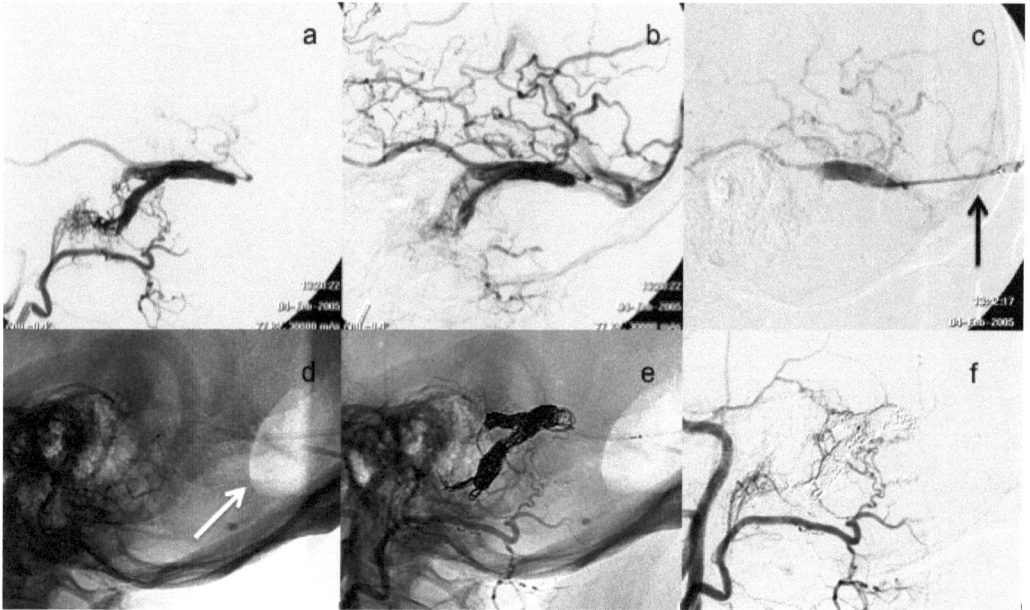

Figure 4: (a) and (b) DAVF of the "isolated" transverse-sigmoid sinus, draining into cortical veins. (c) Contrast injection through the catheter of the peripheral access needle (arrow) used to puncture the sinus after its surgical exposure. (d) The tip of the microcatheter is in the distal end of the occluded sinus; the arrow points to the edge of the craniotomy. (e) and (f) Complete coil occlusion of the sinus and of the fistula. (Courtesy of Dr. E. Boccardi).

DAVFs can involve the whole cavernous sinus or just a part of it; they can also involve the intercavernous sinus, the basilar sinus and the clival sinus, which are sometimes difficult to discriminate angiographically. DAVFs can also involve both cavernous sinuses.

Clinical symptoms can be related to impaired venous drainage of the orbit, the inflammatory action on the cranial nerves that pass through the cavernous sinus and the increase of blood flow in the vascular structures of the region.

Fistulas that drain mainly into the ophthalmic veins (more frequently into the superior vein) impair the venous drainage of the orbit, causing conjunctival chemosis, visual loss, exophthalmos and glaucoma. Orbital venous drainage may also be impaired by thrombosis of the ophthalmic veins due to the extension of the thrombophlebitis of the cavernous sinus associated with the fistula; these fistulas are frequently small and with slow flow and the associated symptoms are also due to cranial nerve impairment (diplopia and headache) [15].

If the DAVF of the cavernous sinus drains mainly into the inferior petrosal sinus it can be almost asymptomatic or cause a bruit due to the increased blood flow near the middle ear. DAVFs of the cavernous sinus that drain laterally or posteriorly can involve cortical veins of the middle cranial fossa (*i.e.* the Sylvian vein) or the infratentorial veins, sometimes into the perimedullary spinal veins (type V fistulas of Cognard's classification). Although type II DAVFs of the cavernous sinus seem to be less aggressive than type II fistulas in other locations, they do require treatment.

Ocular symptoms of DAVFs of the cavernous sinus can improve with medical therapy using corticoids and anticoagulation [16]. In cases of DAVFs of the cavernous sinus without cerebral venous drainage, we usually attempt to reduce the symptoms with medical therapy and reserve endovascular treatment to those patients who do not benefit from the medical therapy.

The endovascular treatment of DAVFs of the cavernous sinus is preferentially done *via* transvenous occlusion of the cavernous sinus [17]; both coils and liquid embolic agents can be used to occlude the fistula. It is, therefore, recommended that a DMSO-compatible microcatheter is used because frequently the embolization starts with detachable coils and is completed with Onyx to ensure total occlusion of the fistula.

The cavernous sinus can be reached either through the inferior petrosal sinus or through the superior ophthalmic vein (Fig. **5**) [18]. When patent, the inferior petrosal sinus is easy to catheterize and offers a rapid and stable route for coil embolization of the cavernous sinus. The superior ophthalmic vein is frequently approachable through the facial vein with a femoral access [19]; in these cases, we prefer to use a distal access guiding catheter that can reach the facial vein near the orbit. In some cases direct puncture of the facial or frontal vein is required: an 18 gauge peripheral venous catheter is used to access the frontal or facial vein and a 2.4 French microcatheter is passed through it to navigate the superior ophthalmic vein up to the cavernous sinus (Fig. **6**).

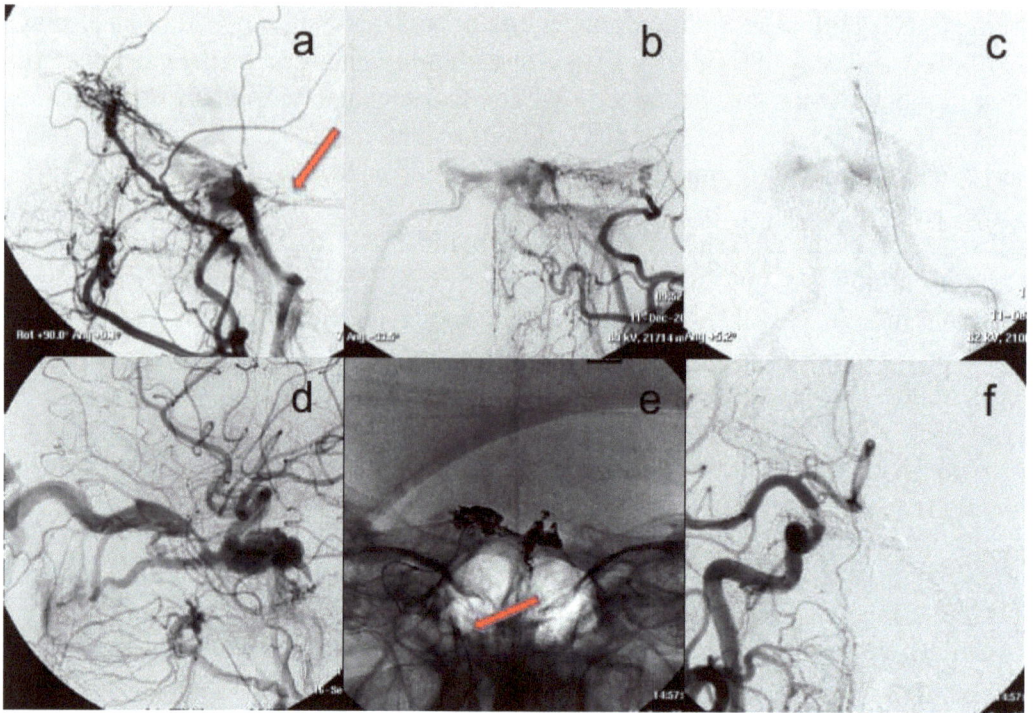

Figure 5: (a) A DAVF of the cavernous sinus draining into both the inferior petrosal sinuses and the left superior petrosal sinus (red arrow). (b) The same patient in an anteroposterior view showing both inferior petrosal sinuses injected by the fistula. (c) The same patient: the microcatheter is in the left cavernous sinus passing through the left inferior petrosal sinus. (d) Another patient with a DAVF of the right cavernous sinus and intercavernous sinus draining into the right ophthalmic vein; (e) and (f) The same patient as in (d) at the end of the procedure. (e) The red arrow points to the tip of the distal access catheter in the facial vein at the medial edge of the orbit; the Onyx cast is in the right cavernous sinus and the intercavernous sinus. (f) Right common carotid artery injection showing complete obliteration of the fistula.

In past years surgical exposure of the superior ophthalmic vein was used frequently and this is still a good approach in difficult cases [19-21]. Venous access through the superior petrosal sinus can also be attempted, but it is more difficult [22].

In some cases both the inferior petrosal sinus and the superior ophthalmic vein are occluded and the fistula drains into cortical veins or into small partially thrombosed orbital veins. In these cases endovascular occlusion of the fistula is difficult because of the lack of any venous access to the cavernous sinus. The first attempt in such situations is to pass through the occluded inferior petrosal sinus (Fig. 7), with a good chance of reaching the point of the fistula [18]. Some authors proposed percutaneous transorbital extra-conic puncture of the cavernous sinus in cases of lack of any venous route [23-25]. Direct puncture of the cortical vein after craniotomy was even suggested [26].

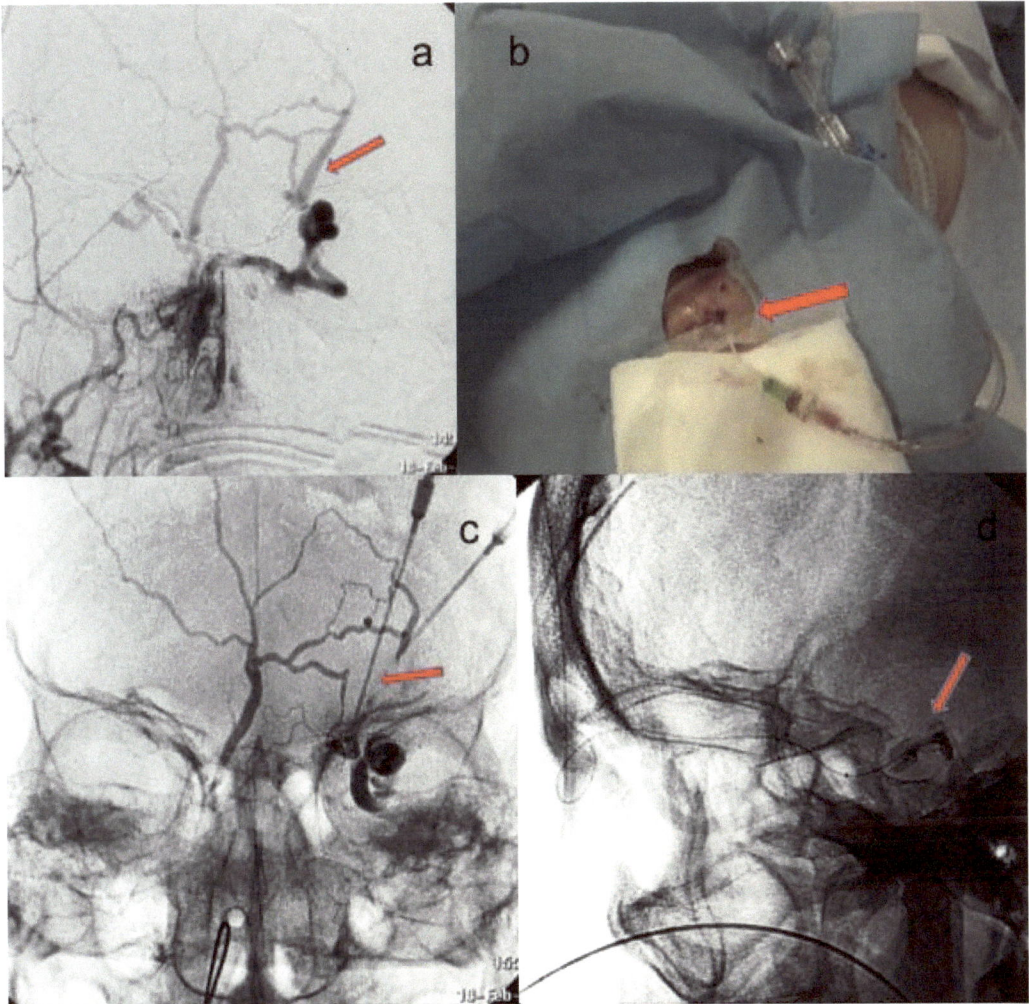

Figure 6: (a) DAVF of the left cavernous sinus and intercavernous sinus draining into the ophthalmic vein and frontal vein (arrow). (b) and (c) Puncture of the frontal vein (arrow) with the catheter attached to a Y connector to allow the transit of the microcatheter. (d) The tip of the microcatheter in the cavernous sinus (arrow).

The transarterial injection of Onyx to occlude a DAVF of the cavernous sinus is limited by possible embolic complications related to the numerous anastomoses between the most frequent arterial feeders of the fistula (middle meningeal artery, accessory meningeal artery, internal maxillary artery and neuromeningeal branch of the ascending pharyngeal artery) and the carotid siphon or the ophthalmic artery through their meningeal branches. Moreover there is the risk of cranial nerve palsies due to compression in osseous foramina or to ischemic injury related to the occlusion of the vasa nervorum [16, 27]. Nevertheless in some selected cases transarterial Onyx injection can give good results; in our experience, the preferred route is the superior pharyngeal branch of the ascending pharyngeal artery (Fig. **8**).

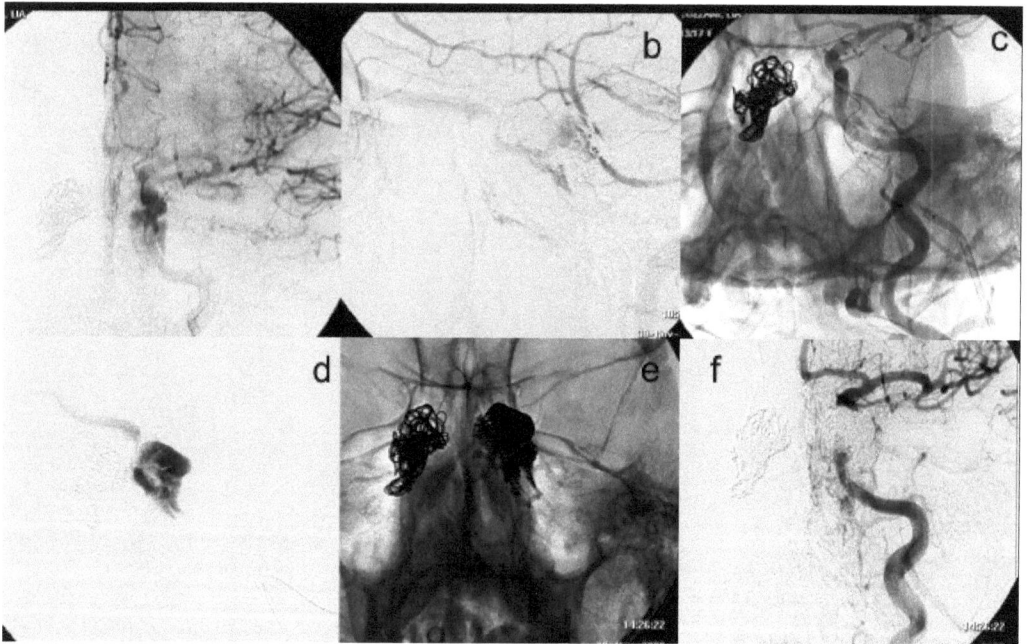

Figure 7: (a) and (b) DAVF of the left cavernous sinus in a patient previously treated for a DAVF of the right cavernous sinus; the fistula has slow flow and drains into the superior ophthalmic vein without access from the facial vein. (c) A microcatheter reached the cavernous sinus passing through the chronically occluded inferior petrosal sinus. (d) A control angiogram from the microcatheter to confirm its correct position. (e) and (f) The fistula was completely occluded with coils and Onyx.

In this case the tip of the microcatheter is placed in the apex of the vault of the nasopharynx and the Onyx is injected into the really tiny transclival arteries that reach the fistula through the trabecular bone of the clivus; this access, in our experience, had several benefits because catheterization of the superior pharyngeal branch of the ascending pharyngeal artery is easier and safer than catheterization of its neuromeningeal branch or the cavernous branches of the middle or accessory meningeal arteries. Moreover there are fewer arterial anastomoses with dural branches of the ICA and the vertebral artery, reducing the risk of embolic complications.

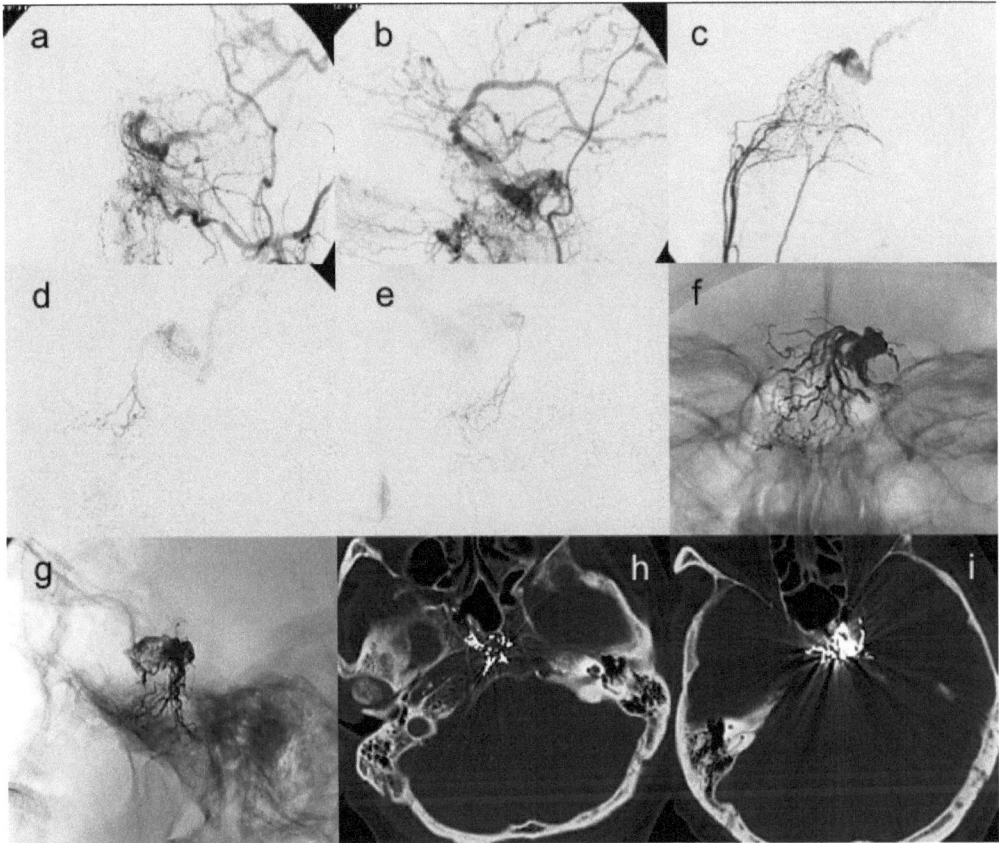

Figure 8: (a) and (b) DAVF of the left cavernous sinus draining into the cortical veins, with partial thrombosis of the superior ophthalmic vein. (c) Frontal view of injection of the ascending pharyngeal artery. (d) and (e) Frontal and lateral views of microcatheter injection from the superior pharyngeal branch of the ascending pharyngeal artery. (f) to (i) The cast of Onyx at the end of the procedure.

Dural Arteriovenous Fistulas of the Superior Sagittal Sinus

DAVFs of the superior sagittal sinus frequently drain into cortical veins either directly (type III of Borden's classification) or indirectly (type II of Borden's classification) and are frequently high flow fistulas [9].

Transarterial Onyx embolization is the treatment of choice in most cases; in type II fistulas a remodeling balloon may be required to avoid occlusion of the sinus (Fig. **9**).

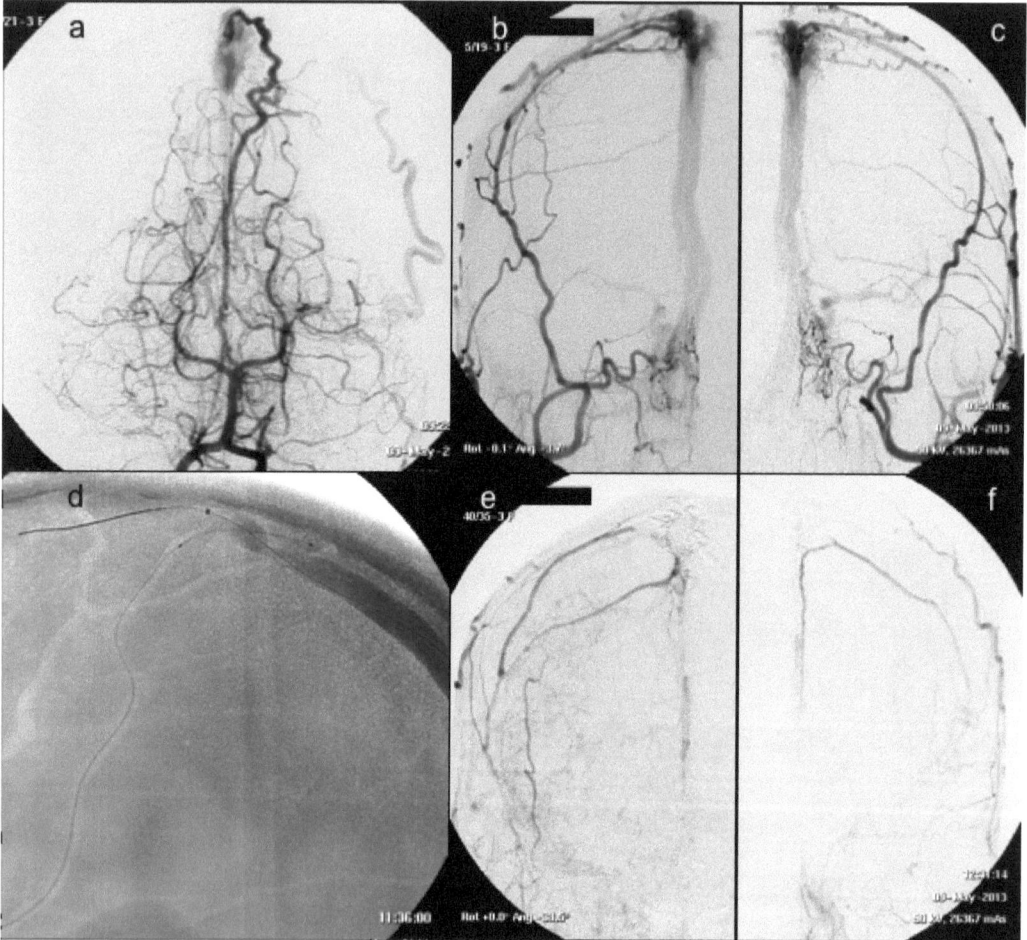

Figure 9: Tipe I DAVF of the superior sagittal sinus, fed by the posterior meningeal artery (a) and both the middle meningeal arteries (b) and (c), was occluded by Onyx injection from the left middle meningeal artery with a remodelling balloon Copernic 8 x 80 mm (d) inflated in the sinus to preserve its patency. (e) and (f) show the complete occlusion of the fistula. (Courtesy of Dr. L. Valvassori).

The arterial route is usually an easy access because the main feeding branches frequently come from the middle meningeal arteries.

Dural Arteriovenous Fistulas of the Tentorium

Tentorial DAVFs need to be divided into fistulas of the falco-tentorial junction (or of the vein of Galen region or of the straight sinus) and fistulas of the superior petrosal sinus. Fistulas in both locations are characterized by a high frequency of aggressive clinical presentation because the venous drainage is almost always into cerebral veins [3, 9, 28].

Fistulas of the falco-tentorial junction drain toward the vein of Galen with frequent retrograde outflow in the internal cerebral veins and basal veins, causing aggressive clinical features, such as hemorrhage, focal neurological deficits, seizure, and myelopathy. These fistulas can cause basal ganglia impairment with motor and sensory disturbances, cognitive decline and hyper-somnolence [29].

DAVFs of the falco-tentorial junction frequently have a pial supply from distal branches of the superior cerebellar arteries or posterior cerebral arteries; this arterial supply increases the risk of hemorrhage following endovascular occlusion of the fistula (Fig. **10**) [30].

The treatment of choice of DAVFs of the falco-tentorium is transarterial Onyx embolization which, in most of cases, provides complete occlusion of the fistula. Sometimes transarterial occlusion of the fistula cannot be achieved and transvenous occlusion of the vein of Galen and the fistula is the only endovascular possibility (Fig. **11**).

Branches of the middle meningeal arteries and tentorial branches of the posterior meningeal arteries are the most frequent supplies of DAVFs of the falco-tentorial junction and the former often provide the route for the endovascular occlusion of such fistulas.

Both the posterior cerebral artery (artery of Davidoff and Schechter) [31] and the superior cerebellar artery [32] can give dural branches directed to the tentorium and the falco-tentorial junction; in cerebral angiograms these branches have a course similar to that of the posterior half of the tentorial branch of Bernasconi and Cassinari arising from the carotid syphon. Both these arteries can be catheterized and are easy and safe routes for obtaining transarterial occlusion of DAVFs of the falco-tentorial junction by Onyx injection (Fig. **12**).

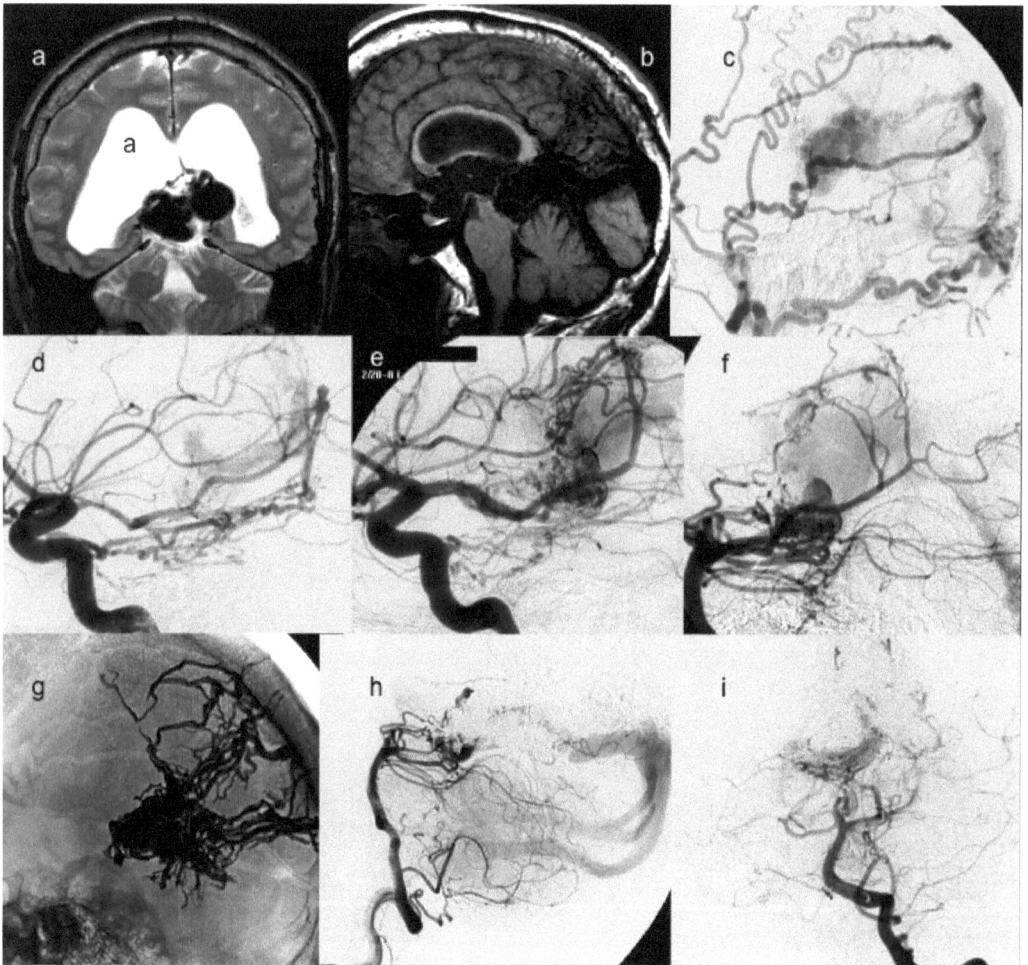

Figure 10: DAVF of the falco-tentorial junction with large venous ectasia of the vein of Galen (a, b, c) with several pial feeding branches (d, e, f, g). The cast of Onyx at the end of the second endovascular procedure with some residual flow from the pial branches (h, i). The patient died two months later of cerebral hemorrhage from those pial branches (no images available). (Courtesy of Dr. L. Valvassori).

DAVFs of the superior petrosal sinus typically drain into the petrosal vein, and from here into the lateral mesencephalic vein, the basal vein and the vein of Galen, so they are usually type III fistulas that can present with intracranial hemorrhage. They can also cause trigeminal neuralgia and temporal seizures.

Until the advent of the Onyx their treatment was almost always surgical because the disconnection of the draining vein is relatively easy and has a low morbidity. Nowadays transarterial Onyx embolization through the meningeal branches of the external carotid artery is the treatment of choice; if the draining vein is neither too tortuous nor ectatic, the transvenous route can be attempted but it is essential that the vein is occluded at its origin from the superior petrosal sinus (Fig. **13**).

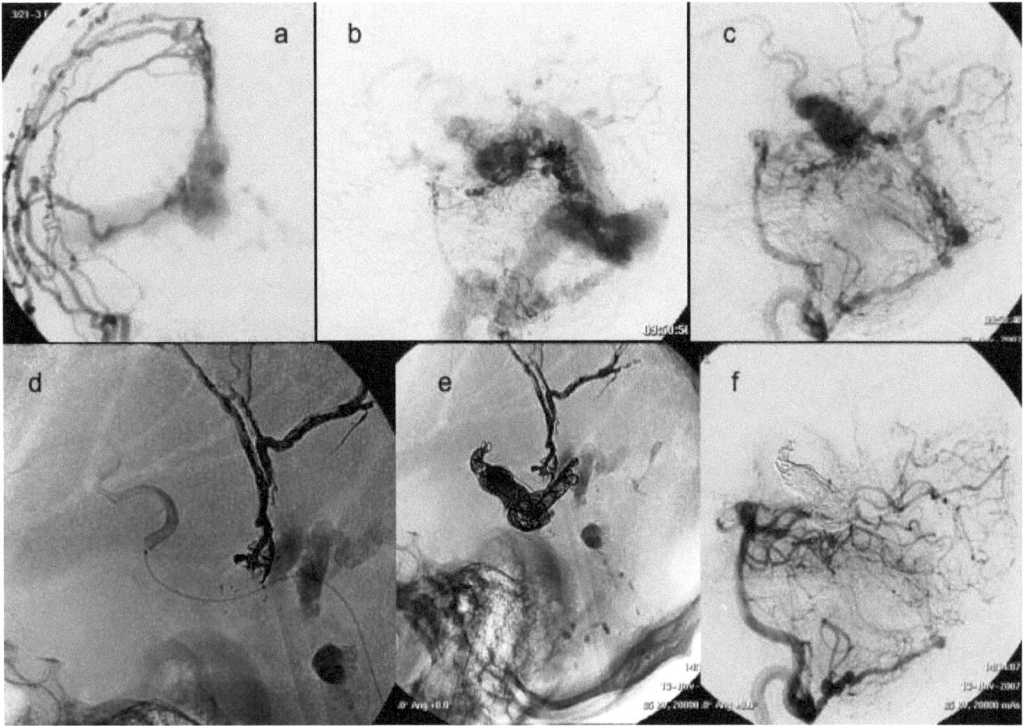

Figure 11: (a) and (b) DAVF of the falco-tentorial junction with venous drainage into the straight sinus and the cortical veins. (c) After three transarterial procedures, the drainage of the DAVF toward the cerebral veins increased. (d) A microcatheter was advanced into the internal cerebral vein and the treatment started with occluding both internal cerebral veins with coils. (e) The internal cerebral veins and the vein of Galen were occluded with coils and cyanoacrylate with complete obliteration of the fistula (f). (Courtesy of Dr. E. Boccardi).

Dural Arteriovenous Fistulas of the Anterior Cranial Fossa

DAVFs in the anterior cranial fossa are mainly located in the olfactory fossa or near the apophysis of the crista galli, where the olfactory and frontopolar veins enter the anterior edge of the superior sagittal sinus; they are usually type III fistulas. Their arterial supply comes from the ethmoidal branches of the ophthalmic and internal maxillary arteries or from the anterior meningeal artery. DAVFs of the anterior cranial fossa typically present with hemorrhage or seizure.

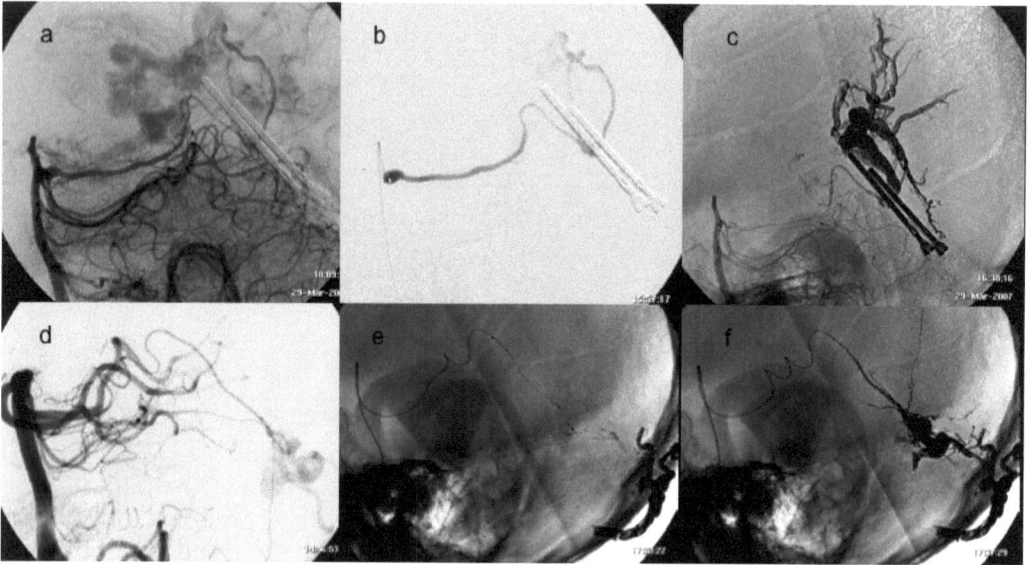

Figure 12: Two different DAVFs of the falco-tentorial junction treated by Onyx injection through the Davidoff and Schechter artery. (a), (b) and (c) This patient had undergone a previous, unsuccessful surgical attempt to occlude the fistula; an early tentorial branch of the posterior cerebral artery was catheterized leading to successful occlusion of the fistula. (d), (e) and (f) A DAVF of the inferior wall of the straight sinus receiving a tentorial branch of the P2 segment of the posterior cerebral artery; a first attempt to occlude the fistula through the occipital artery was performed in an other center without success. Complete occlusion of the fistulas was achieved in both patients. (Courtesy of Dr. E. Boccardi).

Surgical disconnection of the draining vein allows complete occlusion of the fistula and is associated with a low rate of morbidity so it is the usual treatment of DAVFs of the anterior cranial fossa. Sometimes the angio-architecture of the fistula allows a low-risk endovascular approach to the fistula from the anterior meningeal artery, through its connection with the middle meningeal artery (Fig. **14**) or transvenously by retrograde catheterization of the draining vein (Fig. **15**). Transarterial embolization through the ophthalmic artery is at high risk of thromboembolic complications in the central artery of the retina which can cause blindness.

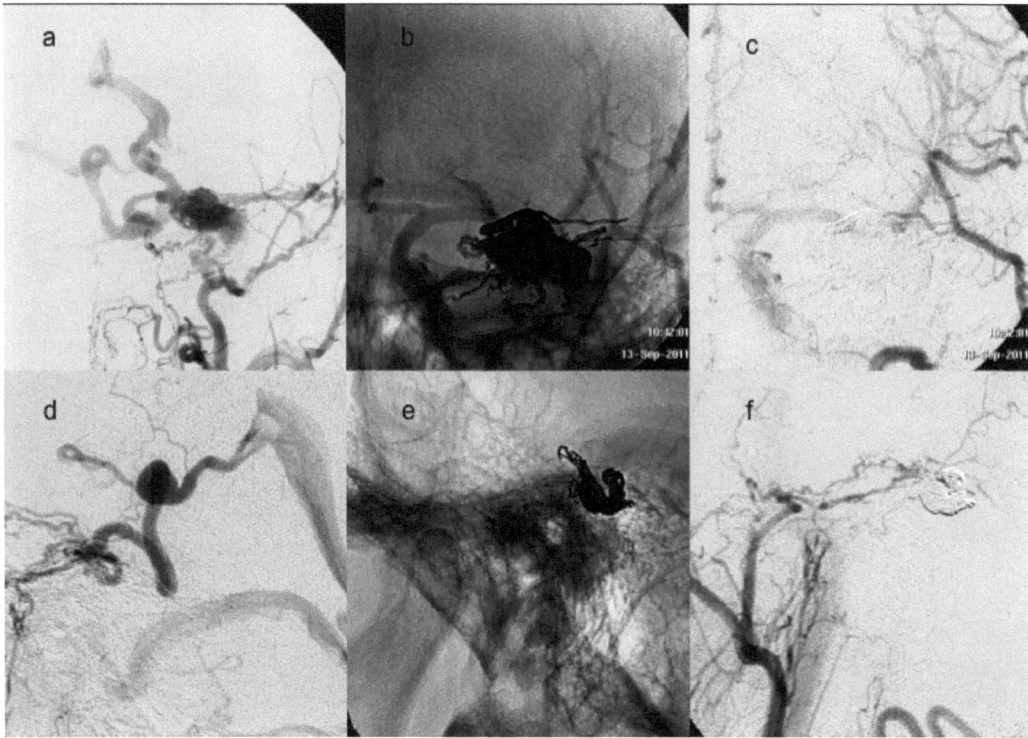

Figure 13: Two cases od DAVF of the superior petrosal sinus. (a) Frontal view of an angiogram of the left external carotid artery showing the fistula of the superior petrosal sinus draining into the petrosal vein toward the vein of Galen. (b) and (c) The cast of Onyx and the control angiogram of the common carotid artery demonstrating the complete obliteration of the fistula. (d) Lateral view of an angiogram of the left external carotid artery showing the fistula and its venous drainage. (e) and (f) After several attempts to reach the fistula through the branches of the middle meningeal artery, the point of the fistula was reached transvenously and coiling the draining vein achieved complete occlusion of the fistula. (Courtesy of Dr. E. Boccardi).

DIRECT ARTERIOVENOUS FISTULAS

Direct arteriovenous fistulas are communications between one or more arteries and a single vein without an intervening nidus. They can be spontaneous or post-traumatic. Spontaneous arteriovenous fistulas are more frequent in children whereas traumatic fistulas can occur in children and adults and involve mainly dural vessels. A CCF is the most common type of direct arteriovenous fistula.

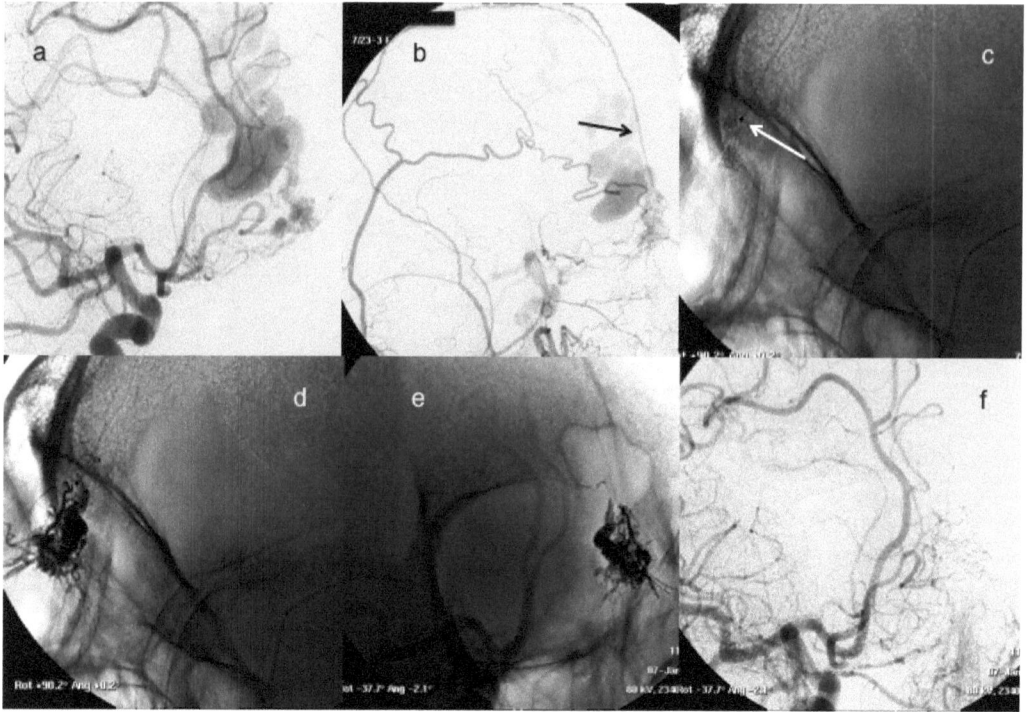

Figure 14: A DAVF of the anterior cranial fossa treated by transarterial Onyx injection. (b) The arrow points out the anterior meningeal artery filling the fistula through its anastomosis with the branches of the middle meningeal artery. (c) The tip of the microcatheter reached the fistula through the anterior meningeal artery. (d) and (e) The cast of Onyx in lateral and oblique views. (f) Right common carotid artery injection demonstrating the complete occlusion of the fistula. (Courtesy of Dr. M. Piano).

Carotid-cavernous Fistulas

CCFs can be spontaneous and post-traumatic. Spontaneous CCFs occur mainly in the elderly and are often due to the rupture of an aneurysm of the cavernous segment of the ICA; other causes of spontaneous CCFs are fibromuscular dysplasia, arterial dissection, and collagen deficiency syndromes.

Post-traumatic CCFs are the consequence of accidental blunt craniofacial trauma. The cavernous ICA is tightly adherent to the dura of the skull base, especially the walls of the sphenoid sinus that are frequently damaged by craniofacial trauma. Fractures of the walls of the sphenoid sinus can tear the ICA, which evolves into a pseudo-aneurysm and later into an arteriovenous fistula; in comatose patients CCFs frequently appear several days after the craniofacial trauma when the blood flow is high enough to induce the signs related to the impaired venous drainage of the orbit and the deep cerebral venous system.

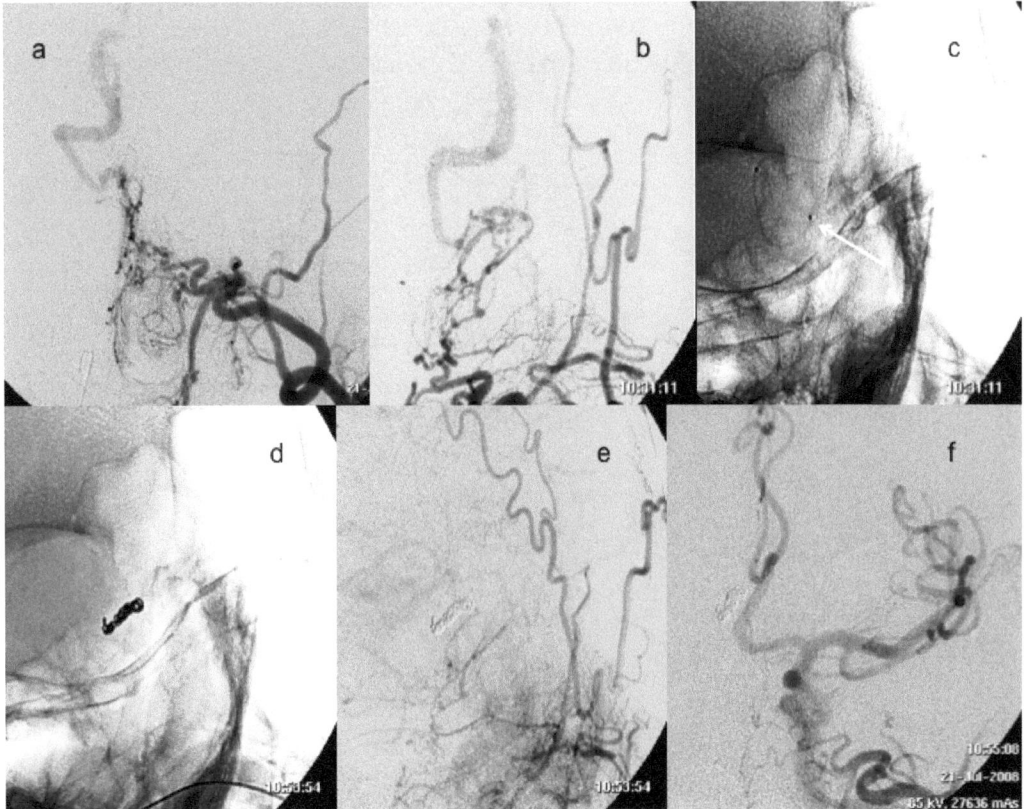

Figure 15: A DAVF of the anterior cranial fossa treated by transvenous coiling of the draining vein. (a) and (b) Frontal and oblique views of an angiogram of the left external carotid artery showing the fistula with a short and non-tortuous cortical vein draining into the superior sagittal sinus. (c) The microcatheter reached the foot of the vein. (d), (e) and (f): The cast of coils in the vein completely obliterating the fistula. (Courtesy of Dr. E. Boccardi).

Iatrogenic trauma during trans-sphenoidal hypophysectomy or other intracranial surgery is another cause of CCF; in these cases a massive hemorrhage may occur necessitating emergency endovascular treatment.

Symptoms related to CCFs are mainly bruit, proptosis and chemosis of the conjunctiva. The increased intraorbital venous pressure can also cause loss of vision and glaucoma. Diplopia due to cranial nerve palsy may occur. Intracranial hemorrhage is rare but can develop if the venous drainage is directed into the sphenoparietal sinus and from there into the cortical veins.

The angiographic assessment of CCFs requires a six-vessel angiography, completed by manual compression of the ipsilateral ICA to understand the exact location of the breach in the wall of the ICA, to assess the possibility of a safe occlusion of the ICA and to exclude the coexistence of fistulas from the meningeal branches of the external carotid artery (Fig. **16**).

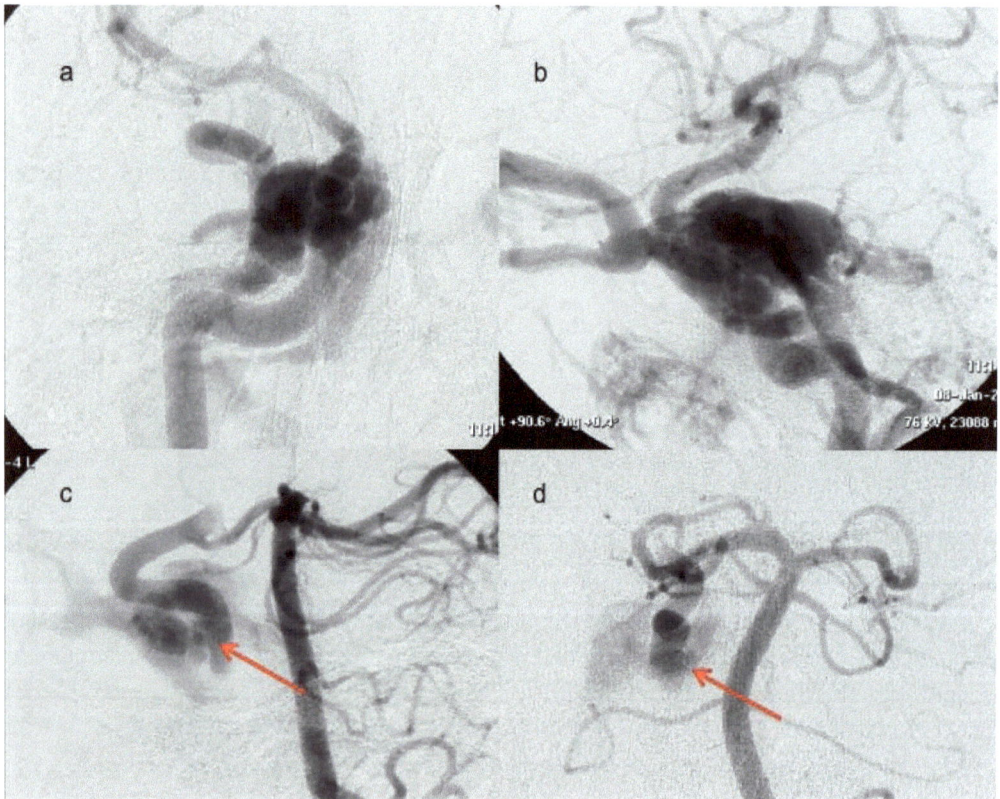

Figure 16: (a) and (b) A right CCF is shown by injection of the ICA. The venous drainage is into the ophthalmic veins, the inferior petrosal sinus and cortical veins; the exact location of the breach in the wall of the ICA is not clear. (c) and (d) Injection of the posterior circulation during manual compression of the carotid artery clearly shows the location of the fistula. (Courtesy of Dr. L. Valvassori).

CCFs are treated by occluding the connection between the ICA and the cavernous sinus. CCFs were one of the groundbreaking neurovascular pathologies amenable to endovascular treatment using the detachable endovascular balloons introduced and developed by Serbinenko and Debrun between the 1970s and 1980s [33-37].

A detachable balloon, mounted on the tip of a microcatheter and partially inflated, is floated through the fistula pushed by the high flow through the fistulous connection. Once inside the cavernous sinus the balloon is inflated and occludes the arterial breach from the venous sinus. Pulling on the microcatheter the balloon in detached and, if it maintains its position, the fistula is occluded (Fig. **17**).

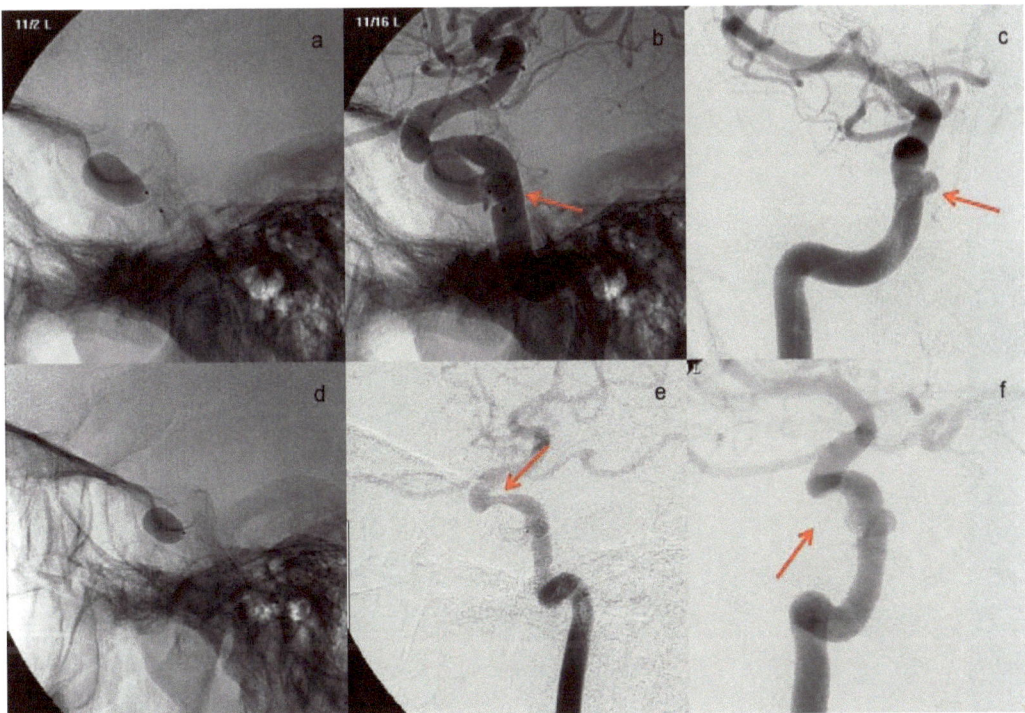

Figure 17: The same patient as in Fig. **16**. (a), (b) and (c) A Goldbal 1 detachable balloon (Balt Extrusion) is inflated inside the cavernous sinus completely occluding the fistula, with residual visualization of a small sector of the cavernous sinus (arrow in b and c). (d) The balloon has been detached. (e) and (f) Control angiography shows complete occlusion of the fistula with minimal reduction of the lumen of the ICA due to the pressure of the inflated balloon (arrows). (Courtesy of Dr. L. Valvassori).

Simple inflation and deflation of the balloon can also help to understand the exact site of the fistula and its characteristics. Despite this, the use of detachable balloons is, at times, associated with technical problems such as early detachment, deflation of the balloon within the first few hours after the procedure, or rupture of the balloon caused by its contact with bone fragments. These balloons can also cause distension of the site of the fistula or of the cavernous sinus itself.

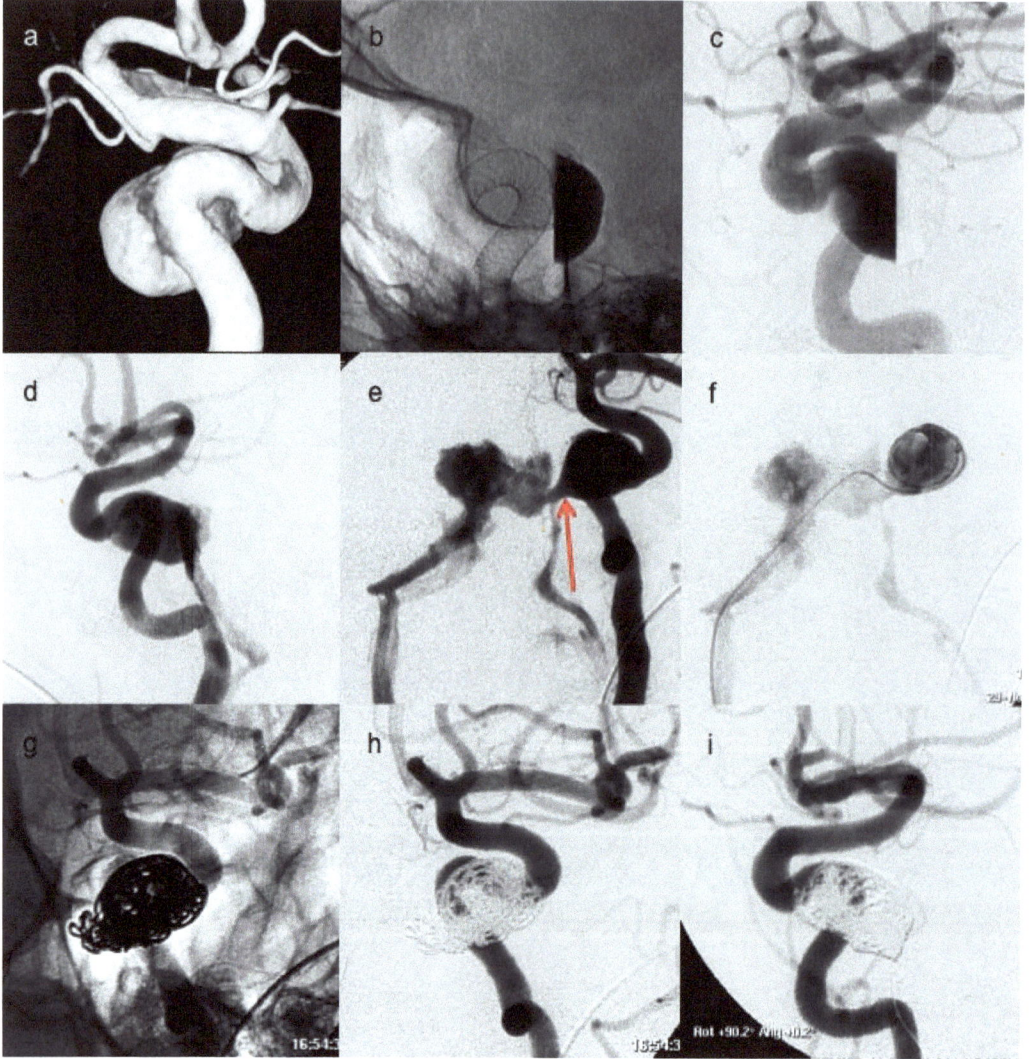

Figure 18: Transvenous coil embolization of a CCF. (a), (b) and (c) An intracavernous aneurysm of the left ICA was treated with a flow diverter stent (Pipeline, EV3). (d) and (e) Some days later the patient reported the onset of a bruit and angiography showed a CCF due to the rupture of the intracavernous aneurysm. (f) to (i) The fistula was treated by coil embolization of the aneurysm through its point of rupture, passing into the contralateral inferior petrosal sinus.

With the obvious improvements due to the progress of materials, in many centers around the world the treatment of choice of CCFs remains the occlusion of the fistula with detachable balloons. However, detachable balloons are, unfortunately, not so widely used they were in the past because many neurointerventionists are more familiar with the use of coils than with detachable balloons; moreover in recent years procurement of the balloons has become really difficult because only Balt Extrusion still produce them and in minimal amounts. Nevertheless, balloon occlusion of CCFs is still cheaper and faster than other endovascular techniques.

Transarterial and transvenous coil embolization involves packing the cavernous sinus near the fistula. Coil embolization is now the most widespread technique for endovascular occlusion of CCFs [38] (Figs. **18** and **19**), but this procedure is not always easy to complete and has high costs.

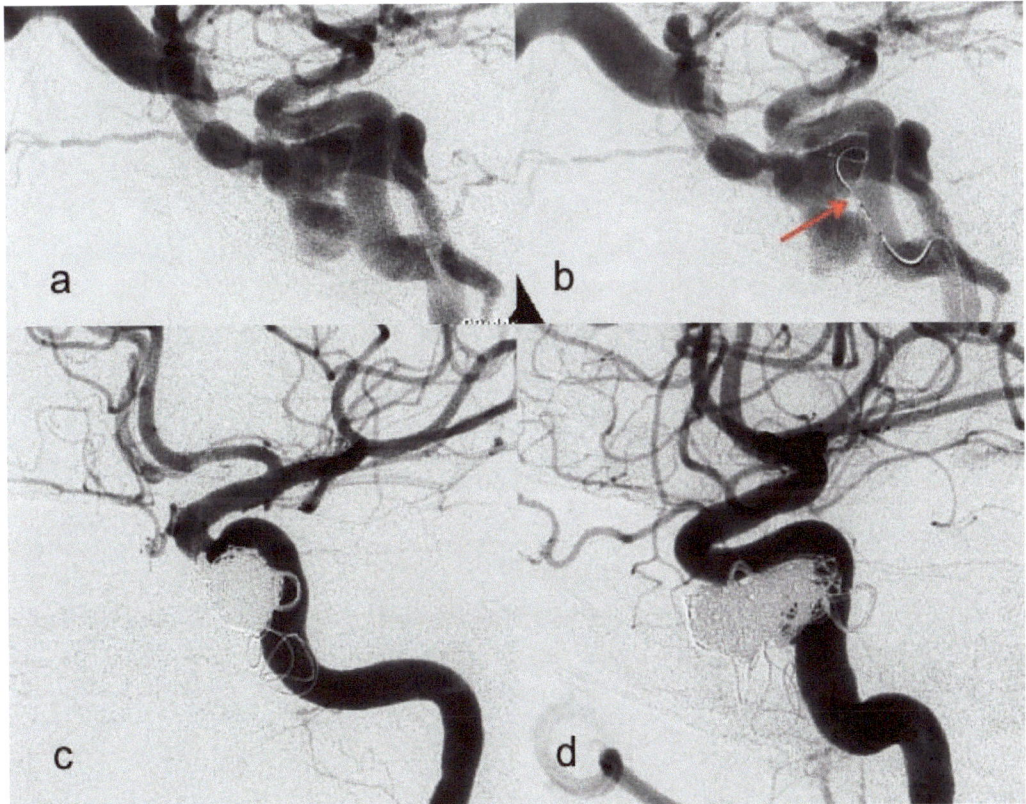

Figure 19: Transarterial coil embolization of a CCF. (a) Left ICA angiogram showing a CCF. (b) A microcatheter was placed in the cavernous sinus passing through the breach in the wall of the ICA. (c) and (d) Complete occlusion of the fistula by coiling the cavernous sinus.

Stent-grafts (covered stents) can be used to occlude CCFs; no covered stent is specifically dedicated for neurovascular use but such stents have been used in many cases to occlude CCFs or intracranial aneurysms (Fig. **20**). Their main drawback is the stiffness of both the stent and its delivery system [39].

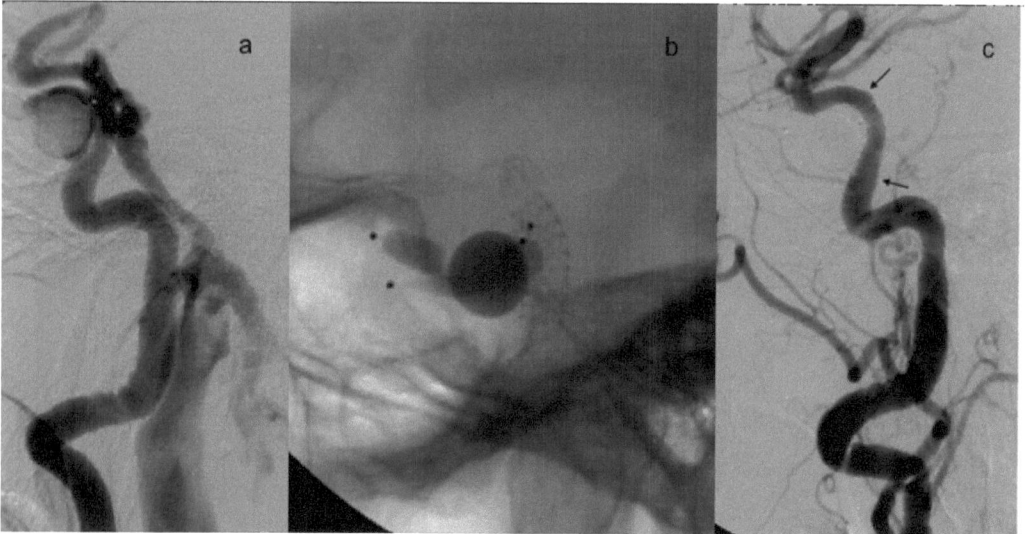

Figure 20: (a) A CCF was previously treated with several detachable balloons but the fistula is still patent. (b) A Jostent stent graft was placed covering the site of the fistula. (c) The fistula is completely occluded at the end of the procedure. (Courtesy of Dr. E. Boccardi).

When tolerated, endovascular occlusion of the ICA is still a good treatment; it is essential to trap the breach of the artery completely, especially distally, to avoid a persistent CCF being filled by reverse flow in the distal ICA (Fig. **21**).

Traumatic direct arteriovenous fistulas between dural arteries of the cavernous sinus and the sinus itself are rare but the differential diagnosis with DAVFs can be difficult (Fig. **22**). Obviously, a correct diagnosis is required in order to select the appropriate treatment strategy.

Pial Arteriovenous Fistulas

Pial arteriovenous fistulas (PAVFs) are rare arteriovenous shunts composed of one or more arterial feeders and one vein; they result in high venous blood flow with the risk of varix formation and subsequent hemorrhage (Fig. **23**). PAVFs are mainly congenital (frequently as part of syndromes such as Rendu-Osler-Weber or Ehlers-Danlos syndrome) but can also be post-traumatic or iatrogenic [40, 41].

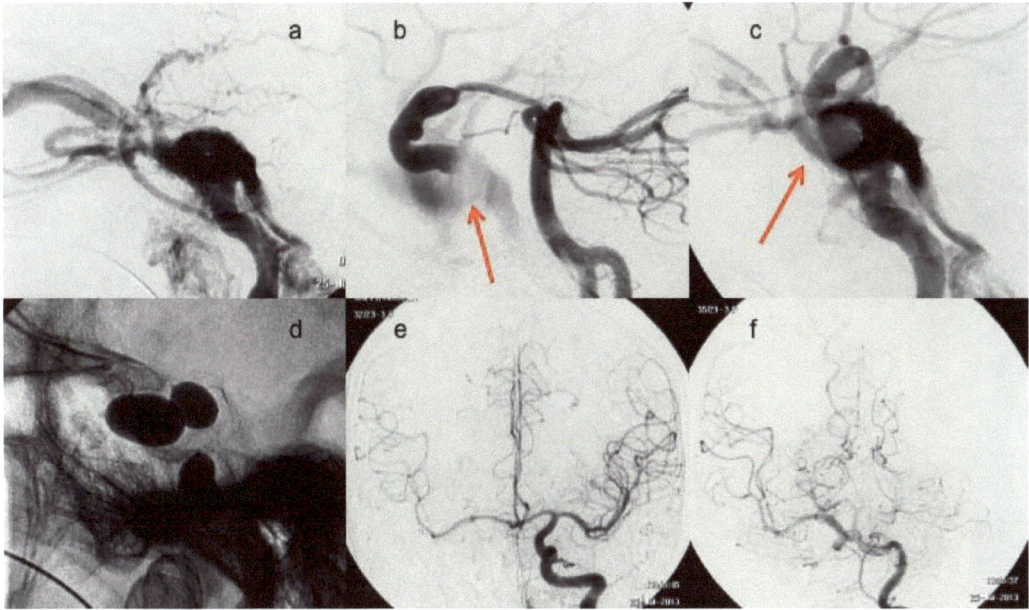

Figure 21: (a) A spontaneous CCF of long duration which steals the whole flow of the ICA, with venous drainage into cerebral cortical veins, the superior ophthalmic vein and the inferior petrous sinus. (b) The CCF causes inversion of the flow in the ICA distal to the fistula; injection of the vertebral artery clearly shows the hole in the artery (arrow). (c) A Goldbal 1 balloon (arrow) was inflated in the cavernous sinus through the fistula but the fistula persisted. (d) Two more detachable balloons were released into the ICA to occlude it. (e) and (f) Injections of the left ICA and the left vertebral artery showing the occlusion of the fistula with good flow in the right hemisphere. (Courtesy of Dr. M. Piano).

Clinical symptoms of PAVFs are headache, hemorrhage, intracranial hypertension and focal neurological signs. Neonates with high-flow fistulas can present with heart failure as can patients with vein of Galen aneurysmal malformation.

The aim of treatment is to disconnect the feeding artery from the draining vein, which requires clear identification of the point of the fistula: too proximal occlusion may result in persistence of the fistula still supported by small collateral arterial branches that cannot be catheterized; too distal occlusion of the draining vein can cause venous hypertension in small collateral veins increasing the risk of hemorrhage.

The best strategy is, therefore, to try to occlude the fistula point with the last segment of the feeding artery and the first segment of the draining vein.

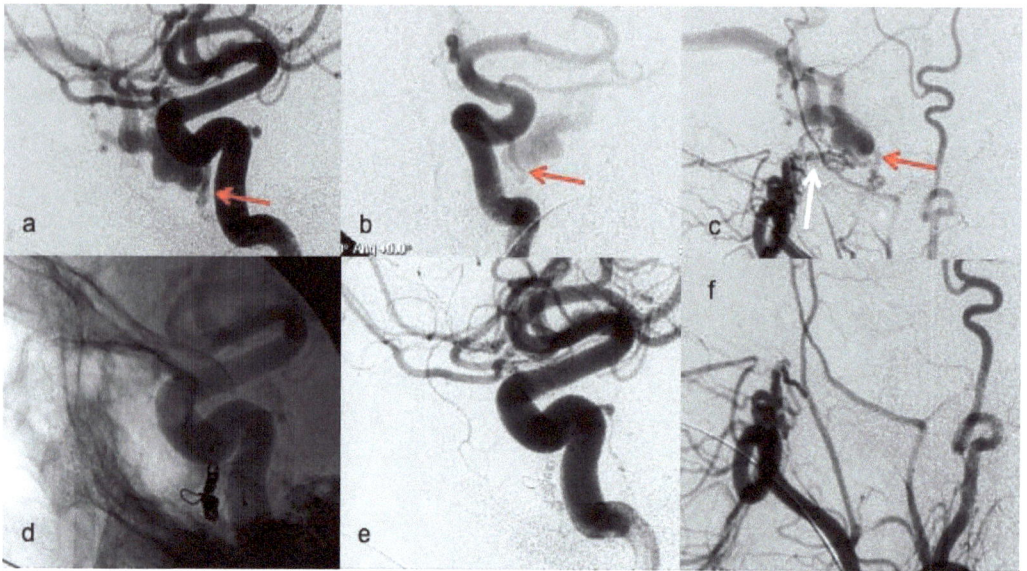

Figure 22: Direct post-traumatic arteriovenous fistula between the meningo-hypophyseal trunk and the cavernous sinus. (a) and (b) Injections of the ICA show the arteriovenous fistula filled by the enlarged meningo-hypophyseal trunk (red arrows). (c) Injection of the external carotid artery shows that the feeders of the fistula come from the accessory meningeal artery and the artery of the foramen rotundum (white arrow) that merge with the feeder from the ICA immediately before entering the fistula. (d) The cast of coils at the end of procedure with the microcatheter still in place in the meningo-hypophyseal trunk. (e) and (f) Injections from the internal and external carotid arteries show complete obliteration of the fistula. (Courtesy of Dr. E. Boccardi).

The endovascular occlusion of the fistula can be achieved using both liquid embolic agents (n-BCA or Onyx) and coils and detachable balloons (Fig. **24**). In very high-flow fistulas, coils are frequently deployed at the start of the procedure to reduce the flow and allow safer injection of n-BCA or Onyx without distal migration. Non-detachable balloons can currently be inflated proximally to the tip of the microcatheter arresting the flow and allowing safer formation of the embolic plug.

The injection of Onyx in neonates or very young children could be dangerous because of the possible harmful action of DMSO on the lungs. The phenomenon of normal perfusion pressure breakthrough has been reported after successful obliteration of PAVFs, causing bleeding and cerebral edema [42].

Angiographic follow-up is also required because *de novo* DAVFs have been reported in children with completely occluded PAVFs [40].

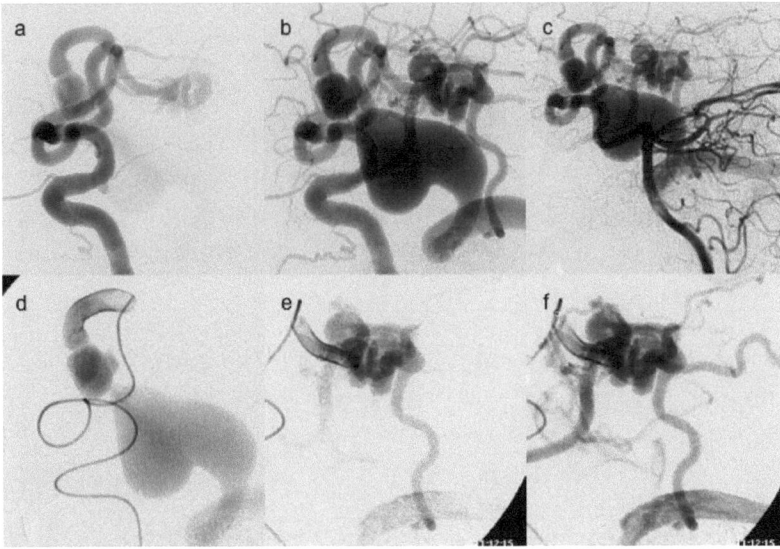

Figure 23: A 27-year old female with headache and a pial arteriovenous fistula. The fistula is composed of two different arteriovenous shunts, as shown by the selective microcatheterization. (d) The first arteriovenous shunt is directed in the vein of Labbé with a venous varix. (e) and (f) The second shunt is drained by various temporal cortical veins. (Courtesy of Dr. E. Boccardi).

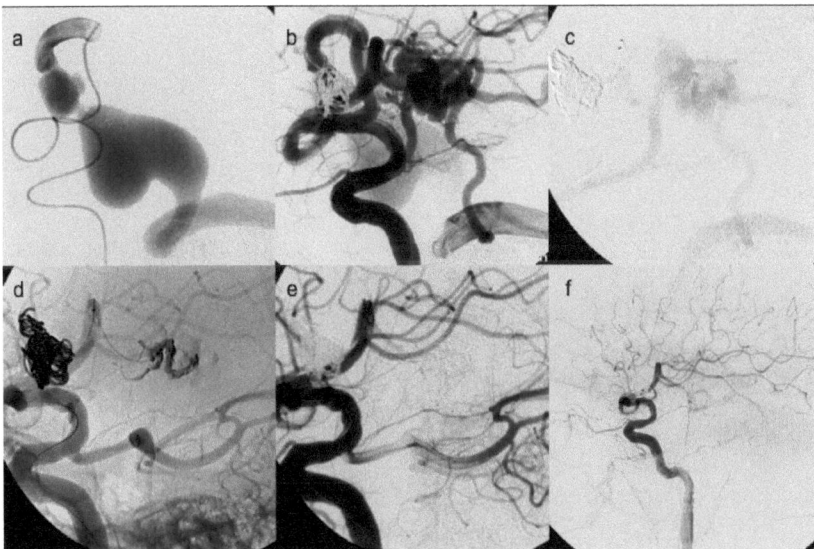

Figure 24: The same patient as in Fig. **23**. (a) Selective injection of the middle cerebral artery branch feeding the first arteriovenous shunt. (b) The first fistula was occluded with coils and the architecture of the second shunt became clearer. (c) The second shunt was catheterized. (d) The casts of coils and Onyx occluding both shunts. (e) and (f) ICA injections demonstrating the obliteration of the fistula with normal blood flow in the cerebral hemisphere. (Courtesy of Dr. E. Boccardi).

CONCLUSION

The current treatment of choice of most arteriovenous fistulas, both dural and pial, is endovascular. This always requires clear understanding of the vascular architecture of the fistula (feeding arteries, point of fistula and draining veins). The aim of the treatment is to occlude the fistula point, disconnecting arteries and veins; this frequently requires occlusion of the closest segments of both feeding arteries and draining veins.

A fistula can be occluded with different materials and techniques depending on the characteristics of the fistula and the confidence of the operator with the materials and techniques.

ACKNOWLEDGEMENTS

This chapter is the result of the daily work of all the staff of the Neurointerventional team of the Neuroradiology Department of Niguarda Ca' Granda Hospital in Milan.

Mariangela Piano, Luca Quilici, Luca Valvassori and Dodi Boccardi, my colleagues of the Neurointerventional team, have kindly allowed me to reproduce clinical images from their cases.

I personally thank Luca Valvassori and Dodi Boccardi for their hard work in teaching me neurointerventional skills over the last decade.

CONFLICT OF INTEREST

The author confirms that this chapter contents have no conflict of interest.

REFERENCES

[1]   Chaichana KL, Coon AL, Tamargo RJ, Huang J. Dural arteriovenous fistulas: epidemiology and clinical presentation. Neurosurg Clin N Am 2012; 23: 7-13.
[2]   Gomez J, Amin AG, Gregg L, Gailloud P. Classification schemes of cranial dural arteriovenous fistulas. Neurosurg Clin N Am 2012; 23: 55-62.
[3]   Cognard C, Gobin YP, Pierot L, *et al*. Cerebral dural arteriovenous fistulas: clinical and angiographic correlation with a revised classification of venous drainage. Radiology 1995; 194: 671-80.
[4]   Borden JA, Wu JK, Shucart WA. A proposed classification for spinal and cranial dural arteriovenous fistulous malformations and implications for treatment. J Neurosurg 1995; 82: 166-79.
[5]   Djindjian R, Merland JJ, Rey A, Thurel J, Houdart R. [Super-selective arteriography of the external carotid artery. Importance of this new technic in neurological diagnosis and in embolization]. [In French] Neurochirurgie 1973: 165-71.

[6]   Shah MN, Botros JA, Pilgram TK, *et al*. Borden-Shucart type I dural arteriovenous fistulas: clinical course including risk of conversion to higher-grade fistulas. J Neurosurg 2012; 117: 539-45.

[7]   Luciani A, Houdart E, Mounayer C, Saint Maurice JP, Merland JJ. Spontaneous closure of dural arteriovenous fistulas: report of three cases and review of the literature. AJNR Am J Neuroradiol 2001; 22: 992-6.

[8]   Schumacher M, Szczeponik N. Successful treatment of dural AV fistulas by manual compression: a matter of perseverance. Neuroradiology 2007; 49: 495-8.

[9]   Oh JT, Chung SY, Lanzino G, *et al*. Intracranial dural arteriovenous fistulas: Clinical characteristics and management based on location and hemodynamics. J Cerebrovasc Endovasc Neurosurg 2012; 14: 192-202.

[10]   Rezende MT, Piotin M, Mounayer C, Spelle L, Abud DG, Moret J. Dural arteriovenous fistula of the lesser sphenoid wing region treated with onyx: Technical note. Neuroradiology 2006; 48: 130-4.

[11]   Ong CK, Ong MT, Le K, *et al*. The trigeminocardiac reflex in onyx embolisation of intracranial dural arteriovenous fistula. J Clin Neurosci 2010; 17: 1267-70.

[12]   Jittapiromsak P, Ikka L, Benachour N, Spelle L, Moret J. Transvenous balloon-assisted transarterial onyx embolization of transverse-sigmoid dural arteriovenous malformation. Neuroradiology 2013; 55: 345-50.

[13]   Chapot R, Stracke P, Velasco A, *et al*. The pressure cooker technique for the treatment of brain AVMs. J Neuroradiol 2014; 41: 87-91.

[14]   Spiotta AM, Hughes G, Masaryk TJ, Hui FK. Balloon-augmented onyx embolization of a dural arteriovenous fistula arising from the neuromeningeal trunk of the ascending pharyngeal artery: technical report. J Neurointerv Surg 2011; 3: 300-3.

[15]   Choi BS, Park JW, Kim JL, *et al*. Treatment strategy based on multimodal management outcome of cavernous sinus dural arteriovenous fistula (CSDAVF). Neurointervention 2011; 6: 6-12.

[16]   Zhang J, Lv X, Jiang C, Li Y, Yang X, Wu Z. Transarterial and transvenous embolization for cavernous sinus dural arteriovenous fistulae. Interv Neuroradiol 2010; 16: 269-77.

[17]   Théaudin M, Saint-Maurice JP, Chapot R, *et al*. Diagnosis and treatment of dural carotid-cavernous fistulas: a consecutive series of 27 patients. J Neurol Neurosurg Psychiatry 2007; 78: 174-9.

[18]   Long XA, Karuna T, Zhang X, Luo B, Duan CZ. Onyx 18 embolisation of dural arteriovenous fistula *via* arterial and venous pathways: preliminary experience and evaluation of the short-term outcomes. Br J Radiol 2012; 85: e395-403.

[19]   Venturi C, Bracco S, Cerase A, *et al*. Endovascular treatment of a cavernous sinus dural arteriovenous fistula by transvenous embolisation through the superior ophthalmic vein *via* cannulation of a frontal vein. Neuroradiology 2003; 45: 574-8.

[20]   Singh J, Morris PP. Superficial temporal vein: route to embolization of cavernous dural arteriovenous fistula. J Neuroimaging 2011; 21: 251-4.

[21]   Kim MJ, Shin YS, Ihn YK, *et al*. Transvenous embolization of cavernous and paracavernous dural arteriovenous fistula through the facial vein: report of 12 cases. Neurointervention 2013; 8: 15-22.

[22]   Mounayer C, Piotin M, Spelle L, Moret J. Superior petrosal sinus catheterization for transvenous embolization of a dural carotid cavernous sinus fistula. AJNR Am J Neuroradiol 2002; 23: 1153-5.

[23]   Amiridze N, Zoarski G, Darwish R, Obuchowski A, Solovevchic N. Embolization of a cavernous sinus dural arteriovenous fistula with onyx *via* direct puncture of the cavernous sinus through the superior orbital fissure: Asystole resulting from the trigeminocardiac reflex. A case report. Interv Neuroradiol 2009; 15: 179-84.

[24]   Mehrzad H, Alam K, Rennie A. The treatment of a dural carotid cavernous fistula (CCF) using onyx *via* a transorbital approach: a technical note. Neuroradiology 2011; 53: 895-8.

[25]   Dashti SR, Fiorella D, Spetzler RF, Albuquerque FC, McDougall CG. Transorbital endovascular embolization of dural carotid-cavernous fistula: Access to cavernous sinus through direct puncture: case examples and technical report. Neurosurgery 2011; 68(1 Suppl Operative): 75-83; discussion 83.

[26]   Chaudhary N, Lownie SP, Bussière M, Pelz DM, Nicolle D. Transcortical venous approach for direct embolization of a cavernous sinus dural arteriovenous fistula: technical case report. Neurosurgery 2012; 70(2 Suppl Operative): 343-8.

[27]   Gandhi D, Ansari SA, Cornblath WT. Successful transarterial embolization of a barrow type D dural carotid-cavernous fistula with ethylene vinyl alcohol copolymer (onyx). J Neuroophthalmol 2009; 29: 9-12.

[28]   Wajnberg E, Spilberg G, Rezende MT, Abud DG, Kessler I, Mounayer C, Association of Rothschild Foundation Alumni (ARFA). Endovascular treatment of tentorial dural arteriovenous fistulae. Interv Neuroradiol 2012; 18: 60-8.

[29]   Morparia N, Miller G, Rabinstein A, Lanzino G, Kumar N. Cognitive decline and hypersomnolence: thalamic manifestations of a tentorial dural arteriovenous fistula (dAVF). Neurocrit Care 2012; 17: 429-33.

[30]   Hatano T, Bozinov O, Burkhardt JK, Bertalanffy H. Surgical treatment of tentorial dural arteriovenous fistulae located around the tentorial incisura. Neurosurg Rev 2013; 36: 429-35.

[31]   Hart JL, Davagnanam I, Chandrashekar HS, Brew S. Angiography and selective microcatheter embolization of a falcine meningioma supplied by the artery of Davidoff and Sschechter. Case report. J Neurosurg 2011; 114: 710-3.

[32]   Weil AG, McLaughlin N, Denis D, Bojanowski MW. Tentorial branch of the superior cerebellar artery. Surg Neurol Int 2011; 2: 71.

[33]   Debrun GM, Viñuela F, Fox AJ, Davis KR, Ahn HS. Indications for treatment and classification of 132 carotid-cavernous fistulas. Neurosurgery 1988; 22: 285-9.

[34]   Debrun G, Lacour P, Vinuela F, Fox A, Drake CG, Caron JP. Treatment of 54 traumatic carotid-cavernous fistulas. J Neurosurg 1981; 55: 678-92.

[35]   Debrun G, Lacour P, Caron JP, *et al.* [Treatment of arteriovenous fistulas and of aneurysms using an inflatable and releasable balloon. Experimental principles. Application to man]. Nouv Presse Med 1975; 4: 2315-8.

[36]   Serbinenko FA. Balloon catheterization and occlusion of major cerebral vessels. J Neurosurg 1974; 41: 125-45.

[37]   Alaraj A, Wallace A, Dashti R, Patel P, Aletich V. Balloons in endovascular neurosurgery: history and current applications. Neurosurgery 2014; 74(Suppl 1): S163-90.

[38]   De Renzis A, Nappini S, Consoli A, *et al.* Balloon-assisted coiling of the cavernous sinus to treat direct carotid cavernous fistula. A single center experience of 13 consecutive patients. Interv Neuroradiol 2013; 19: 344-52.

[39]   Archondakis E, Pero G, Valvassori L, Boccardi E, Scialfa G. Angiographic follow-up of traumatic carotid cavernous fistulas treated with endovascular stent graft placement. AJNR Am J Neuroradiol 2007; 28: 342-7.

[40]   Hetts SW, Keenan K, Fullerton HJ, *et al.* Pediatric intracranial nongalenic pial arteriovenous fistulas: clinical features, angioarchitecture, and outcomes. AJNR Am J Neuroradiol 2012; 33: 1710-9.

[41]   Jabbour P, Tjoumakaris S, Chalouhi N, *et al.* Endovascular treatment of cerebral dural and pial arteriovenous fistulas. Neuroimaging Clin N Am 2013; 23: 625-36.

[42]   Giller CA, Batjer HH, Purdy P, Walker B, Mathews D. Interdisciplinary evaluation of cerebral hemodynamics in the treatment of arteriovenous fistulae associated with giant varices. Neurosurgery 1994; 35: 778-82; discussion 782-4.

CHAPTER 3

Arteriovenous Malformations

Marco Cenzato* and Alberto Debernardi

Department of Neurosurgery, Niguarda Cà Granda Hospital, Milan, Italy

Abstract: Arteriovenous malformations of the brain are one of neurosurgery's most fascinating and challenging pathologies. These malformations were initially described in 1854 by Luschka and in 1863 by Virchow; subsequently several other scientists including Giordano, Spetzler and Martin, Ponce and Lawton described the pathogenesis, clinical presentation and medical treatments of cerebral arteriovenous malformations in detail. The clinical presentation of these malformations is extremely varied: they can present with hemorrhage, seizures or focal neurological deficits with a close correlation between the anatomical location of the malformation and its presenting symptoms. Unruptured and ruptured malformations are distinct pathological entities with different natural histories and multimodal treatment risks. The estimated generic bleeding risk of an unruptured arteriovenous malformation is between 3% and 4% per year; this risk of bleeding increases to 6% in the first year after a hemorrhagic episode and returns, after 5 years, to the same value as that of a corresponding unruptured malformation. Cerebral arteriovenous malformations are very complex entities and for this reason the first and major clinical dilemma is whether or not to treat a patient with such a malformation; the second issue is how to treat them. Each treatment is tailored to the individual patient, drawing a careful balance between efficacy and risks. In brief, a variable combination of three methods of treatment, endovascular, surgical and radiosurgical, can be considered. Each has specific indications and contraindications but all have the same aim: complete elimination of the malformation.

Keywords: Arteriovenous malformation, cerebrovascular disease, surgery.

INTRODUCTION

General Considerations and Natural History

Arteriovenous malformations (AVMs) of the brain are one of neurosurgery's most fascinating and challenging pathologies. AVMs were initially described in 1854 by Luschka [1] and in 1863 by Virchow [2]. In 1889 Giordano [3] performed the first surgical exposure of an AVM and the first successful surgical extirpation.

---

*Corresponding author Marco Cenzato: Department of Neurosurgery, Niguarda Cà Granda Hospital, Milan, Italy; Tel: 0264442401; Fax: 0264442053; E-mail: marco.cenzato@ospedaleniguarda.it

Simone Peschillo (Ed.)

In the mid-1900s some scientific reports reviewed the use of pre-operative exsanguination to decrease bleeding during intracranial surgery [4]. The treatment of AVMs changed radically in the 1970s with the introduction of microsurgery, with Yasargil being one of the major promoters of this innovation. In 1976 he published the details of the first series of ten AVM patients treated with microsurgical techniques with no mortality and minimal morbidity [5].

As microsurgery became increasingly accepted as a management option for AVMs, identifying those malformations that could be resected safely became a priority. In 1986 Spetzler and Martin published a grading scale that became used worldwide [6]; subsequently Lawton *et al.* proposed a supplementary grading scale which introduced additional parameters that affect the outcome of AVM surgery, such as the patient's age, hemorrhagic presentation, nidal diffuseness, and deep perforating artery supply [7]. Spetzler and Ponce then presented a variation of the original Spetzler-Martin scale; their modified three-tier classification divided AVMs into three classes: class A, including grade I and II AVMs of the Spetzler-Martin classification; class B, including grade III AVMs; and class C, including grade IV and V AVMs [8].

Cerebral AVMs are a complex tangle of abnormal blood vessels with three morphological components: (i) the dysplastic core (nidus), where there is a direct connection between arteries and veins, (ii) the feeding arteries, and (iii) the draining veins. The nidus lacks normal high resistance arteriolar and capillary beds and is often well circumscribed from the cerebral parenchyma. Nidus vessels usually have markedly attenuated walls, due to a deficient muscularis layer. Arterial feeders and draining veins are not exclusively devoted to the AVM and also supply normal brain parenchyma; vascular shunts can therefore induce changes in the normal vasculature adjacent to the malformation.

AVMs have generally been regarded as congenital lesions, representing inborn errors of embryonic vascular morphogenesis caused by malfunction of the embryonic process of capillary maturation [9, 10]; however several studies seem to suggest post-natal development [11, 12].

The natural history of cerebral AVMs is difficult to predict: they may remain stable over time, grow, or even regress or recur [13-16]. The fact that AVMs can regrow after negative post-operative angiograms, especially in children, may be a consequence of the relatively immature cerebral vasculature and may involve active angiogenesis mediated by humoral factors [17].

Genetic mechanisms could contribute to the development and subsequent biological behavior of cerebral vascular malformations. Germline mutations affecting distinct angiogenic pathways have been suggested to be the underlying cause of a variety of vascular malformations including AVMs [18]. Apoptotic cell death and vascular remodeling also play important roles in the development and maintenance of malformations [19-21].

Although once considered static malformations, AVMs are now seen as dynamic lesions whose nature can potentially change radically over time. Despite multiple studies, several classifications and the great interest of the scientific community, the selection of patients for treatment of AVMs remains challenging.

Epidemiology and Clinical Presentation

The exact incidence of cerebral AVMs is not known. Indeed, given the rarity of the disease and the existence of asymptomatic patients, it has not been possible to establish a true prevalence. The scientific literature reports incidences between 0.02% and 0.5%, with the rate probably influenced by geographical and racial factors [22-24]. In 1948, Olivecrona *et al.* reported that the incidence of cerebral AVMs detected in a large autopsy series was 1.4% [25]. Given the variation in the detection rate of asymptomatic AVMs, Berman *et al.* argued that the most reliable estimate for the occurrence of the disease was the detection rate of 0.94 per 100,000 person-years for symptomatic lesions [26].

Cerebral AVMs seem to occur slightly more frequently in males (male-to-female ratio of 1.4:1) and it appears that the majority of these malformations become symptomatic before the age of 40 [27]. As a general rule it can be said that approximately 50% of AVMs present with hemorrhage, 25% with seizures, and 25% with other clinical manifestations such as headache and/or progressive loss of mental or neurological function [28]. There is, obviously, a close correlation between the anatomical location of an AVM and its presenting symptoms. For instance, AVMs in the frontal lobe, temporal lobe or hippocampal structures in the temporal lobe more often present with seizures, whereas AVMs in the basal ganglia, corpus callosum, choroid plexus, brain stem, and the cerebellum more often present with hemorrhage [29].

Hemorrhage

Spontaneous cerebral hemorrhage is one of the two major presenting clinical symptoms of symptomatic AVMs: the frequency of intacranial hemorrhage from ruptured AVMs ranges from 32% to 82% [30]. It is not unusual that old bleeds and hemosiderin deposits are detected on magnetic resonance images, during open surgery or at autopsy series [31].

The reported risk of hemorrhage as the initial symptom in cerebral AVM is 2% to 4% per year [32-35] and the risk of an AVM bleed increases after the first hemorrhagic event; in fact, the rate of repeat bleeding is 33% in the first year and then falls to 11% in subsequent years with an average annual rate of 18% [36, 37].

Cerebral hemorrhage after rupture of an AVM appears to be associated with less morbidity and mortality with respect to that of other intracranial vascular malformations, such as aneurysms. The mortality rate associated with the first hemorrhage has been estimated to be about 10% to 15% and the overall morbidity about 50% [33, 38]; in one study parenchymal hemorrhage resulted in a neurological deficit in 52% of patients [39].

Several scientific studies have tried to explain the cause of hemorrhage from AVMs and determine the risk factors predisposing to this spontaneous event. Factors that may increase the risk of hemorrhage include high intranidal pressure due to high pressure in the feeding arteries or restrictions in venous outflow [40, 41], the presence of intranidal aneurysms [42, 43], a deep periventricular or intraventricular location [43, 44], and small size [45, 46]. Recently, several authors and our group have focused on the venous outflow of AVMs and the presence of intra-nidal aneurysms as mechanisms related to hemorrhage [40, 41, 47]. It has been found that the risk of hemorrhage is high in AVMs with a single drainage vein, severely impaired venous drainage and exclusive deep venous drainage.

Another important issue is the association between cerebral AVMs and aneurysms, which could increase the risk of acute AVM bleeding. Our group published a report on this association, with the aim of identifying priorities and indications for treatment of arterial and venous "aneurysms" associated with brain AVMs [47]. We analyzed 34 patients with 45 arterial and venous aneurysms extrapolated from a global series of 400 treated AVMs and concluded that different subtypes of aneurysms had different clinical behaviors. The bleeding risk of unrelated and flow-related, remote types was almost the same as that of any other unruptured aneurysm. This means that the bleeding risk of these aneurysms should just take into account the ISUIA parameters (location, size and morphology). Conversely, the flow-related, adjacent types and intra-postnidal types ("venous aneurysms") had a significantly higher hemorrhagic potential.

The relationship between the size of an AVM and its propensity to bleed is unclear and a matter of continuous discussion. Several studies showed that small AVMs have higher pressures in feeding arteries than do larger AVMs [42, 48]. Miyasaka *et al.* measured intra-operative feeding artery pressure and drainage vein pressure in 30 patients with cerebral malformations, using direct puncture of the vessels [49, 50]. They found that small nidus size and only one drainage vein increased the risk of hemorrhage. However, some authors reject this theory and sustain that there is no relationship between AVM size and bleeding risk [33, 34] or between size and pressure in feeding arteries [51]. They consider that the increased risk of bleeding of cerebral AVMs is a misinterpretation and sustain that small AVMs are less likely to cause any other symptoms and are, therefore, less likely to be diagnosed unless they bleed.

Seizures

A seizure is a common presenting symptom of cerebral AVMs and may also represent a clinical manifestation of a small hemorrhage from such malformations. Seizures are the first symptoms of cerebral AVMs in 16% to 67% of patients [28, 29, 52]. These electrical manifestations are usually associated with frontal and temporal lobe malformations, especially those in the hippocampal area [52, 53].

In 1995, Turjman *et al.* identified [54] several anatomical and functional parameters that seem to be predictors of epilepsy. The anatomical parameters are considered to be cortical location, especially in the temporal and frontal lobes, the presence of a varix in the venous drainage, and association with related and/or unrelated arterial aneurysms. The functional parameters are considered to be feeding vessels through the carotid artery and middle cerebral artery and the cortical location of the feeders [55].

Focal Neurological Deficits

Focal neurological signs can be the first manifestation of a cerebral AVM, although it is rare that progressive focal neurological deterioration occurs and results in a dramatic clinical syndrome. Usually, such a syndrome is associated with large AVMs with a high flow, several feeding arteries and several drainage veins [56-59].

Progressive neurological deterioration is obviously not caused by hemorrhagic mechanisms, but the pathogenesis is not completely understood. There are several hypotheses on the pathophysiological mechanisms in the scientific literature. At first, the neurological deterioration was presumed to be caused by the vascular steal phenomenon, in which cerebral arterial hypotension leads to ischemia in brain areas adjacent to the lesion [30, 60]. This concept is supported by the fact that occlusion of feeding arteries can ameliorate symptoms. In further support of this theory, in 1999 Kaminaga *et al.* reported the findings of a study of hemodynamic changes around cerebral AVMs before and after embolization [61]. Using positron emission tomography, the authors found a decrease in regional cerebral blood flow in the ipsilateral hemisphere in patients with focal symptoms before embolization and also found that the improvement in symptoms after endovascular treatment corresponded with the recovery of regional blood flow, as measured by positron emission tomography.

Despite the reports and the theoretical logical hemodynamic consequence of high-flow AVMs on the cerebral vascular circulation, this concept has recently been challenged. Given a lack of relation between feeding artery pressure, flow velocity and focal neurological deficits, several authors concluded that the steal phenomenon cannot be considered an established mechanism of clinical deterioration in the vast majority of AVM patients. AVMs can certainly induce a certain degree of cerebral hypotension in the normal brain parenchyma around the malformation, but definite proof of a causal link with neurological symptoms is lacking.

Several non-hemorrhagic mechanisms have been proposed to explain the phenomenon of focal neurological deficits, such as venous hypertension due to arterialization of the venous system [62], a mass effect [63, 64], perifocal edema [63, 65] and obstructive hydrocephalus from ventricular compression by dilated deep veins [66].

Other Manifestations

A common but very generic symptom of unruptured cerebral AVMs is headache, which is the most common presenting symptom in 7%-48% of patients: these headaches do not have distinctive features in terms of frequency, duration, or severity [30, 36]. Patients with unruptured cerebral AVMs can develop new-onset headache, have progressive headaches or headaches with a significant change in pattern, headaches that never alternate sides, and headaches associated with any neurological finding or seizures [67]. Scientific studies indicate a strong relationship between AVMs in the occipital lobe and migraine-like symptoms with visual phenomena and headaches [68]; large AVMs with a prominent meningeal artery supply frequently produce unilateral headaches [55].

Some authors sustain that complete surgical removal of the malformation resolves the clinical symptoms immediately, whereas others do not support the relationship between cerebral malformations and headache [69, 70].

Cerebral malformations may cause neuropsychiatric disturbances and progressive intellectual deterioration [70, 71]. In 1988, Wenz *et al.* reported the pre-therapeutic evaluation of 79 patients with AVMs and revealed marked deviations from the normal population; 24% had deficits in intelligence, attention (35%) and memory (48%) [72]. Moreover, developmental learning disorders have been documented in 66% of adults with AVMs [73]. The cognitive deterioration can be attributed to cerebral steal or seizures and seems to improve after surgical or endovascular treatment.

The Pathogenesis of Arteriovenous Malformations: A Response-to-injury Paradigm

In the past, cerebral AVMs were considered congenital lesions. Recently, however, the scientific community has proposed new theories about the pathogenesis and development of these malformations. Clinical research studies of AVM patients and animal models suggest a novel paradigm, the so-called "response-to-injury", to explain the pathogenesis of malformations [12].

Modest injury from an otherwise unremarkable episode of trauma, infection, inflammation, or irradiation, or a mechanical stimulus such as compression may be at the base of a "response-to-injury" mechanism for AVM formation. It is thought that when a cerebral "stimulus" occurs on an underlying structural defect, such as a microscopic developmental venous anomaly or some sort of venous outflow restriction in a microcirculatory bed, or on an underlying genetic background such as mutations in key angiogenic genes, the normal injury response is shifted towards an abnormal dysplastic response.

Several scientific studies have been conducted on cerebral AVM tissue; these studies suggest an active angiogenic and inflammatory lesion with over-expression of several growth factors and cytokines, such as vascular endothelial growth factor, myeloperoxidase, interleukin 6 and matrix metalloproteinase [74-78]. A cerebral "stimulus" can cause the recruitment of progenitor cells, which may influence AVM growth. Endothelial progenitor cells, CD133, SDF-1 and CD68 may mediate pathological vascular remodeling [79-81].

The pathogenesis of brain AVMs unquestionably has a genetic influence. For example, AVMs are highly prevalent in patients with hemorrhagic telangiectasia, which can be caused by mutations in the genes for endoglin (*ENG*) and activin-like kinase 1 (*ALK1* or *ACVLR1*) [82, 83]. A genetic predisposition was also identified in patients with high-risk AVMs, with blood biomarkers for intracerebral hemorrhage.

In brief, the mechanisms of AVM initiation are currently unknown, but may involve a mechanical insult or a structural aberration, with the subsequent growth and behavior of the lesion being influenced by genetic variation.

UNRUPTURED AND RUPTURED CEREBRAL ARTERIOVENOUS MALFORMATIONS: NATURAL HISTORY, PROPOSED TREATMENTS AND RISKS

Cerebral AVMs are complex vascular entities with peculiar vascular patterns, precise anatomical localizations and selected choices of treatment. It is important to understand the natural history of these malformations and, in particular, that there is a profound difference between the natural history of AVMs that have bled and unruptured AVMs.

In 1983, Graf *et al.* published an evaluation of 200 cases of unruptured AVM with a follow-up of six years. It was concluded that small malformations have a higher risk of bleeding [84]. The study with the largest population to date is that by Ondra *et al.* [35], published in 1990, in which 1616 patients were analyzed for a period of 24 years. The patients in this study had a 4% annual risk of bleeding and 1% annual mortality risk. Hernesniemi *et al.* [85] published a report of 238 cases of AVMs and stated that the risk of bleeding in this cohort was quite similar to that in the other studies. However, they found some factors that increased the risk of bleeding above the standard value of 4%, such as a previous hemorrhage, a deep location, the presence of deep vein discharges, exclusively deep venous drainage, presence of an ectasia before a stenosis on the venous side, and aneurysms on arterial feeders [84, 85]. According to these authors' research, AVM size does not seem to influence the risk of bleeding significantly, while location does, with infratentorial malformations being associated with a markedly higher risk of bleeding than supratentorial ones.

According to the international literature the estimated generic risk of bleeding of an unruptured AVM is between 3% and 4% per year with an annual mortality risk of around 1%; this risk increases in the presence of the factors described. Furthermore, cerebral AVMs are extremely heterogeneous with regards to location and size as well as the characteristics of the nidus and the afferent and efferent vessels.

As far as concerns ruptured AVMs, a Finnish study on the natural history of AVMs, published in 2008, clearly showed that the risk of bleeding was higher in the first years after the hemorrhagic episode, by an average value of 2-4% a year and up to as much as 6% a year, before returning, after 5 years, to the same value as that of a corresponding unruptured AVM [85].

It is important to emphasize that very often the risk of bleeding is considered to overlap the risk of neurological damage. It is commonly considered that the risk of bleeding from an AVM is significantly lower than the risk of bleeding from an aneurysm and, therefore, that bleeding from an AVM does not have such a poor outcome as generally thought. This assumption also underlies the ARUBA study [86].

Multimodal management of cerebral AVMs requires precise knowledge of the risks of the individual treatments and these should be compared with the risk of the natural history of the malformations. Obviously there are fundamental differences in treatment risks between AVMs that have bled and unruptured AVMs. Unfortunately, however, the literature compares the risks of mutimodal treatment and natural history without making a clear distinction between ruptured AMVs and unruptured ones, since most of the reports present mixed case studies.

While there is a general consensus that an already ruptured AVM puts the patient at a higher risk of further bleeding, the arguments for treating unruptured malformations are certainly more complex and the literature is equivocal. The recently published ARUBA study is a randomized study that compared the risks of treating unruptured AVMs and those of the natural evolution of the condition. The study was stopped early because it became evident that the risk of treatment was higher than that of the natural course of the malformations [86]. This study was based on an assumption that the natural history of intact AVMs is less dangerous than commonly considered; the risk of any treatment is not, therefore, justified. The ARUBA study did, however, raise several criticisms, the main one concerning the nature of the treatment that was compared with natural history: no distinction was made between kinds of treatment, which were mostly endovascular, a type of treatment that is known to have several complications. In a case study of 200 patients evaluated, only 18 were treated surgically.

In an unpublished, multicenter, consecutive series of 450 AVMs treated surgically in Italy it was clear that the outcome of the AVMs was quite different depending on whether they were operated on when intact or after bleeding. Bleeding had a strong impact on clinical outcome, greater than surgery when indications were correct. As a result of the bleeding almost all the patients underwent surgery: 20% remained with a moderate disability and 17% with a severe disability. Among those who bled, from 10% to 25% died. Patients operated upon after bleeding had serious neurological deficits that derived from the bleeding rather than from the surgery, while patients operated upon before bleeding had a better outcome at the follow-up evaluation than might generally have been expected, as we will define later. Unruptured AVMs treated surgically and evaluated after a follow-up of at least 6 months were associated with severe disability in less than 2% of cases, moderate disability in 5.5 % of the cases, and no deaths.

All the discussion on indications must, therefore, be evaluated in a statistical fashion, considering the risk of bleeding for that specific AVM and the risk of surgery for that specific AVM.

To summarize, the risk of bleeding is between 2% and 4%, and may increase if the AVM has some of the anatomical features mentioned above. The ARUBA study [86] confirmed that the risk of bleeding in a collection of case studies was around 3% per year in unruptured malformations.

We personally agree with Lawton's statements, who essentially said that it is not fair to "Wait for the AVM to do the harm." Although the cautious approach embodies sound judgment and experienced selection of patients, it is a management decision that may also be viewed with suspicion because it exposes a patient to hemorrhagic risk, if not outright hemorrhage. Furthermore, by extending the logic of waiting to its extreme, a neurosurgeon who selects only patients with ruptured AVMs for surgery is likely to have favorable outcome data crediting him or her with patients' neurological recovery rather than accurately reflecting the true risks of surgery.

THE TREATMENT OF ARTERIOVENOUS MALFORMATIONS

Cerebral AVMs are very complex vascular malformations and for this reason the first and major medical dilemma is whether or not to treat a patient with these malformations; the dilemma on how to treat them is, therefore, secondary. The treatment of an AVM must be tailored to the individual patient, drawing a careful balance between efficacy and risk of a specific treatment or multiple treatments. Indeed, a variable combination of three methods of treatment can be considered for the management of cerebral AVMs: endovascular, surgical and radiosurgical treatment. Each treatment has specific indications and contraindications but all have the same aim of completely eliminating the malformation.

A malformation can only be considered healed when early venous drainage and residues of the nidus are no longer observable at post-treatment angiography. The literature suggests that a partially closed AVM does not always have a lower risk of bleeding; on the contrary, it is believed that modification of AVM flow, induced either by endovascular partial occlusion or partial surgical removal of the malformation, can potentially expose the patient to a much higher risk of AVM rupture. Indeed, Miyamoto *et al.* [87] recently found that, after incomplete treatment of cerebral AVMs, the hemorrhage rate increased to 17% and the treatment-related morbidity and mortality rates increased to 23% and 9.3%, respectively

Endovascular Treatment

At the end of the 1990s and in the early years of the 21st century, endovascular procedures had a considerable success, especially following the introduction of Onyx, a material that was promised to close AVMs in a more comprehensive manner than could be achieved with either glue or coils. Onyx is a mellow, cohesive material without fragments, which is a great advantage because when injected slowly it can close the nidus of the malformation without causing early occlusion of the venous side.

The introduction of this material towards the end of the 1990s channeled the treatment of AVMs mainly toward endovascular techniques. However, as experience accumulated and the populations treated increased, it was observed that the great expectations regarding this material in the treatment of AVMs were substantially not met. The medical possibility of closing AVMs completely and exclusively with an endovascular treatment has not proven as effective as hoped.

The advantage of treating AVMs with Onyx is that of keeping the endovascular material within the nidus, with a low risk of premature closure of the venous district. However, the goal of endovascular treatment must be considered a reduction in the volume of the nidus, since complete obliteration of the AVM is seldom achieved. In most cases the occlusion is not complete and hence there is the possibility of a relapse; in any case, the risk of bleeding is not decreased and is, in fact, potentially increased. Another disadvantage of endovascular treatment is that the injection of Onyx is in some ways unpredictable: the slow flow injection introduces the embolic material within the nidus in an often erratic and uncontrollable pattern.

The type of material used for an endovascular procedure is obviously also relevant to a theoretical associated surgical procedure. From a surgical point of view Onyx can be considered a good material; it is less rigid than cyanoacrylic glue and can be removed piecemeal with scissors from a packed AMV.

Sometimes a neuroradiologist will overfill the nidus in the attempt to close an AVM, but if the closure is not obtained and the patient has to be operated upon, the volume of the AVM is often bigger than it was originally. Sometimes the Onyx fills the AVM but small deep perforating vessels coming from deep white matter can remain open; these are the most difficult feeders to close surgically and they can grow following the endovascular procedure. Finally, Onyx may close the superficial part of the malformation leaving the deep part, surgically more difficult to close, behind a bulky mass of rubbery material.

Role of Endovascular Treatment before or in Alternative to Surgery

An endovascular procedure for cerebral AVMs is rarely considered a treatment option *per se*, but can be considered above all as an emergency treatment for a ruptured AVM and in multi-staged management with subsequent surgery or radiosurgery.

A patient with a ruptured AVM undergoes emergency angiography to exclude the presence of an AVM-associated aneurysm and/or endoventricular choroidal feeder, which can be responsible for the bleeding. Occluding such an aneurysm with glue can prevent further bleeding from the AVM. If no aneurysm can be found, the goal is to close the main fistulas to reduce the shunt and the stress on the venous side of the AVM.

As previously shown, endovascular treatment can be a very good method of occluding the deep feeders of an AVM, which are more difficult to reach for the surgeon and which supply the AVM from the opposite side with respect to the surgical approach. Obviously, from a surgical point of view there is no need to close superficial feeders that can be safely and easily closed directly during surgery. Grade 1 and 2 AVMs can be operated upon without embolization. However, endovascular treatment is mandatory before surgery for large AVMs in which a multi-stage flow reduction can reduce the brain edema and hemorrhage after surgery (Figs. **1** and **2**).

Endovascular treatment can be followed by Gamma Knife treatment, in particular when surgery is not feasible for anatomical, dynamic or generic patient-related reasons. Thus, close cooperation between surgeons and neuroradiologists is essential, with a "strategy" to deal with the malformations being the key to success. An incorrect strategy could, in fact, expose the patients to several risks secondary to repeated procedures without a real advantage

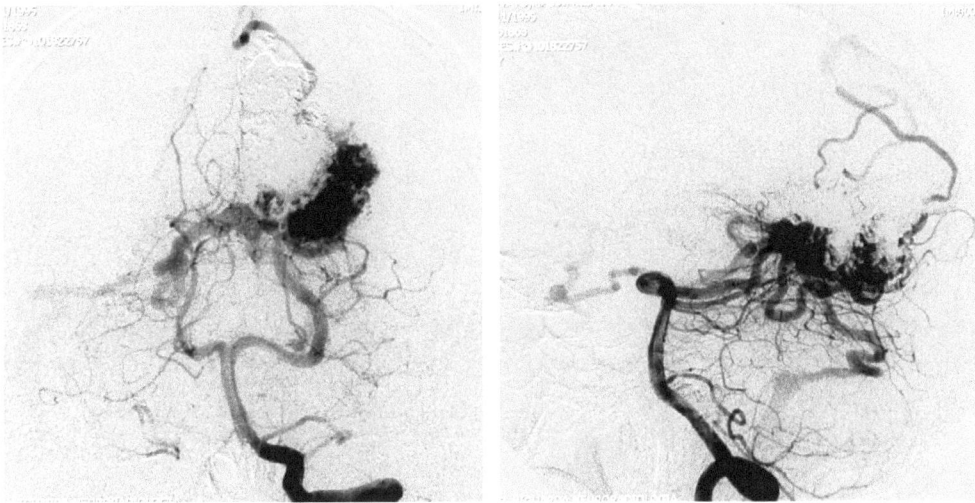

Figure 1: From a surgical point of view this way of embolizing an occipital AVM is not useful. All the deep feeders are left unchanged and the surgeon has a mass of rubber in front of the feeders.

As stated by Lawton "It is notable that embolization, either alone or in combination, was linked with substantially increased mortality risk, and for this reason should be undertaken with care and full knowledge of implications..."

In conclusion the surgeon's requests to his or her endovascular colleague can be summarized as follows: that the endovascular embolization is performed the day before the planned surgery and that the patient is kept in the intensive care unit until entering the operating room; that deep vessels on the side opposite the surgical view are selectively embolized; that the endovascular treatment does not fill the AVM; and that Onyx is used rather than glue. This last request is due to an unpleasant experience in a single case in which cyanoacrylic glue was used for embolization in a patient with large veins. A thin layer of glue escaped in the venous side of the AVM. This thin layer acted as a blade and cut the venous wall during surgery (Fig. **3**).

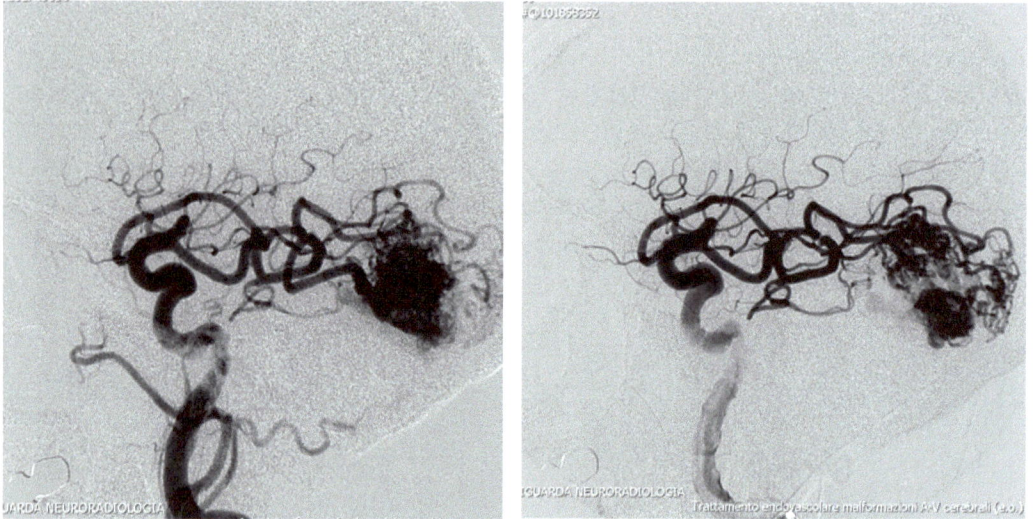

Figure 2: This way of embolizing is more useful for the surgeon than that shown in Fig. **1**. In a similar AVM the main deep feeder is closed and the more superficial and accessible feeders are left unchanged. The AVM is not rigid.

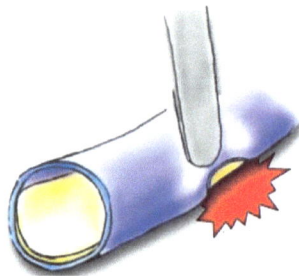

Figure 3: In a single case a thin layer of cyanoacrylic glue, used to embolize an AVM in a patient with large venous vessels, escaped in the venous side of the AVM. During surgery this thin layer acted as a blade and cut the venous wall when the vein was surgically reclined.

Radiosurgery

Radiosurgery is an important tool for the treatment of AVMs. The mechanism of action is to focus a high dosage of gamma rays on the nidus of the malformation.

With focused beams, radiation to brain tissue surrounding the AVM can be minimized. As demonstrated by surgical specimens the inflammatory processes driven by the radiation cause progressive obliteration of the vessel lumen and thereby occlude the AVM. This process can take several months and is generally considered completed after 3 years. During this time span the patient cannot be considered protected by the treatment from further bleeding. It is generally thought that the bleeding risk is unchanged until the AVM has completely disappeared.

Indications for Radiosurgery for Arteriovenous Malformations

Several studies (level V evidence) indicate that radiosurgery provides good cures for AVMs with low rates of complications. Radiosurgery is generally indicated for small AVMs, less than 4 cm in diameter, which have few indications for surgery, such as small malformations and those in eloquent cortex.

In accordance with patients' wishes, some authors also use radiosurgery in superficial, small grade 1 or 2 AVMs for which surgery has a very low risk [88,89]. Although the rates of complications of radiosurgery are very low, the obliteration rate (the angiographic disappearance of the AVM) is around 80% within 2 or 3 years, a result that is stratified by AVM size. Small AVMs respond better. It is not fair to suggest radiosurgery as a comparable alternative to surgery: the patient must be aware that the obliteration rate following radiosurgery is not 100% and that the risk of bleeding remains unchanged for 2-3 years. Furthermore, radiosurgery carries a low risk of radiation necrosis, a risk that has been estimated to be around 2%. Therefore, the patient treated with radiosurgery runs the risks of incomplete obliteration, bleeding and radionecrosis, while the rate of complications associated with surgery for grade 1 AVMs is less than 2% and the outcome is excellent with a 100% cure rate at long-term follow-up.

Candidates for radiosurgery are selected on the basis of the site and volume of the AVM, and an assessment of the surgical risk. Age also plays a role.

There is evidence that staged radiosurgery for large AVMs that are not suitable for surgical treatment is a promising alternative where other techniques fail. After a careful evaluation of the different compartments of a large AVM, radiosurgery can be focused on a single compartment at a time (Figs. **4** & **5**).

The treatment is administered in various sessions at 6-month intervals, causing progressive reduction of the AVM [90, 91]. Although not yet defined as a standard, the preliminary results have been really surprising in some cases. Some large, deep inoperable AVMs have literally disappeared with several treatments distributed over the years. We now propose this kind of treatment for grade V deep AVMs, including ruptured AVMs after endovascular obliteration of a possible aneurysm on a deep feeder.

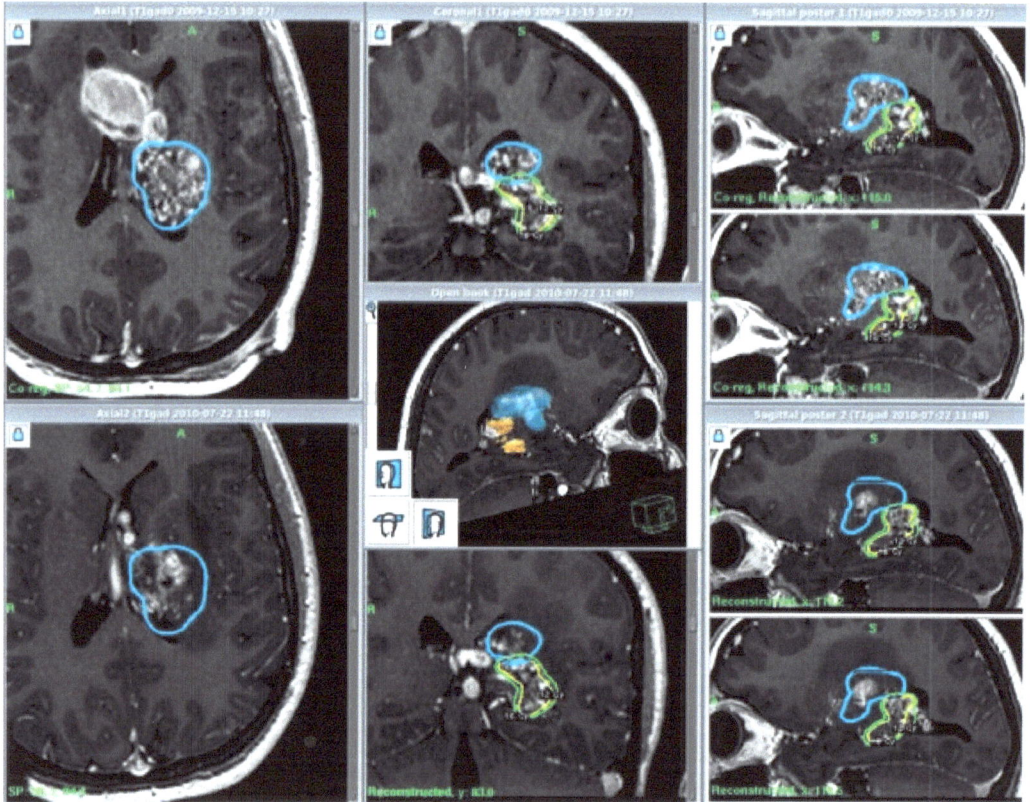

Figure 4: Planning multistage Gamma Knife treatment for a large, deep AVM.

Endovascular treatment and radiosurgery

Endovascular treatment may be necessary before radiosurgery to reduce high flow shunts or to close deep aneurysms on feeders but embolization with Onyx or glue before radiosurgery is generally not advisable [92, 93]. Embolization material is radio-opaque and if scattered within the AVM nidus it may make it more difficult to provide a conformal dose plan at the time of planning radiosurgery. Moreover the nidus is rarely shrunken by the endovascular treatment and there is no evidence that flow reduction alone without reduction of the volume of the AVM provides any benefit before radiosurgery.

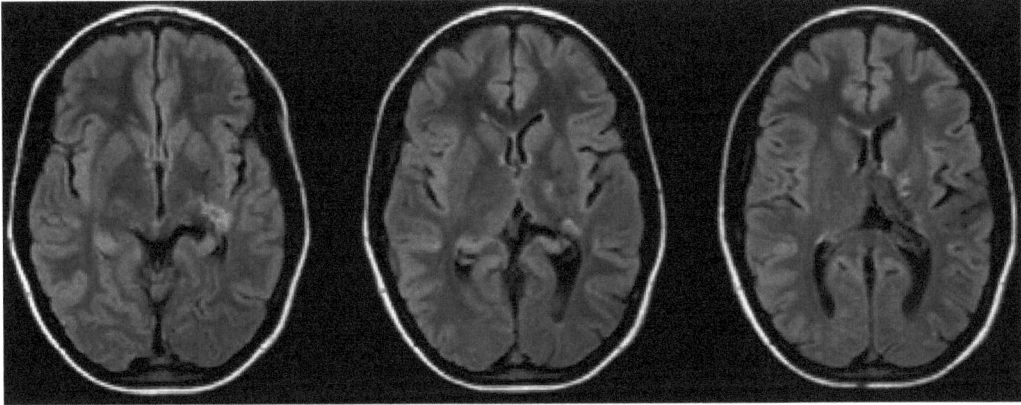

Figure 5: The same patient as in Fig. **4**, 24 months after radiosurgery.

In patients with unruptured AVMs the sequence can be inverted: the patient first undergoes radiosurgical treatment then if, after 3 years, a residual malformation is still evident, it can be treated by endovascular occlusion or, possibly, by surgical resection. Surgery after radiosurgery is often easier. The nidus is less vascularized and more fibrotic and hemostasis is easier. Prior radiosurgery thus facilitates surgical resection.

Surgery

The most difficult part of surgery is to define which AVMs can be treated surgically and which cannot. Surgery of AVMs is risky for two main reasons: (i) rebleeding after surgery due to residual AVM or to the failure of the venous wash-out effect; (ii) direct damage of functional neural tissue. The pre-surgical evaluation of the risk of AVM surgery is, therefore, of paramount importance.

In 1986, Spetzler and Martin created a well-known scale for grading AVMs based on three radiological parameters [6]. It is now considered the most widely used system and has been validated both prospectively and retrospectively as a practical and reliable method for operative risk assessment and outcome prediction after AVM microsurgery. Spetzler and Martin found that three malformation parameters were statistically significant in predicting surgical outcome: size of the AVM, proximity of eloquent cerebral cortex, and exclusive deep venous drainage. The scores of the scale range from 1 to 5. The classification is used universally and is currently applied to define the risk of AVM surgery and therefore to group AVM series in a homogeneous manner. The scale gives an immediate estimate of the complexity of AVMs and is, therefore, also widely adopted for the communication of clinical information.

Low- and high-grade AVMs require different surgical management and have different morbidity and mortality rates. According to published reports, patients with grade I AVMs have a high probability (92% to 100%) of a favorable outcome, while those with grade II malformations have a 95% chance of an excellent or good outcome. For grade III lesions, the rate of excellent or good outcomes was reported to be 68.2% in the short-term and then increased to 88.6% at the late follow-up. Thus, although patients with grade III AVMs may have a less than ideal immediate outcome, when re-evaluated after 6 months most have regained an excellent clinical condition. The rate of excellent outcomes in patients with grade IV lesions is lower than 75%. Finally, the reported rate of good/excellent outcomes in patients with grade V AVMs was 57.1%, with a 14.3% rate of poor outcome and a 4.8% mortality rate in longer-term follow-up. Therefore, the surgical outcome of grade I and II AVMs is extremely good with no mortality and very low morbidity; in contrast, grade IV and V AVMs have a high rate of poor outcomes and surgery is not, therefore, recommended for unruptured grade IV and V AVMs.

Grade III AVMs are the most difficult to define. The grade assignment can be the result of the sum of points for a small AVM in eloquent cortex with a deep vein, or for a larger AVM in non-eloquent cortex with a deep vein or for a large AVM in eloquent cortex. In 2003, Lawton [94] defined a further sub-classification of the third Spetzler-Martin grade, dividing grade III AVMs into three sub-categories: IIIA (large AVM in a non-eloquent cerebral area), IIIB (small AVM, eloquent cerebral area and with a deep vein), and IIICc (large AVM in an eloquent cerebral area). Grade IIIA AVMs can be assimilated with the grade I and II AVMs, while grade IIIC AVMs can be considered as grade IV or V AVMs. Grade IIIB malformations must be judiciously selected for surgery; in fact the presence of cerebral AVM in an eloquent area of the brain makes the difference.

In 2010 Lawton *et al.* [7] further refined the Spetzler-Martin scale, integrating the classification with a supplementary score determined from the patient's age, hemorrhagic presentation, nidal diffuseness, and deep perforating arterial supply. This scale has proven to have better predictive power for forecasting the possibility of complications after surgical treatment of an AVM.

As is evident from the several scales presented, numerous parameters can influence the surgical decision. Size, nidus diffuseness, perforating arteries, age, eloquent area involved, and deep venous drainage are all parameters that must be taken into account when deciding whether to manage an AVM surgically.

Nidus diffuseness is an important predictor determining the difficulty of resecting an AVM. Highly diffuse AVMs have a nidus without clear anatomical dissection planes and so it is challenging to identify the right dissection distance around such malformations [95]. In some cases, the dissection is performed too close to the nidus, which can cause bleeding or may leave behind abnormal portions of the nidus. In other cases, the dissection is performed too far away from the nidus, which results in complete AVM resection, but may remove more brain tissue than is necessary.

When suggesting surgery to a patient with an unruptured AVM, a statistical evaluation of the hypothetical future risk of bleeding must be weighed against the present risk of surgery-induced brain injury. This requires an honest evaluation of the results of the person performing the surgery and his or her confidence with such a difficult kind of surgery.

Dealing with a patient with a ruptured AVM is completely different: often the hematoma has already created a cleavage between the AVM and brain tissue and the prognosis is totally different. The outcome of a patient with a ruptured malformation is mostly determined by the hemorrhage itself, while surgery has a lesser impact on conditioning the outcome.

Timing of Surgery in Hemorrhagic Arteriovenous Malformations

It is generally preferable to resect an AVM in an elective setting. This is challenging surgery and it is better to operate on relaxed brain tissue. The most difficult part of surgery is hemostasis and edematous brain tissue complicates control of hemostasis, especially of the thin vessels in deep white matter. If the AVM has bled and the hematoma is not too big, as in most cases, it is advisable to wait a few days, generally a week, before surgery. If the hematoma is life - threatening then the blood clot should be removed, but resection of the AVM can be delayed until the acute phase is overcome, again generally after a week.

Decompressive craniectomy with or without partial evacuation of the hematoma may improve outcomes by reducing intracranial pressure and protecting the surrounding brain.

Surgical Tips

Neuro-endovascular treatment has evolved, but so has surgery. In the last years various improvements have been introduced. Surgery has become less invasive and the use of neuronavigation, tractography and functional magnetic resonance imaging is now more widespread. Neurophysiological understanding is increasing and intraoperative fluorangiography is more diffuse. Furthermore, there are new surgical instruments available, such as non-stitch bipolar and laser equipment.

Planning the surgical treatment of an AVM requires a careful evaluation of the radiological images, with identification of all the main arterial AVM feeders and the main venous drainages. Three-dimensional reconstruction angiography can often be useful for understanding the location of the main vessels.

The surgical treatment of cerebral AVMs can be summarized as follows. A large skin and bone flap is preferred to expose the surrounding brain and to facilitate understanding of the incoming and outgoing vessels on the surface of the brain. Being too close to the margins of the AVM can be unsatisfactory because of less control of the vessels.

A microscope with fluoroangiography and intraoperative Doppler are extremely useful and are considered by some to be essential tools. Indocyanine green angiography is useful at the beginning of surgery. In fact, before opening the dura, the luminescence of the AVM and the main venous vessels can be seen through the dura, which can guide the surgeon and enable correct opening of the dura thereby avoiding damage to the malformation and especially to the veins. Once the AVM has been exposed, fluoroangiography is extremely useful for identifying the inflow and outflow vessels. Early identification and early occlusion of the main feeders can reduce the tightness of the AVM and facilitate resection around the borders of the malformation.

Cerebral AVMs often receive deep arterial feeders from the choroid arteries through the ventricle. These generally reach the tip of the conus of the AVM at the opposite part with respect to the surgeon's view. It is important to deal with these feeders, which are often large and have a high flow, carefully at the end of the resection of the malformation. Coagulation in these vessels is usually simpler after a wide ventricular wall opening.

Often the tiny vessels that surround the AVM nidus in the deep white matter are just a loop of small vessels that come out from the AVM and after a few millimeters re-enter the malformation. Sometimes it is better to follow them and retract them rather than coagulate them [96].

Non-stitch bipolar forceps are another essential tool. Coagulation of the deep, tiny vessels within the white matter is the main challenge of AVM surgery. These vessels are extremely fragile; their walls are disproportionally thin compared to the diameter of the vessel which is expanded by the low resistance of the AVM. Thus the protein content of these vessel walls is not sufficient to ensure safe coagulation. Great patience is often required when coagulating these vessels, especially with stitch bipolar forceps and trying to follow these vessels in the eloquent white matter to coagulate them is one of the causes of neurological damage. A precise, efficient method of coagulation is therefore extremely useful and non-stitch bipolar forceps facilitate this process. One surgical tip when coagulating feeders is to catch a small portion of the surrounding brain tissue as well in order to have more proteins between the tip of the bipolar forceps and thereby obtain more efficient coagulation [97]. Another valid alternative is to use a thulium laser to coagulate these tiny vessels. The advantages of thulium are that it does not penetrate tissues and that it can also be used in a wet surgical field.

At the end of the resection careful exploration of the surgical field is essential, because the chance of leaving a residual is high. We suggest that the surgical field is re-evaluated with indocyanine green angiography looking for the precocious appearance of a vein which is expression of a residual. The limitation of intraoperative fluoroangiography is that it does not enable visualization of features hidden by the brain tissue, thus a small, deep residual will not be picked up. Exploring the whole surgical field with intraoperative Doppler can help to detect high flow signals behind a thin wall of white matter.

Although intraoperative angiography is extremely useful for guaranteeing complete removal of an AVM, it sometimes may not be able to provide the resolution necessary to understand whether there is a small residual or whether the resection is complete. We recommend an immediate postoperative angiography for possible early visualization of a precocious vein or a true residual.

Postoperative Management

After a negative postoperative control angiography with evidence of complete removal of the AVM we generally prefer to keep the patient in an intensive care unit and maintain anesthesia for a few hours to permit slow awakening with complete control of the blood pressure. Blood pressure control is important in the postoperative period after AVM resection because the tiny deep white matter vessels that have been coagulated are more fragile and can bleed if exposed to a high blood pressure. Moreover, surrounding brain tissue may be prone to hemorrhage until autoregulation has been restored.

OUTCOME

Grade III and IV AVMs are more prone to surgical complications because they are large, residual nidus may be left and postoperative bleeding and reoperation are both possible. Hyperemia and edema have also been observed and described. The patient and relatives must be informed that the first 48 hours are critical and that the patient is at risk of rebleeding and, possibly, of reoperation. Nevertheless if the patient is followed in an intensive care unit and monitored carefully, the chance of serious neurological damage in the long-term is low. A bleed after surgery for a large AVM often occurs in the space of the resected AVM, thus some time passes before the intracranial pressure reaches a critical level: if the patient is taken back to the operating room immediately, serious consequences may be avoided. Patients who have a troublesome postoperative period are often found to have achieved a good outcome when re-evaluated a few months after discharge.

CONCLUSION

In conclusion, we do not agree with the concept of waiting for an unruptured AVM to rupture before treating it, because pre-emptive surgery is effective and not as dangerous. The current selection of patients seems to be correct and surgery should be presented as the first choice. Embolization should be pre-surgical and should be planned with the neurosurgeon. Management with a Gamma Knife is a second choice and endovascular treatment alone is not an option.

ACKNOWLEDGEMENTS

Declared none.

CONFLICT OF INTEREST

The authors confirm that this chapter contents have no conflict of interest.

REFERENCES

[1]   von Luschka H. Die Adergeflechte des menschlichen Gehirnes: eine Monographie 1855.

[2]   Virchow R. Handbuch der speciellen Pathologie und Therapie 1856.

[3]   Yasargil MG. Microneurosurgery: Thieme Classics 1987.

[4]   Bilsland WL. Controlled hypotension by arteriotomy in intracranial surgery. Anesthesia 1951; 6: 20-5.

[5]   Yasargil MG, Jain KK, Antic J, Laciga R. Arteriovenous malformation of the splenium of the corpus callosum: microsurgical treatment. Surg Neurol 1976; 5: 5-14.

[6]   Spetzler RF, Martin NA. A proposed grading system for arteriovenous malformations. J Neurosurg 1986; 65: 476-83.

[7]   Lawton MT, Kim H, McCulloch CE, Mikhak B, Young WL. A supplementary grading scale for selecting patients with brain arteriovenous malformations for surgery. Neurosurgery 2010; 66: 702-13.

[8]   Spetzler RF, Ponce FA. A 3-tier classification of cerebral arteriovenous malformations: clinical article. J Neurosurg 2011; 114: 842-9.

[9]   Mullan S, Mojtahedi S, Johnson DL, Macdonald RL. Cerebral venous malformation-arteriovenous malformation transition forms. J Neurosurg 1996; 85: 9-13.

[10]   Padget DH. Cranial venous system in man in reference to development, adult configuration, and relation to arteries. Am J Anat 1956; 98: 307-55.

[11]   Lasjaunias P. Vascular diseases in neonates, infants and children: interventional neuroradiology management. Springer 1997.

[12]   Kim H, Su H, Weinsheimer S, Pawlikowska L, Young WL. Brain arteriovenous malformation pathogenesis: a response-to-injury paradigm. Acta Neurochir Suppl 2011; 111: 83-92.

[13]   Enam SA, Malik GM. Association of cerebral arteriovenous malformations and spontaneous occlusion of major feeding arteries: clinical and therapeutic implications. Neurosurgery 1999; 45: 1105-11.

[14]   Gabriel EM, Sampson JH, Wilkins RH. Recurrence of a cerebral arteriovenous malformation after surgical excision. Case report. J Neurosurg 1996; 84: 879-82.

[15]   Hino A, Fujimoto M, Iwamoto Y, Takahashi Y, Katsumori T. An adult case of recurrence arteriovenous malformation after "complete" surgical excision: a case report. Surg Neurol 1999; 52: 156-8.

[16]   Pellettieri L, Svendsen P, Wikholm G, Carlsson CA. Hidden compartments in AVMs – a new concept. Acta Radiol 1997; 38: 2-7.

[17]   Kader A, Goodrich JT, Sonstein WJ, Stein BM, Carmel PW, Michelsen WJ. Recurrent cerebral arteriovenous malformations after negative post-operative angiograms. J Neurosurg 1996; 85: 14-8.

[18]   Stapf C, Mohr JP. New concepts in adult brain arteriovenous malformations. Curr Opin Neurol 2000; 13: 63-7.

[19]   Bennett MR, Evan GI, Schwartz SM. Apoptosis of human vascular smooth muscle cells derived from normal vessels and coronary atherosclerotic plaques. J Clin Invest 1995; 95: 2266-74.

[20]   Geng YJ, Libby P. Evidence of apoptosis in advanced human atheroma. Colocalization with interleukin-1 beta-converting enzyme. Am J Pathol 1995; 147: 251-66.

[21]   Takagi Y, Hattori I, Nozaki K, Ishikawa M, Hashimoto N. DNA fragmentation in central nervous system vascular malformations. Acta Neurochir 2000; 142: 987-94.

[22]   Jellinger K. Vascular malformations of the central nervous system: a morphological overview. Neurosurg Rev 1986; 9: 177-216.

[23]   McCormick WF. Pathology of vascular malformations of the brain. In: Wilson CB, Stein BM, eds. Intracranial Arteriovenous Malformations. Baltimore: Williams and Wilkinson 1984; 44-63.

[24] Valavanis A, Yasargil MG. The endovascular treatment of brain arteriovenous malformations. Adv Tech Stand Neurosurg 1998; 24: 131-214.

[25] Olivecrona H, Riives J. Arteriovenous aneurysms of the brain: their diagnosis and treatment. Arch Neurol Psychiatry 1948; 59: 567-603.

[26] Berman MF, Sciacca RR, Pile-Spellman J, *et al*. The epidemiology of brain arteriovenous malformations. Neurosurgery 2000; 47: 389-96.

[27] Mingrino S. Supratentorial arteriovenous malformations of the brain. Adv Tech Stand Neurosurg 1978; 5: 93-123.

[28] Hofmeister C, Stapf C, Hartmann A, *et al*. Demographic, morphological, and clinical characteristics of 1289 patients with brain arteriovenous malformation. Stroke 2000; 31: 1307-10.

[29] Martin NA, Vinters HV. Arteriovenous malformations. In: Carter LP, Spetzler RF (eds) Neurovascular surgery. McGraw-Hill, New York, 1995; 875-903.

[30] Mast H, Mohr JP, Osipov A, *et al*. "Steal" is an unestablished mechanism for the clinical presentation of cerebral arteriovenous malformations. Stroke 1995; 26: 1215-20.

[31] Prayer L, Wimberger D, Stiglbauer R, *et al*. Haemorrhage in intracerebral arteriovenous malformations: detection with MRI and comparison with clinical history. Neuroradiology 1993; 35: 424-7.

[32] Auger RG, Wiebers DO. Management of unruptured intracranial arteriovenous malformations: a decisional analysis. Neurosurgery 1992; 30: 561-9.

[33] Brown RD Jr, Wiebers DO, Forbes G, *et al*. The natural history of unruptured intracranial arteriovenous malformations. J Neurosurg 1988; 68: 352-7.

[34] Crawford PM, West CR, Chadwick DW, Shaw MD. Arteriovenous malformations of the brain: natural history in unoperated patients. J Neurol Neurosurg Psychiatry 1986; 49: 1-10.

[35] Ondra SL, Troupp H, George ED, Schwab K. The natural history of symptomatic arteriovenous malformations of the brain: a 24-year follow-up assessment. J Neurosurg 1990; 73: 387-91.

[36] The Arteriovenous Malformation Study Group. Arteriovenous malformations of the brain in adults. N Engl J Med 1999; 340: 1812-8.

[37] Brown RD Jr. Epidemiology and natural history of vascular malformations of the central nervous system. In: Jafar J, Awad I, Rosenwasser R, eds. Vascular malformations of the central nervous system. Philadelphia: Lippincott Willimans & Wilkins 1999; 129-47.

[38] Brown RD Jr, Wiebers DO, Torner JC, O'Fallon WM. Frequency of intracranial hemorrhage as a presenting symptom and subtype analysis: a population-based study of intracranial vascular malformations in Olmsted Country, Minnesota. J Neurosurg 1996; 85: 29-32.

[39] Hartmann A, Mast H, Mohr JP, *et al*. Morbidity of intracranial hemorrhage in patients with cerebral arteriovenous malformation. Stroke 1998; 29: 931-4.

[40] Mansmann U, Meisel J, Brock M, Rodesch G, Alvarez H, Lasjaunias P. Factors associated with intracranial hemorrhage in cases of cerebral arteriovenous malformation. Neurosurgery 2000; 46: 272-9.

[41] Norbash AM, Marks MP, Lane B. Correlation of pressure measurements with angiographic characteristics predisposing to hemorrhage and steal in cerebral arteriovenous malformations. AJNR Am J Neuroradiol 1994; 15: 809-13.

[42] Doung DH, Young WL, Vang MC, *et al*. Feeding artery pressure and venous drainage pattern are primary determinants of hemorrhage from cerebral arteriovenous malformations. Stroke 1998; 29: 1167-76.

[43] Hirai S, Mine S, Yamakami I, Ono J, Yamaura A. Angioarchitecture related to hemorrhage in cerebral arteriovenous malformations. Neurol Med Chir Tokyo [Suppl] 1998; 38: 165-70.

[44] Marks MP, Lane B, Steinberg GK, Chang PJ. Hemorrhage in intracerebral arteriovenous malformations: angiographic determinants. Radiology 1990; 176: 807-13.

[45] Kader A, Young WL, Pile-Spellman J, *et al*. The influence of hemodynamic and anatomic factors on hemorrhage from cerebral arteriovenous malformations. Neurosurgery 1994; 34: 801-7.

[46]   Pollock BE, Flickinger JC, Lunsford LD, Bissonette DJ, Kondziolka D. Factors that predict the bleeding risk of cerebral arteriovenous malformations. Stroke 1996; 27: 1-6.

[47]   D'Aliberti G, Talamonti G, Cenzato M, *et al*. Arterial and venous aneurysms associated with arteriovenous malformations. World Neurosurg [in press].

[48]   Nataf F, Meder JF, Roux FX, *et al*. Angioarchitecture associated with haemorrhage in cerebral arteriovenous malformations: a prognostic statistical model. Neuroradiology 1997; 39: 52-8.

[49]   Miyasaka Y, Yada K, Ohwada T, Kitahara T, Kurata A, Irikura K. An analysis of the venous drainage system as a factor in hemorrhage from arteriovenous malformations J Neurosurg 1992; 76: 239-43.

[50]   Miyasaka Y, Kurata A, Irikura K, Tanaka R, Fujii K. The influence of vascular pressure and angiographic characteristics on haemorrhage from arteriovenous malformations. Acta Neurochir 2000; 142: 39-43.

[51]   Hassler W, Steinmetz H. Cerebral hemodynamics in angioma patients: an intraoperative study. J Neurosurg 1987; 67: 822-31.

[52]   Heros RC. Arteriovenous malformations of the medial temporal lobe. Surgical approach and neuroradiological characterization. J Neurosurg 1982; 56: 44-52.

[53]   Yeh HS, Tew JM Jr, Gartner M. Seizure control after surgery on cerebral arteriovenous malformations. J Neurosurg 1993; 78: 12-18.

[54]   Turjman F, Massoud TF, Vinuela F, Sayre JW, Guglielmi G, Duckwiler G. Aneurysms related to cerebral arteriovenous malformations: superselective angiographic assessment in 58 patients. AJNR Am J Neuroradiol 1994; 15: 1601-5.

[55]   Heros RC, Tu YK. Unruptures arteriovenous maformations: a dilemma in surgical decision making. Clin Neurosurg 1986; 33: 187-236.

[56]   Batjer HH, Devous MD Sr, Seibert GB, *et al*. Intracranial arteriovenous malformation: relationships between clinical and radiographic factors and ipsilateral steal severity. Neurosurgery 1988; 23: 322-8.

[57]   Batjer HH, Devous MD Sr, Seibert GB, *et al*. Intracranial arteriovenous malformation: controlateral steal phenomena. Neurol Med Chir Tokyo 1989; 29: 401-6.

[58]   Feindel W, Garretson H, Yamamoto L, Perot P, Rumin N. Blood flow patterns in the cerebral vessels and cortex in man studies by intracarotid injection of radioisotopes and Coomassie Blue dye. J Neurosurg 1965; 23: 12-22.

[59]   Feindel W, Yamamoto JL, Hodge CP. Red cerebral veins and the cerebral steal syndrome. Evidence from fluorescein angiography and microregional blood flow by radioisotopes during excision of an angioma. J Neurosurg 1971; 35: 167-79.

[60]   Krauss JK, Kiriyanthan GD, Borremans JJ. Cerebral arteriovenous malformations and movement disorders. Clin Neurol Neurosurg 1999; 101: 92-9.

[61]   Kaminaga T, Hayashida K, Iwama T, Nishimura T. Hemodynamic changes around cerebral arteriovenous malformation before and after embolization measured with PET. J Neuroradiol 1999; 26: 236-41.

[62]   Vinuela F, Nombela L, Roach MR, Fox AJ, Pelz DM. Stenotic and occlusive disease of the venous drainage system of deep brain AVM's. J Neurosurg 1985; 63: 180-4.

[63]   Kumar AJ, Vinuela F, Fox AJ, Rosenbaum AE. Revisited old and new CT findings in unruptured larger arteriovenous malformations of the brain. J Comput Assist Tomogr 1984; 8: 648-55.

[64]   Mendelowitsch A, Radue EW, Gratzl O. Aneurysm, arteriovenous malformation and arteriovenous fistula in posterior fossa compression syndrome. Eur Neurol 1990; 30: 338-42.

[65]   Miyasaka Y, Yada K, Kurata A, Tokiwa K, Tanaka R, Ohwada T. An unruptured arteriovenous malformation with edema. AJNR Am J Neuroradiol 1994; 15: 385-8.

[66]   Pribil S, Boone SC, Waley R. Obstructive hydrocephalus at the anterior third ventricle caused by dilated veins from an arteriovenous malformation. Surg Neurol 1983; 20: 487-92.

[67]   Frishberg BM. Neuroimaging in presumed primary headache headache disorders. Semin Neurol 1997; 17: 373-82.

[68]   Troost BT, Newton TH. Occipital lobe arteriovenous malformations. Clinical and radiological features in 26 cases with comments on differentiation from migraine. Arch Ophthalmol 1975; 93: 250-6.

[69]   Kurita H, Ueki K, Shin M, *et al.* Headaches in patients with radiosurgically treated occipital arteriovenous malformations. J Neurosurg 2000; 93: 224-8.

[70]   Stabell KE, Nornes H. Prospective neuropsychological investigation of patients with supratentorial arteriovenous malformations. Acta Neurochir 1994; 131: 32-44.

[71]   Farnham FR, Ritchie CW, James DV, Kennedy HG. Pathology of love. Lancet 1997; 350: 710.

[72]   Wenz F, Steinvorth S, Wildermuth S, *et al.* Assessment of neuropsychological changes in patients with arteriovenous malformation (AVM) after radiosurgery. Int J Radiat Oncol Biol Phys 1998; 42: 995-9.

[73]   Lazar RM, Connaire K, Marshall RS, *et al.* Developmental deficits in adult patients with arteriovenous malformations. Arch Neurol 1999; 56: 103-6.

[74]   Hashimoto T, Lawton MT, Wen G, *et al.* Gene microarray analysis of human brain arteriovenous malformations. Neurosurgery 2004; 54: 410-23.

[75]   Rothbart D, Awad IA, Lee J, Kim J, Harbaugh R, Criscuolo GR. Expression of angiogenic factors and structural proteins in central nervous system vascular malformations. Neurosurgery 1996; 38: 915-24.

[76]   Chen Y, Fan Y, Poon KY, *et al.* MMP-9 expression is associated with leukocytic but not endothelial markers in brain arteriovenous malformations. Front Biosci 2006; 11: 3121-8.

[77]   Chen Y, Pawlikowska L, Yao JS, *et al.* Interleukin-6 involvement in brain arteriovenous malformations. Ann Neurol 2006; 59: 72-80.

[78]   Hashimoto T, Wen G, Lawton MT, *et al.* Abnormal expression of matrix metalloproteinases and tissue inhibitors of metalloproteinases in brain arteriovenous malformations. Stroke 2003; 34: 925-931.

[79]   Gao P, Chen Y, Lawton MT, *et al.* Evidence of endothelial progenitor cells in the human brain and spinal cord arteriovenous malformations. Neurosurgery 2010; 67: 1029-35.

[80]   Hao Q, Chen Y, Zhu Y, *et al.* Neutrophil depletion decreases VEGF-induced focal angiogenesis in the mature mouse brain. J Cereb Blood Flow Metab 2007; 27: 1853-60.

[81]   Nuki Y, Matsumoto MM, Tsang E, *et al.* Roles of macrophages in flow-induced outward vascular remodelling. J Cereb Blood Flow Metab 2009; 29: 495-503.

[82]   Abdalla SA, Letarte M. Hereditary haemorrhagic telangectasia: current views on genetics and mechanisms of disease. J Med Genet 2006; 43: 97-110.

[83]   Gallione CJ, Richards JA, Letteboer TG, *et al.* SMAD4 Mutations found in unselected HHT patients. J Med Genet 2006; 43: 793-7.

[84]   Graf CJ, Perret GE, Torner JC. Bleeding from cerebral arteriovenous malformations as part of their natural history. J Neurosurg 1983; 58: 331-7.

[85]   Hernesniemi JA, Dashti R, Juvela S, Vaart K, Niemela M, Laakso A. Natural history of brain arteriovenous malformations: a long-term follow-up study of risk of hemorrhage in 238 patients. Neurosurgery 2008; 63: 823-9.

[86]   Mohr JP, Parides MK, Stapf C, *et al.* Medical management with or without interventional therapy for unruptured brain arteriovenous malformations (ARUBA): a multicentre, non-blinded, randomised trial. Lancet 2014; 383: 614-21.

[87]   Miyamoto S, Hashimoto N, Nagata I, *et al.* Posttreatment sequelae of palliatively treated cerebral arteriovenous malformations. Neurosurgery 2000; 46: 589-94.

[88]   Fokas E, Henzel M, Witting A, Grund S, Engenhart-Cabillic R. Stereotactic radiosurgery of cerebral arteriovenous malformations: long-term follow-up in 164 patients of a single institution. J Neurol 2013; 260: 2156-62.

[89]   Ding D, Yen CP, Xu Z, Starke RM, Sheehan JP. Radiosurgery for patients with unruptured intracranial arteriovenous malformations. J Neurosurg 2013; 118: 958-66.

[90] Kim HY, Chang WS, Kim DJ, *et al.* Gamma Knife surgery for large cerebral arteriovenous malformations. J Neurosurg 2010; 113: 2-8.

[91] Yamamoto M, Akabane A, Matsumaru Y, Higuchi Y, Kasuya H, Urakawa Y. Long-term follow-up results of international 2-stage Gamma Knife surgery with an interval of at least 3 years for arteriovenous malformations larger than 10 cm3. J Neurosurg 2012; 117: 126-34.

[92] Miyachi S, Negoro M, Okamoto R, Otsuka G, Suzuki O, Yoshida J. Embolization of arteriovenous malformations prior to radiosurgery. Interv Neuroradiol 2000; 6: 131-7.

[93] Pierot L, Kadziolka K, Litre F, Rousseaux P. Combined treatment of brain AVMs with use of Onyx embolization follow by radiosurgery. AJNR Am J Neuroradiol 2013; 34: 1395-400.

[94] Lawton MT, UCSF Brain Arteriovenous Malformation Study Project. Spetzler-Martin grade III arteriovenous malformations: surgical results and a modification of the grading scale. Neurosurgery 2+003; 52: 740-8.

[95] Du R, Keyoung HM, Dowd CF, Young WL, Lawton MT. The effects of diffuseness and deep perforators arterial supply on outcomes after microsurgical removal of brain arteriovenous malformations. Neurosurgery 2007; 60: 638-46.

[96] Hashimoto N, Nozaki K, Takagi Y, Kikuta K, Mikuni M. Surgery of cerebral arteriovenous malformations. Neurosurgery 2007; 61: 375-87.

[97] Hernesniemi J, Romani R, Lehecka M, *et al.* Present state of microneurosurgery of cerebral arteriovenous malformations. Acta Neurochir Suppl 2010; 107: 71-6.

CHAPTER 4

Complex Aneurysms From Endovascular and Surgical Points of View

D. Cannizzaro[*], R. Delfini, A. Caporlingua and A. Santoro

Department of Neurology and Psychiatry, Neurosurgery, "Sapienza" University of Rome, Rome, Italy

Abstract: Large aneurysms (more than 25 mm in diameter) or aneurysms in particular positions inside the skull base are defined complex. They are associated with a high risk of subarachnoid or intracranial hemorrhage and neurological deficits. We discuss this particular class of aneurysms which, given their peculiar characteristics, require a complex therapeutic approach, including synergistic treatment with surgical and endovascular modalities.

Keywords: Bypass, complex aneurysm, endovascular treatment, revascularization, vascular neurosurgery.

INTRODUCTION

The continuous evolution of endovascular techniques for the treatment of vascular diseases has led to a significant reduction of cerebral aneurysms that are candidates for surgical treatment [1-3]. Endovascular or surgical procedures now allow us to treat most cerebral aneurysms. However, the presence of thrombotic phenomena, intramural calcification, or vessels originating from the aneurysmal sac, large aneurysms and those in specific locations or with particular projections prevent conventional aneurysm management from being used. Such aneurysms are, therefore, defined as complex. Although the definition of complex aneurysms has changed over time, the following parameters are of particular importance in the description of these vascular abnormalities: (i) the location of the aneurysmal sac, which determines the surgical accessibility of the lesion, (ii) the presence of thrombotic phenomena and calcification of the wall of the aneurysm, which make it difficult to position a single clip; and (iii) the size of the aneurysm, which, if large, reduces access to afferent and efferent vessels and these vessels require particular handling. For these reasons, complex aneurysms are treated with

Corresponding author Delia Cannizzaro: Department of Neuroscience "Sapienza" University, Rome, Italy; Tel: 00390649979111; Fax: 00390649979111; E-mail: delia.cannizzaro@gmail.com

indirect approaches: trapping techniques, multiclipping, closure of the afferent vessel, occlusion and distal revascularization.

SURGICAL TREATMENT OF COMPLEX ANEURYSMS

Anterior and Posterior Circulation

When possible, surgery should be considered the first choice to treat complex aneurysms: in most cases careful selection of the cases, preparation of a pre-operative plan with the help of three-dimensional angiography, and radiological techniques to facilitate the choice of the appropriate surgical strategy allow good results to be obtained [4].

Complex Aneurysms of the Anterior Circulation – Surgical Technical Notes

The majority of complex aneurysms are found in the anterior circulation, in particular in the supraclinoid tract of the internal carotid artery (ICA) (Fig. **1**). The pterional approach provides excellent exposure of aneurysms of the anterior circulation (Fig. **2**). A fronto-temporal-orbital-zygomatic approach should be reserved for complex aneurysms of the internal carotid supraclinoid tract.

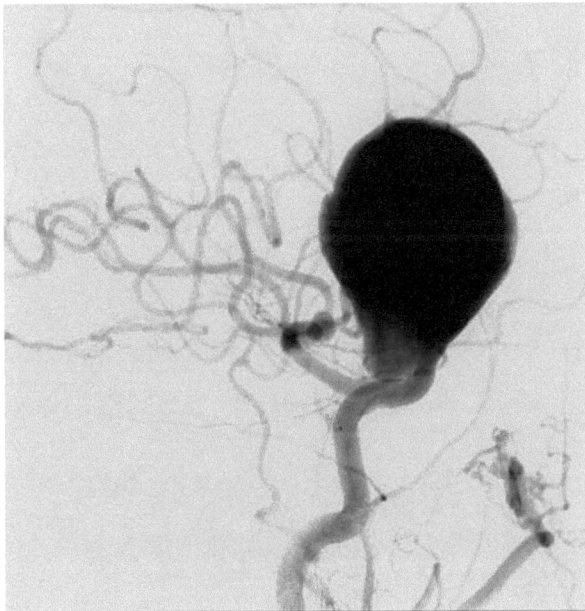

Figure 1: Giant carotid ophthalmic aneurysm.

Pterional Approach

The patient should be placed in the supine position with the head rotated sideways by about 30° to the contralateral side of the aneurysm. Once the operculum bone has been opened, the great wing of the sphenoid bone must be removed to expose the anterior surface of the temporal lobe and the sylvian fissure. The opening of the dura mater should be sufficient to expose the frontal and temporal lobes. The sylvian fissure is then opened. The temporal lobe must be retracted in order to expose the distal middle cerebral artery, which is wider in the case of ICA aneurysms.

The basic steps during the surgical procedure for aneurysms of the supraclinoid tract are clinoidectomy, incision of the dural ring, resection of the lateral wall of the optic canal, and then opening of the optic fissure.

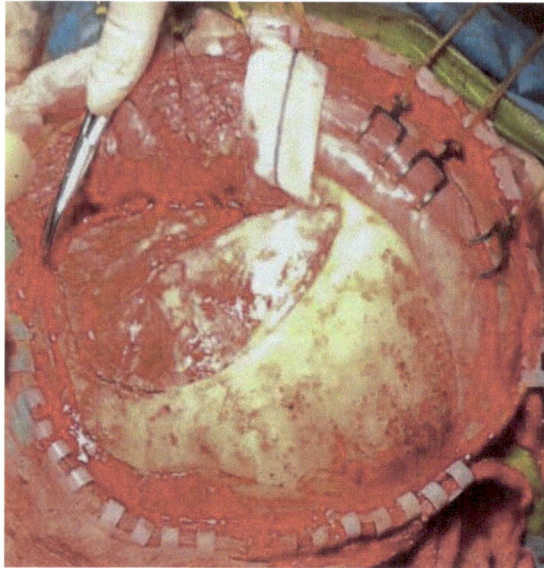

Figure 2: Pterional approach.

Complex Aneurysms of the Posterior Circulation – Surgical Technical Notes

Positions and Approaches

The choice of the exact surgical approach and the best position of the patient are key elements for obtaining good surgical results. This is particularly the case for surgery of the posterior fossa.

There are four main positions to consider: (i) prone/Concorde, (ii) park-bench, (iii) supine with head rotation; and (iv) sitting [5].

Prone Position and Concorde

These positions are mainly used for disorders in which it is necessary to approach the midline. However, even for a far lateral approach, these positions have some advantages over a lateral position. In the prone position, the patient's face is downwards on the table. The chest, the pelvis and the legs are supported gently. In this way the abdominal wall is not compressed. A U-shaped cushion is placed under the thorax. The head can be supported by a pillow or horseshoe, or fixed with a Mayfield frame (Fig. **3**).

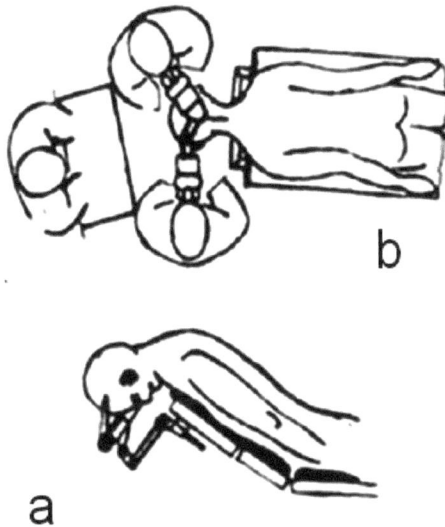

Figure 3: A Concorde position, b surgeon's position.

Lateral Decubitus and the "Park-Bench" Position

Careful support of the chest is needed, leaving the lower arm dependent and a modest decline in the upper one. The sides must be carefully constrained and fixed in this position, to avoid sudden slipping or rotation. The head is supported by a Mayfield frame, the neck can be flexed if necessary. The main advantage is that rotation of the neck is minimized. Risks associated with this position are ventilation-perfusion mismatch, and stretching of the brachial plexus of the dependent limb (Fig. **4**).

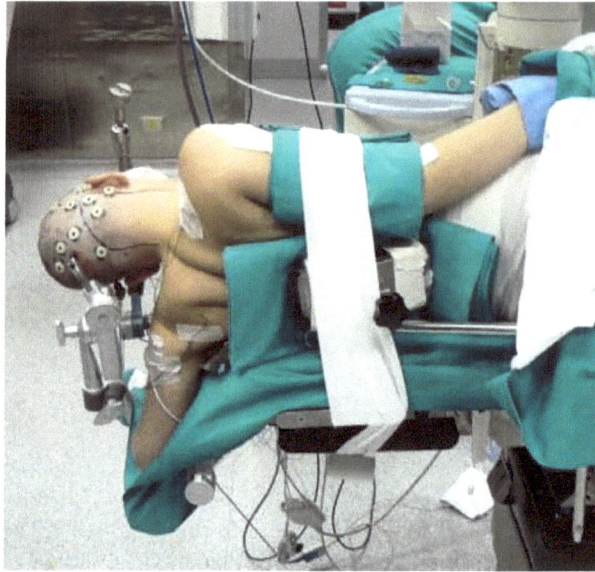

Figure 4: Park bench position.

Supine Position with Rotation of the Head

For lateral vascular lesions in the posterior fossa, a supine position with the head fixed in a Mayfield frame and rotated from one side is adequate. This offers advantages over the lateral position. Correct flexion of the neck is important to avoid excessive compression of the jugular vein and to optimize access to the posterior fossa. Venous congestion must be avoided and can be decreased greatly by raising the head or the whole upper part of the table a few degrees (Fig. **5**).

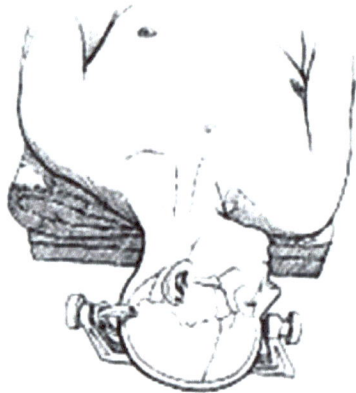

Figure 5: Supine position.

Sitting Position

The main advantage of this position is better visualization of the middle portion of the tentorium and it is, therefore, ideal for a supracerebellar infratentorial approach. The disadvantages are the risk of pulmonary gas embolism: in the 10% of patients with an unknown patent foramen ovale there is also the risk of air embolism in the cerebral circulation. Pre-operative planning is fundamental and should include in-depth cardiac investigations to exclude the presence of a patent foramen ovale. Measures should be taken to prevent thrombus formation in the lower limbs (Fig. **6**).

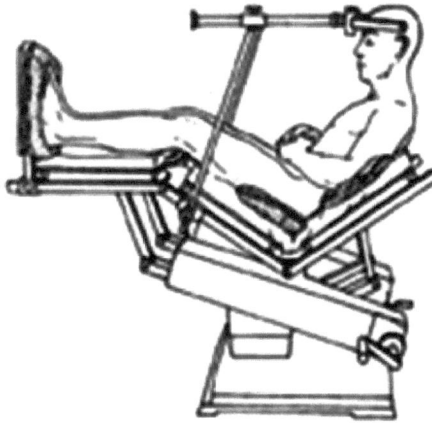

Figure 6: Sitting position.

Midline Approach

After a midline incision of the skin approximately 2 cm from above the external protuberance to the palpable spinous process of C2, following the median line, the muscles are removed from the underlying bone. A suboccipital craniotomy is then performed. The dura mater is opened with a Y-shaped incision (Fig. **7**).

Far Lateral Approach

For this approach the patient is placed in the prone position. The procedure begins with a standard midline opening, but the skin incision is extended toward the side of the mastoid process of interest. This incision is classically defined as the "hockey stick" incision. Skeletonization of the muscle components is performed to obtain good exposure of the occipital squama, mastoid process, the posterior margin of the foramen magnum, and the atlanto-occipital junction. Particular attention must be paid to the course of the vertebral arteries during the preparation of the C1 and C2 segments. The dural incision extends from the cerebellar hemisphere to C2. The formation of a triangular dural flap provides good lateral exposure (Fig. **8**).

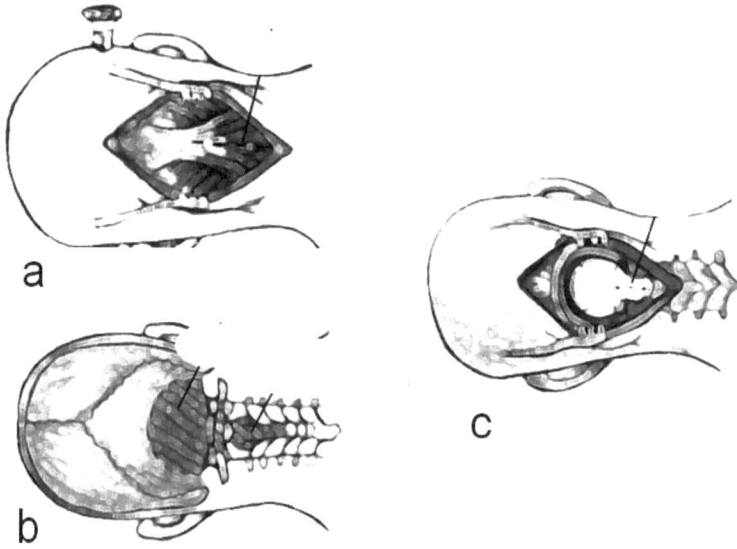

Figure 7: A muscle incision, b craniectomy, c dural incision.

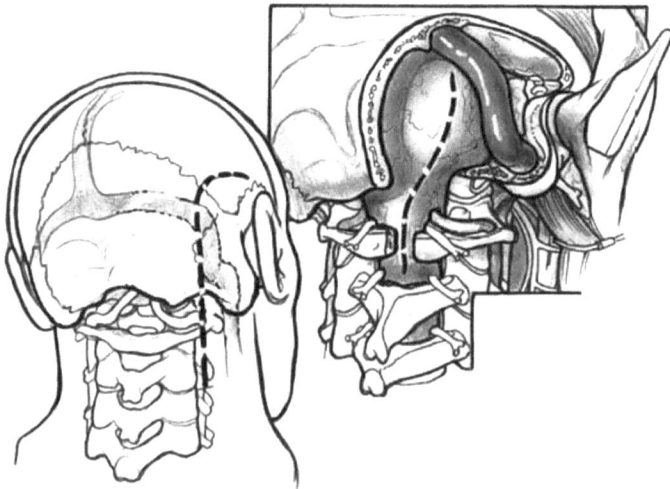

Figure 8: Far lateral approach.

Retrosigmoid Approach

For this approach the patient is placed in the supine position and the head rotated. An S-shaped skin incision is made from behind the top of the ear, to about 5 cm below and behind the palpable mastoid process. Laterally, the first centimeter of the mastoid should be visible, as should be the digastric groove behind and caudal to it. A hole is drilled in the upper part of the exposed bone in the vicinity of the transverse sinus and the craniotomy is then performed. The dura is incised parallel to the mastoid process. The dura is opened with two cuts at the top, resulting in a dural triangle, based on the transverse sinus (Fig. **9**).

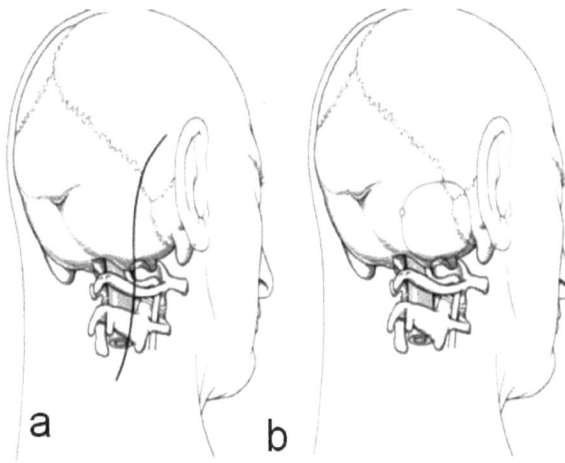

Figure 9: A skin incision, b craniectomy.

Surgical Techniques

Temporary Clipping

A temporary clip is used for intraoperative control of a possible rupture of the aneurysmal sac [6], which can occur during the dissection of the aneurysm and the side branches in the final preparation for positioning the clip. Dissection of an aneurysm involves the control of afferent arteries, identification of the efferent arteries and preparation of the aneurysm neck. Mobilization of the aneurysm involves a high risk of breaking the vascular malformation, which is why temporary clips may need to be placed. In the case of supraclinoid or complex aneurysms of the ICA, temporary clipping is performed at the level of the cervical

ICA. This requires exposure of the common carotid artery and the carotid bifurcation in the neck in the pre-operative phase.

In the case that occlusion of the vessels cannot be tolerated, a few strategies must be used during the temporary clipping: a state of hypothermia (32-33 °C) and the use of anti-edema drugs (mannitol), barbiturates and phenytoin. Temporary clipping has some disadvantages. The temporary clip can hinder the normal dissection of the sac and the placement of the definitive clip, there is a non-negligible risk of cerebral ischemia, time limitations, the lack of a collateral circulation, and mechanical loosening of atheromatous plaques present inside the afferent vessel on which the clip is placed. Motor evoked potentials can be used to monitor the possible development of ischemic injuries and to optimize the time of placement of temporary clips. Despite the disadvantages listed, temporary clipping remains of fundamental importance for the management of cerebral aneurysms, especially complex ones.

Definitive Clipping

The definitive clip is positioned after the final preparation of the neck of the sac of the aneurysm; the afferent and efferent vessels of the sac must be visualized and the presence of perforating branches must always be kept in mind. The neck is well prepared if the clip can be tilted in relation to the afferent vessel and rotated with respect to the vertical axis. Rhoton formulated four rules for the correct positioning of a definitive clip: (i) for aneurysms originating from the branches of a bifurcation, the clip must be positioned parallel to the afferent and efferent branches of the aneurysm and perpendicular to the bifurcation; (ii) for aneurysms that arise from the point of curvature of a vessel at which there is hemodynamic stress, and (iii) for aneurysms originating from portions of the wall where a clear direction of flow can be seen, the definitive clip should be positioned parallel to the parent vessel at the point of curvature of this vessel; and (iv) for aneurysms associated with perforating branches that must be preserved, the clip should be positioned parallel to the perforating vessels crossing the base of the aneurysmal sac. Rhoton's rules cannot be applied to all aneurysms, but careful analysis of the anatomical features of the aneurysmal sac and vessels associated with it enables the most appropriate final clip to be chosen.

The use of a single clip is generally preferred in the treatment of cerebral aneurysms. However, as mentioned previously, in the case of complex aneurysms, it will be necessary to use fenestrated clips or place clips in tandem.

Multiclipping

In the surgical treatment of complex aneurysms a single clip is often not sufficient to exclude the aneurysmal sac completely from the circulation. In such cases multiple clips must be used to remodel the neck and reconstruct the aneurysm.

Pre-operative planning is essential to ensure complete understanding of the anatomy and the three-dimensional configuration of the aneurysm in order to be able to choose the most appropriate clip to apply and its orientation. Careful selection and correct positioning of the first clip can reduce the size of the neck and the sac of the aneurysm, so that the remaining part of the aneurysm and the vessels adjacent to it will be better displayed. The use of a multiclipping technique can exclude the aneurysm from the circulation and reduces the risk of recanalization in complex aneurysms; it can also preserve perforating branches (Fig. **10**).

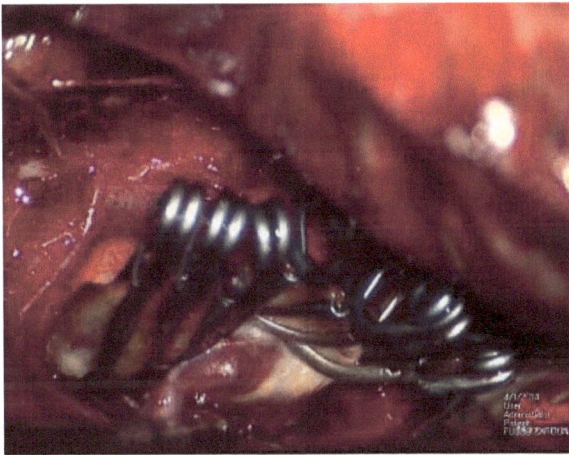

Figure 10: Multiclipping technique.

Trapping

This technique enablesexclusion of the aneurysmal dilatation from the circulation by positioning clips upstream and downstream of the aneurysm. This technique is feasible in the presence of a good collateral circulation. Trapping is mainly used in the case of complex aneurysms of the ICA and middle cerebral artery.

Revascularization

Many bypass techniques have been developed over the years, including low-flow extracranial (EC)-intracranial (IC) bypass, high-flow EC-IC bypass, *in situ* IC-IC bypass.

Low-flow bypasses are the most used type of revascularization. They are created from a single anastomosis between the superficial temporal artery and the middle cerebral artery, or the occipital artery and the cerebellar surface [7]. This category includes bypasses of the superficial temporal artery and the middle cerebral artery or the posterior cerebral artery or anastomoses between the occipital artery and the posterior cerebral artery. High-flow bypass grafts using large-caliber conduits (saphenous vein or radial artery) require two anastomoses: a proximal and a distal one. The *in situ* IC-IC bypass connects two intracranial arteries using a single suture. *In situ* bypasses are included in the sutures after excision of the aneurysmal sac through an end-to-end anastomosis.

The success of revascularization depends on the appropriateness of the selected graft. The choice is between the saphenous vein, radial artery, and the superficial temporal artery (or posterior occipital vessels). The parameters guiding the choice include hemodynamic requirements, diameter, position, accessibility and accessibility of the vessel to use as the graft.

High-Flow Bypasses

High-flow bypasses are used for large caliber vessels: ICA, middle cerebral artery, basilar artery and dominant vertebral artery. A high-flow bypass can be created with an arterial or venous graft: in the former case, the radial artery is used, while in the latter case, the saphenous vein is employed [8].

Radial Artery

The radial artery is removed from the non-dominant arm after performing the Allen test that determines the competence of the collateral circulation in the distal upper limb territories. The diameter of the radial artery is comparable to that of middle cerebral artery and a tract as long as 20 cm can be obtained. Flow through the radial artery is moderate, but this artery can support increased flow rates, making it ideal for high-flow bypasses. The diameter of the radial artery is 3 - 4.55 mm, which makes it perfect for the anastomosis at the level of the middle cerebral or posterior cerebral arteries, which have the same diameter. The arterial graft does not have valves on the inside, so its orientation can be reversed. The radial artery has a linear course and it is easy to access and has a thick muscular wall that facilitates suturing. Finally, its use is associated with a low risk of postoperative infection. The main disadvantage associated with the use of an arterial graft is the high rate of vasospasm, related to the presence of a highly developed muscle layer in the wall of the artery. Many solutions to this problem have been proposed: the use of pressure relaxation after its excision, systemic and local administrationof calcium antagonists during the surgical procedure, as well as the administration of non-steroidal anti-inflammatory drugs and calcium-channel blockers in the postoperative period significantly reduce the risk of vasospasm. The radial artery is obtained by making a linear incision on the volar aspect of the non-dominant arm and then carefully dissecting out about 20 cm of the vessel [9] (Fig. **11**).

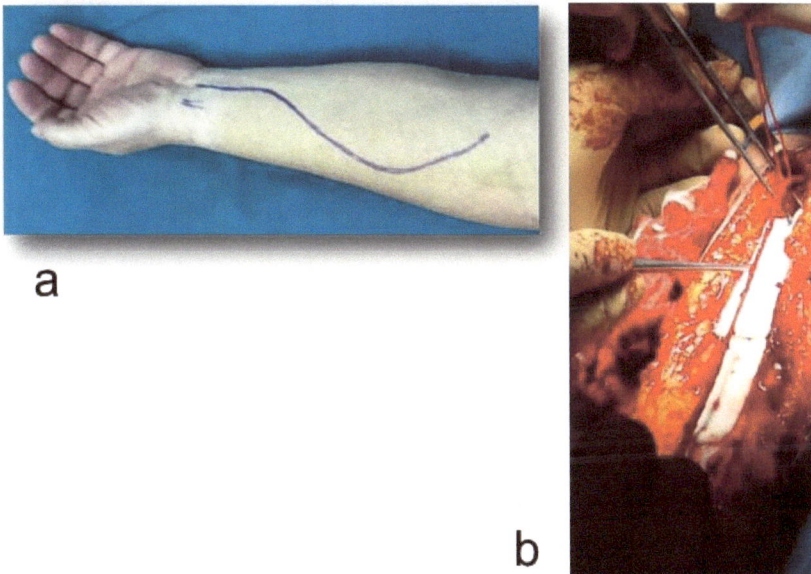

Figure 11: A skin incision, b radial artery.

Saphenous Vein

The territory of the saphenous vein is determined pre-operatively by Doppler of the lower limbs, excluding the presence of thrombotic formations. The vein is identified by stroking and then dissected in a distal to proximal direction: this operation is particularly complicated in obese subjects.

The patient is place in the supine position. The leg from which the vein is to be harvested is rotated externally. The femoral artery and inguinal ligament are identified and a skin incision is performed medially to these structures. The subcutaneous tissue is dissected down to the femoral vein, located medially to the femoral artery. The exposed femoral vein is pulled above the inguinal ligament, and the saphenous vein is identified and dissected along its course. About 30 cm are exposed; the side branches are ligated and resected. The graft takes place under continuous infusion of heparinized solution. Because of the presence of valves within the lumen of the vein, the orientation of the vessel cannot be reversed at the time of creating the by-pass (Fig. **12**).

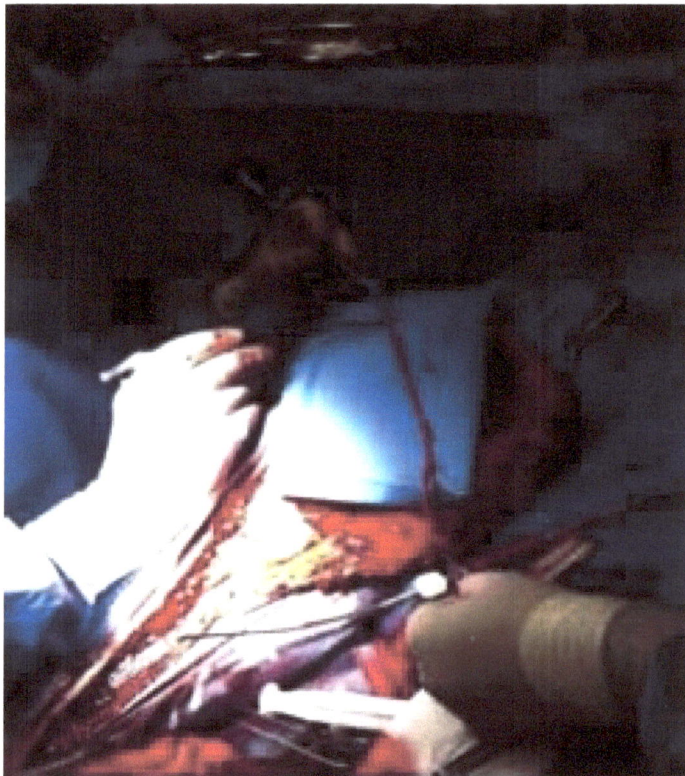

Figure 12: Saphenous vein.

Creating the Bypass

The tunnel that will host the graft begins prior to the root of the zygoma. With the aid of a chamfered tool, the insertion of the temporal muscle in front of the maxillary condyle is penetrated. The tunnel follows the ascending branch of the mandible until the angle of the bone is reached and then penetrates the insertion of the masseter muscle and the parotid fascia until the top edge of the cervical incision is reached. The tunnel thus created will house the graft.

Following the bifurcation of the middle cerebral artery, the frontal and temporal branches are identified, and at that point the branch most suitable for the creation of the anastomosis is selected. The criteria considered are the size and the course of the branch and the presence of adjacent vessels. A subcutaneous tunnel is prepared before the tragus, paying great attention to the course of the facial nerve. The graft is then sutured at the level of the middle cerebral artery. An analysis of angiographic images carried out preoperatively enables identification of the exact level of the bifurcation of the carotid artery in the neck. An incision can, therefore, be made approximately 5 cm anterior to its course and parallel to the sternocleidomastoid muscle. Proceeding with deep dissection the digastric muscle and hypoglossal nerve are identified. At this point the common internal and external carotid arteries can also be identified. The external carotid artery, which will be used for the proximal anastomosis of the EC-IC bypass, is exposed for about 4 cm to allow the temporary clipping and provide enough space to perform the anastomosis. The graft is sutured to the external carotid artery. Once the correct functioning of the graft has been confirmed, the ICA is connected (Fig. **13**). The intracranial anastomosis is generally carried out first, because freedom of the other end of the graft makes handling easier during the suturing. The time required for the intracranial suture is about 30 minutes. The middle cerebral artery has a diameter of approximately3-3.5 mm; in order to fit the lumen of the selected vessel, which in many cases is smaller, a "fish-mouth" cut is performed and sutured with 8 to 10.0 nylon wire. The graft should be flushed continuously with heparinized solution [10].

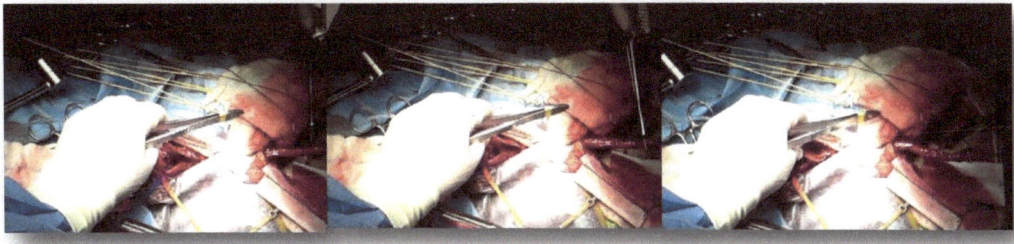

Figure 13: Positioning of the graft.

Arterial Versus Venous Grafts

An arterial graft has several advantages over a venous graft [11], the foremost being the absence of valves within the lumen and the same wall structure that ensures a good response to the pressures present within the arterial circulation. Venous grafts are associated with higher risks of thromboembolism and slower compliance to arterial blood pressure values; nevertheless, the long-term outcomes are positive [12]. The failure rate per annum is 1-1.5%. Arterial grafts carry a higher risk of vasospasm at an early stage. Much attention has been paid to this problem in recent years. Platelet anti-aggregants are administered in the pre-operative period. During surgery the graft is connected to a pump that delivers a continuous infusion of nimodipine while the bypass is prepared. For 72 hours after surgery lysine acetylsalicylate acid is given intravenously. A venous graft is most vulnerable to damage at the time of excision of the vein; a particularly large skin incision is necessary in order to remove it and veins have lower resistance than arteries to twisting and kinking phenomena. The risk of vasospasm is higher in arterial grafts than in venous ones. There is a description of the use of arterial grafts for coronary bypasses; with prophylactic pre-, intra- and post-operative administration of nimodipine, the risk of vasospasm was significantly decreased. We believe that every patient who is a potential candidate for a bypass procedure must be entered into a meticulous preoperative program including careful study of the saphenous veins (right and left) and radial arteries (right and left) in order to select the most suitable donor vessel.

In reports of cardiac surgery series comparing radial artery and saphenous veins grafts, it has been described that patency rates at 1 year are higher with radial artery grafts.

Low–Flow Bypasses

Superficial Temporal Artery

Given its diameter and position, the superficial temporal artery is used for anastomoses with the distal middle cerebral artery for the treatment of M3 and M4 complex aneurysms. Doppler studies enable the course of the superficial temporal artery and its parietal and frontal branches to be traced on the skin. No local anesthesia is used in order to prevent damage to the vessel and to prevent lidocaine-induced vasospasm. The skin incision is made along the parietal branch of the superficial temporal artery extending about 15 cm in the direction of the frontal branch, paying particular attention not to damage it (Fig. **14**). The superficial temporal artery is dissected in a distal to proximal direction with the aid of an electronic microscope [13].

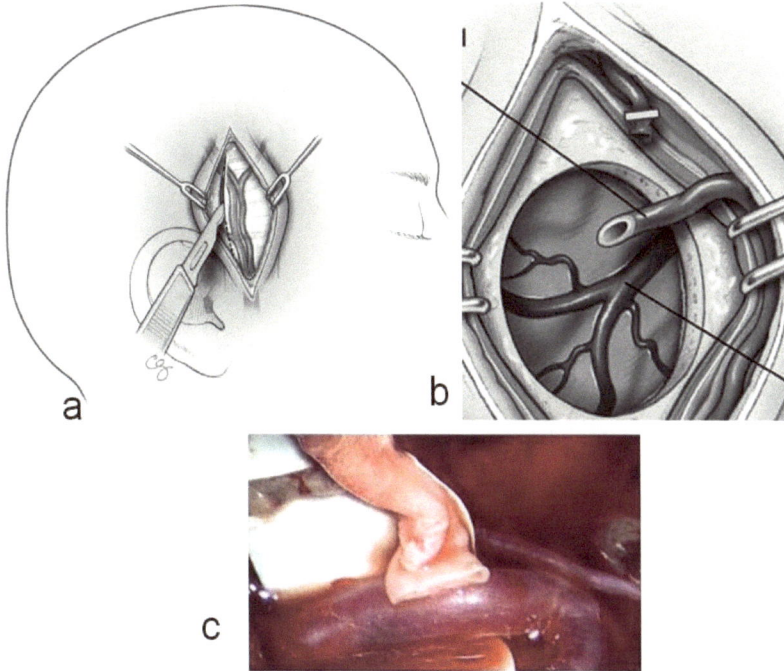

Figure 14: A skin incision, b the superficial temporal artery (STA) is mobilized, c STA is prepared for anastomosis.

Occipital Artery

The occipital artery is used for the treatment of aneurysms of the posterior circulation, although occasionally the superficial temporal artery, which can be anastomosed with the superior cerebellar artery, is used.

The occipital artery can be anastomosed with the posterior inferior cerebellar artery and the posterior cerebral artery. Moreover, if the superficial temporal artery is lacking, the occipital artery can be sutured with the middle cerebral artery. The preparation of the occipital artery is difficult because of its tortuous and deep course through the muscle layers (Fig. **15**). With the help of transcutaneous Doppler, the course of the occipital artery can be determined. The skin incision and median occipital artery dissection extend for about 15 cm [14].

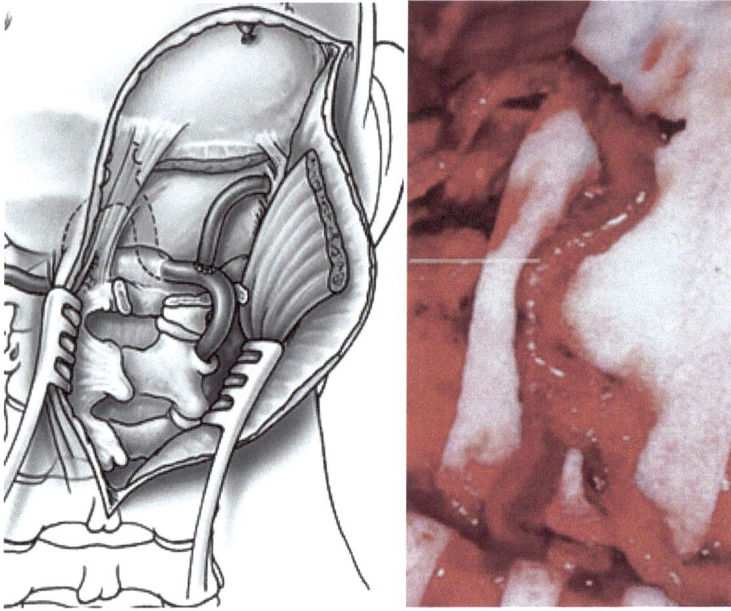

Figure 15: Occipital artery.

In Situ Bypasses

In some cases the treatment of a complex aneurysm may require the sacrifice of a vessel, with trapping and removal of the section of pathological artery. An *in situ* suture can restore normal arterial flow, through the interposition of a vessel adjacent to the aneurysm sac that will replace the compromised circulation. This technique is commonly used at the level of the anterior cerebral and posterior inferior cerebellar arteries. In both districts, the vessels are dissected from the sub-arachnoid space and the clips are positioned 4 mm distal and proximal to the suture which is made at the level of the excess medial surface of the vessel. If an adjacent vessel is not available for the *in situ* anastomosis, a direct end-to-end suture can be used to repair a compromised vessel [15].

Pre-operative Management

A patient selected for a revascularization procedure should undergo a series of instrumental clinical examinations. First, coagulation disorders must be excluded. Patients with deficiency of factor V or a pro-thrombotic risk should not undergo saphenous vein harvesting. Platelet aggregation tests should be carried out to check the individual's response to anti-aggregant agents and enable the lowest effective dose to be administered. The use of proton pump inhibitors should be limited. Patients from whom a radial artery graft will be taken should be administered aspirin at a dose of 325 mg/day, in addition to statins, in the 7 days preceding the surgery. Placing a lumbar drainage reduces the pressure on brain parenchyma and can be combined with the use of anti-edemigenic drugs. Intra-operatively, continuous neurophysiological monitoring with electro-encephalography and somatosensory evoked potentials is essential. During the time required for the suturing, the patient is kept in burst suppression, with particular attention to blood pressure in patients with sub-arachnoid hemorrhage at high risk of vasospasm.

Balloon Occlusion Test

The protocol for performing a balloon occlusion test involves the occlusion of an artery by a balloon mounted on a catheter. The vessel is occluded for 30 minutes with continuous evaluation of the electroencephalographic and neurological status and the development of collateral circulation. A patient who tolerates the occlusion test can be subjected to a vasodilator-induced decrease of as much as 15-20 mmHg below their normal blood pressure value during the surgical intervention. Patients who develop neurological deficits and cannot, therefore, tolerate the test occlusion are candidates for a revascularization procedure [16].

Intra-Operative Management

Doppler and Indocyanine

After suturing, microDoppler can be used to check the presence and validity of the flow within the graft and in the vessels upstream and downstream of the suture (Fig. **16**). Pulsatility of the graft alone is not sufficient to confirm its patency. The use of indocyanine green was introduced into cerebrovascular neurosurgery practice recently. The execution of fluorescein angiography through the administration of indocyanine green as a contrast medium is a safe technique and provides real-time information on the patency of the vessels, the characteristics of the aneurysmal sac, and the relationship of the sac with adjacent vessels. After venous injection of indocyanine green at a dose of 0.2-0.5 mg/kg, the arterial and venous vessels in the area of interest will be visible.

Upon reaching the aneurysmal sac, dissected from adjacent branches, it is advisable to inject indocyanine green before placing the clip and creating the anastomosis. The benefit of early fluorescein angiography is to enable visualization and analysis of the anatomy of the vessels, thereby facilitating selection of the most appropriate clip to apply. Moreover, one can test the flow characteristics of the vessels of interest so as to compare them with the angiographic view obtained immediately after exclusion of the aneurysm and completion of the revascularization procedures. Useful information can be obtained by observing the sac of the aneurysm during fluorescein angiography, which may show calcifications, intramural thrombosis and the flow within the sac [17].

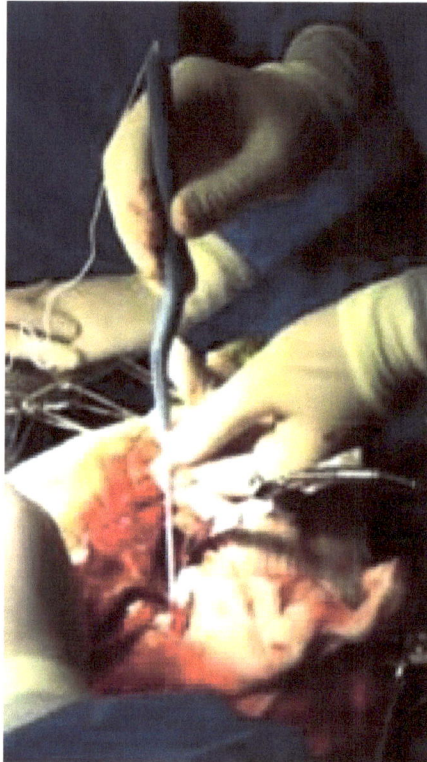

Figure 16: Doppler used to evaluate the validity of the graft.

Post-Operative Management

The monitoring of the graft involves performing Doppler examinations every four hours during the first post-operative day and every eight hours in the second. Cerebral angiography or computed tomography angiography is performed to assess the patency of the graft in the first 36 hours after surgery. In addition, adequate blood pressure must be ensured (about 20 mmHg higher than the patient's blood pressure). Platelet anti-aggregating agents, in association with subcutaneous heparin, should be administered. At discharge the patient is prescribed acetyl salicylic acid 325 mg/day for about three months. In addition, the patient should undergo nuclear magnetic resonance angiography at three months, one year, two years, then at five years, if he or she has no additional symptoms.

ENDOVASCULAR TREATMENT OF COMPLEX ANEURYSMS

When standard surgical clipping is deemed exceedingly hazardous or even impossible, an endovascular approach is often considered in a multidisciplinary consultation involving neurosurgeons, neuroendovascular surgeons and anesthesiologists. Both anatomical and clinical factors contribute to the complexity of intracranial aneurysms eligible for endovascular management [18-22]. Anatomical features include size (giant or small for a clip or coil), shape (fusiform, serpentine), presence of a fresh or laminated thrombus, neck conformation (broad, calcified, surgically inaccessible or involving perforating arteries) and perianeurysmal environment (aneurysms situated deep in the brain, edematous tissues, bony structures or scar tissue from previous surgery). Clinical features comprise neurological factors (poor grade, vasospasm at presentation) and general factors (age, comorbidities). The therapeutic strategy is usually tailored to each specific case, considering the presence of the above mentioned factors, and may be an endovascular approach alone or in combination with surgery. Some of the neurointerventional techniques usually adopted for the management of this peculiar group of cerebral aneurysms are summarized in the following paragraphs.

Endovascular Approach to Giant Aneurysms

Outcomes in patients with giant intracranial aneurysms treated with detachable coils (with or without stent reconstruction of the aneurysm neck) are currently not considered superior to those in patients undergoing open surgery [31]. In a recently published series the mortality and morbidity rates were 31% and 46%, respectively. Furthermore, all the patients presenting with vertebrobasilar junction or midbasilar artery aneurysms died or suffered permanent neurological impairment after endovascular treatment [32].

Incomplete obliteration and aneurysm recanalization are not infrequent. Coil packing in giant aneurysms is extremely challenging even for the most experienced neuroendovascular surgeon. Unacceptable risks, in terms of both distal migration of coils and intraoperative aneurysm rupture, would have to be taken to obtain an adequate coil density. The use of larger diameter coils may be warranted, although their efficacy remains to be investigated further [33].

Blood flow diversion from the aneurysm with so-called flow-diversion devices seems to be a technique well suited for the management of giant anterior circulation and cavernous ICA aneurysms (Figs. **17** and **18**). In contrast, they are not designed for aneurysms located at arterial bifurcations or in the proximity of perforating arterial branches whose occlusion would have disastrous consequences (*i.e.* M2 middle cerebral artery or midbasilar artery giant aneurysms). A recent review of the literature on the subject [31] shows acceptable results in terms of mortality (10%), however the complete obliteration rate was found to be rather low (54%) with an increased tendency to develop thromboembolic complications after treatment in this particular group of aneurysms [34]. Future perspectives for the management of giant intracranial aneurysms could include the introduction of intra-aneurysmal mesh sacs that may avoid recanalization after coil embolization [35, 36], the use of bifurcation stents, already employed by interventional cardiologists [37-39] and non-stent neck reconstruction devices [40].

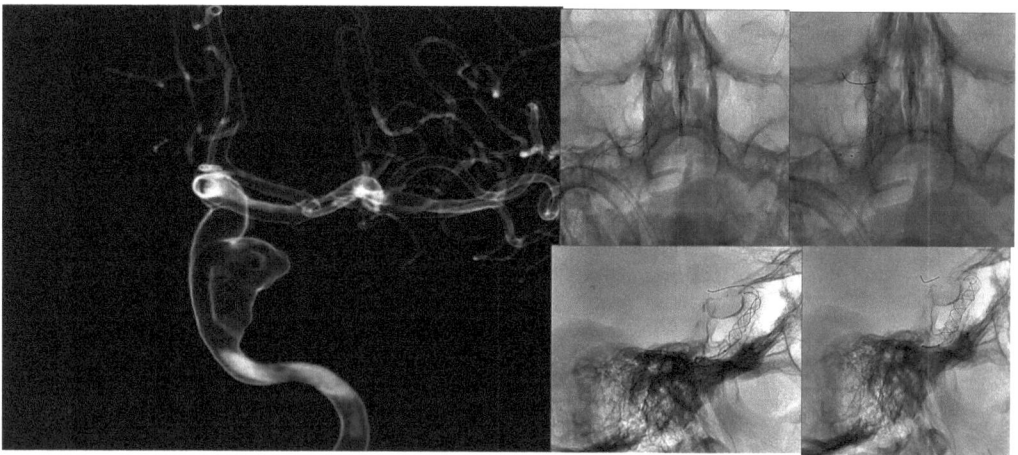

Figure 17: Treatment of a complex aneurysm of the ICA with a double stent.

Endovascular Occlusion of the Parent Vessel

The current treatment of choice for cavernous or posterior ICA aneurysms includes occlusion of the parent vessel, if tolerated. For this purpose the well-known Hunterian ligation technique may be applied, although the effectiveness of arterial ligation decreases as its distance from the aneurysm neck increases. Endovascular balloon occlusion enables the parent vessel to be occluded as proximally as possible to the aneurysm neck thus improving results in terms of thrombotic obliteration of the aneurysm. Moreover, it avoids thromboembolic complications such as the so-called "stump emboli" resulting from standard arterial ligation.

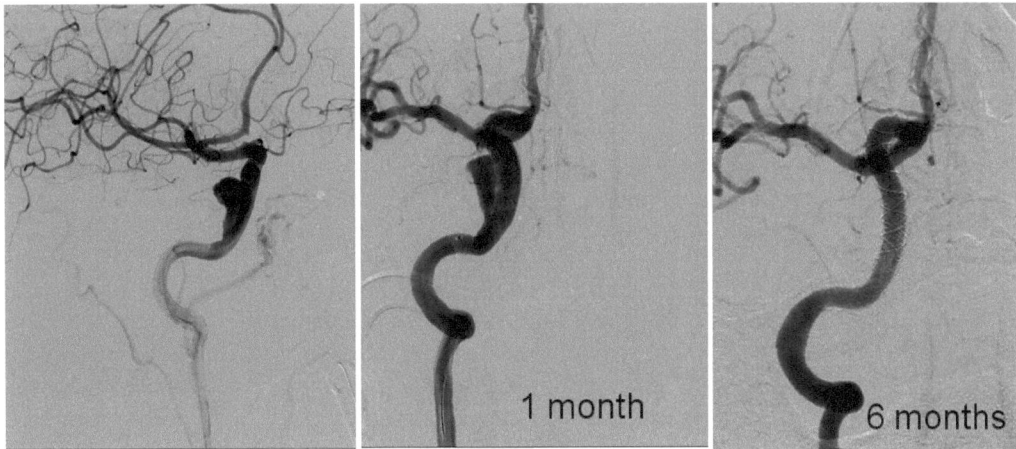

Figure 18: Follow up.

COMBINED SURGICAL AND ENDOVASCULAR APPROACHES

Superselective Angiography

This technique may provide neurosurgeons with more detailed information on the aneurysm's anatomy, which it may not be possible to obtain with standard cerebral angiography. Superselective angiography may play an invaluable role in aneurysms in close relation to or giving rise to perforating arterial branches. Inadvertent thrombus migration and vessel wall perforation are the most common complications encountered during such procedures, although when performed by experts, the risks are often easily outweighed. The results usually help to decide whether to perform surgical clipping or to plan an alternative approach (*i.e.* distal bypass with proximal occlusion for giant unclippable aneurysms, selective distal bypass of the perforating arteries involved in the aneurysm and subsequent aneurysm clipping).

Pre-surgical Coiling or Temporary Intraoperative Balloon Occlusion for Patients with Subarachnoid Hemorrhage at High Risk

The management of patients with subarachnoid hemorrhage with poor clinical and neurological conditions is still debated. Regardless of the peculiarities of the aneurysm and despite documented results, limited to anterior circulation aneurysms, comparing surgical outcomes in patients presenting with either poor or good Hunt and Hess grading on admission [23, 24], surgery is most often avoided in clinical practice, especially in fragile patients with multiple comorbidities. For these reasons, endovascular partial packing of the aneurysm may serve as a "bridging" procedure providing both protection in the acute setting and the opportunity, if adequately performed, for future surgical clipping [25-28]. In selected cases the use of an endovascular balloon, inflated proximally and intraoperatively in the parent vessel, may aid surgical clipping of ruptured giant or broad-necked aneurysms [29].

Intraoperative Temporary Balloon Occlusion for Clipping

Large ophthalmic artery aneurysms as well as large aneurysms of the posteroinferior cerebellar artery or basilar apex might benefit greatly from the use of intraoperative endovascular techniques such as balloon occlusion for the proximal control of, respectively, the cervical ICA and vertebral artery during the clipping phase. The main disadvantage is the need for heparin, which can be a cause of dramatic intraoperative bleeding if the dose is not kept at the minimum possible. On the other hand this combined approach allows immediate control of aneurysmal obliteration after clipping and, for large ophthalmic artery aneurysms, it obviates the need for surgical exposure of the cervical ICA [29].

Post-Clipping Endovascular Embolization

Clipped aneurysms that show unsatisfactory results at control angiography may benefit from post-operative endovascular embolization in order to achieve total obliteration [30].

Endovascular Arterial Occlusion after Bypassing

Giant proximal intradural carotid artery aneurysms require proximal ICA ligation after an evaluation of how well deprivation of carotid artery blood flow is tolerated by means of a balloon occlusion test. For patients who do not tolerate

ICA occlusion during the test, an EC-IC bypass is often considered and coupled with subsequent endovascular parent vessel occlusion.

GIANT ANEURYSMS

Giant aneurysms, defined as aneurysms with a maximum diameter greater than 25 mm, deserve special mention. Such aneurysms account for approximately 3-13% of intracranial aneurysms, with an annual incidence of 5%. Generally presenting with subarachnoid hemorrhage and in a smaller percentage of cases with symptoms related to a mass effect, in 90% of cases giant aneurysms occur in the anterior circulation with a predilection for the ICA. The natural history of giant aneurysms is the result of bleeding, a mass effect, and thromboembolic episodes. These elements, in combination with post-operative complications are determinants of the higher rate of morbidity and mortality associated with giant aneurysms compared with small aneurysms. The risk of rebleeding at 14 days is 18.4%. The mortality rate is 60% within two years and 80% within five years in patients with untreated symptomatic giant aneurysms. When possible, the first line treatment of unrupted giant aneurysms should be placement of a stent, if the symptoms are not related to the presence of a mass effect or seizures uncontrolled by medical therapy. The first line treatment for giant aneurysms that have presented with subarachnoid hemorrhage is surgery. The treatment plan for a patient with a giant aneurysm must take into consideration a number of factors: the clinical presentation, the patient's age, presence of comorbidities, location and characteristics of the aneurysm (saccular, fusiform, mycotic), and hemodynamic factors.

The determination of the anatomical features of the cerebral circulation, an evaluation of the presence of a collateral circulation and patency of the posterior communicating or vertebral artery, as well as detection of abnormalities of the arterial circulation are key elements in deciding the best therapeutic strategy.

CONCLUDING REMARKS

Surgical revascularization procedures remain the only option for the treatment of complex aneurysms. Bypasses are not suitable for a large number of aneurysms, but only for selected cases that are not amenable to conventional treatments. The lowest number of bypass operations for the treatment of complex aneurysms is dependent on the presence of a specialized neurosurgical team. In these cases, endovascular treatment should be considered complementary to the surgical treatment, but cannot replace this latter; endovascular treatment represents a viable alternative for those patients not eligible for surgical treatment, in order to circumvent unfavorable general conditions. However, endovascular treatment cannot be considered a definitive strategy for complex aneurysms.

ACKNOWLEDGEMENTS

Declared none.

CONFLICT OF INTEREST

The authors confirm that this chapter contents have no conflict of interest.

REFERENCES

[1]   Brown RD Jr, Broderich JP. Unruptured intracranial aneurysms: epidemiology, natural history, management options, and familial screening. Lancet Neurol 2014; 13: 393-404.
[2]   Shivashankar R, Miller TR, Jindal G, Simard JM, Aldrich EF, Gandhi D. Treatment of cerebral aneurysms-surgical clipping or endovascular coiling: the guiding principles. Semin Neurol 2013; 33: 476-87.
[3]   Sharma BS, Gupta A, Ahmed FU, Suri A, Mehta VS. Surgical management of giant intracranial aneurysms. Clin Neurol Neurosurg 2008; 110: 674-81.
[4]   Cantore G, Santoro A, Guidetti G, Delfinis CP, Colonese C, Passacantilli E. Surgical treatment of giant aneurysms: current viewpoint. Neurosurgery 2008; 63 (4suppl 2): 270-90.
[5]   Pisapia JM, Walcott BP, Nahed BV, Kahle KT, Ogilvy CS. Cerebral revascularization for the treatment of complex intracranial aneurysms of the posterior circulation: microsurgical anatomy, techniques and outcomes J NeuroIntervent Surg 2011; 3: 249-54.
[6]   Eftekhar B, Morgan MK. Indications for the use of temporary arterial occlusion during aneurysm repair: an institutional experience. J Clin Neurosci 2011; 18: 905-9.
[7]   Amin-Hanjani S, Butler WE, Ogilvy CS, Carter BS, Barker FG 2nd. Extracranial–intracranial bypass in the treatment of occlusive cerebrovascular disease and intracranial aneurysms in the United States between 1992 and 2001: a population-based study. J Neurosurg 2005; 103: 794-804.
[8]   Patel HC, Teo M, Higgins N, Kirkpatrick PJ. High flow extra-cranial to intra-cranial bypass for complex internal carotid aneurysms. Br J Neurosurg. 2010; 24(2): 173-8.
[9]   Kocaeli H, Andaluz N, Choutka O, Zuccarello M. Use of radial artery grafts in extracranial–intracranial revascularization procedures. Neurosurg Focus 2008; 24: E5.
[10]   Jafar JJ, Russell SM, Woo HH. Treatment of giant intracranial aneurysms with saphenous vein extracranial-to-intracranial bypass grafting: indications, operative technique, and results in 29 patients. Neurosurgery 2002; 51: 138-46.
[11]   Baaj AA, Agazzi S, van Loveren H. Graft selection in cerebral revascularization. Neurosurg Focus 2009; 26: E18.
[12]   Quinones-Hinojosa A, Du R, Lawton MT. Revascularization with saphenous vein bypasses for complex intracranial aneurysms. Skull Base 2005; 15: 119-32.
[13]   Lee SC, Ahn JH, Kang HS, Kim JE. Revascularization for symptomatic occlusion of the anterior cerebral artery using superficial temporal artery. J Korean Neurosurg Soc 2013; 54: 511-4.
[14]   Mao Y. Revascularization with the occipital artery to treat aneurysms in the posterior circulation. World Neurosurg 2013; [Epub ahead of print].
[15]   Ramanathan D, Hegazy A, Mukherjee SK, Sekhar LN. Intracranial in situ side-to-side microvascular anastomosis: principles, operative technique, and applications. World Neurosurg 2010; 73: 317-25.
[16]   Elias AE, Chaudhary N, Pandey AS, Gemmete JJ. Intracranial endovascular balloon test occlusion: indications, methods, and predictive value. Neuroimaging Clin N Am 2013; 23: 695-702.

[17]   Roessler K, Krawagna M, Dörfler A. Essentials in intraoperative indocyanine green videoangiography assessment for intracranial aneurysm surgery: conclusions from 295 consecutively clipped aneurysms and review of the literature. Neurosurg Focus 2014; 36: E7.

[18]   Alaraj A, Ti J, Dashti R, Aletich V. Patient selection for endovascular treatment of intracranial aneurysms. Neurol Res 2014; 36: 283-307.

[19]   Standard SC, Guterman LR, Chavis TD, *et al.* Endovascular management of giant intracranial aneurysms. Clin Neurosurg 1995; 42: 267-93.

[20]   Wehman JC, Hanel RA, Levy EI, Hopkins LN. Giant cerebral aneurysm: endovascular challenges. Neurosurgery 2006; 59(5 Suppl 3): S125-38; discussion S3-13.

[21]   Sughrue ME, Saloner D, Rayz VL, *et al.* Giant intracranial aneurysms: evolution of management in a contemporary surgical series. Neurosurgery 2011; 69: 1261-70.

[22]   Hacein-Bey L, Connolly ES Jr, Mayer SA, Young WL, Pile-Spellman J, Solomon RA. Complex intracranial aneurysms: combined operative and endovascular approaches. Neurosurgery 1998; 43: 1304-13.

[23]   Le Roux PD, Elliott JP, Newell DW, Grady MS, Winn HR. The incidence of surgical complications is similar in good and poor grade patients undergoing repair of ruptured anterior circulation aneurysms: a retrospective review of 355 patients. Neurosurgery 1996; 38: 887-95.

[24]   Le Roux PD, Elliott JP, Newell DW, Grady MS, Winn HR. Predicting outcome in poor-grade patients with subarachnoid hemorrhage: a retrospective review of 159 aggressively managed cases. J Neurosurg 1996; 85: 39-49.

[25]   Batjer HH. Aneurysm clipping after endovascular treatment with coils: a report of eight patients. Neurosurgery 1996; 38: 960-1.

[26]   Civit T, Auque J, Marchal JC, Bracard S, Picard L, Hepner H. Aneurysm clipping after endovascular treatment with coils: a report of eight patients. Neurosurgery 1996; 38: 955-61.

[27]   Gurian JH, Martin NA, King WA, Duckwiler GR, Guglielmi G, Viñuela F. Neurosurgical management of cerebral aneurysms following unsuccessful or incomplete endovascular embolization. J Neurosurg 1995; 83: 843-53.

[28]   Kurokawa Y, Abiko S, Okamura T, Watanabe K. Direct surgery for giant aneurysm exhibiting progressive enlargement after intraaneurysmal balloon embolization. Surg Neurol 1992; 38: 19-25.

[29]   Shucart WA, Kwan ES, Heilman CB: Temporary balloon occlusion of a proximal vessel as an aid to clipping aneurysms of the basilar and paraclinoid internal arteries: technical note. Neurosurgery 1990; 27: 116-9.

[30]   Fraser KW, Halbach VV, Teitelbaum GP, *et al.* Endovascular platinum coil embolization of incompletely surgically clipped cerebral aneurysms. Surg Neurol 1994; 41: 4-8.

[31]   Nanda A, Sonig A, Banerjee AD, Javalkar VK. Microsurgical management of giant intracranial aneurysm: a single surgeon experience from Louisiana State University, Shreveport. World Neurosurg 2012; pii: S1878-8750(12)01442-8.

[32]   Jahromi BS, Mocco J, Bang JA, *et al.* Clinical and angiographic outcome after endovascular management of giant intracranial aneurysms. Neurosurgery 2008; 63: 662-75.

[33]   Mascitelli JR, Patel A, Kamath A, Polykarpou M, Moyle M, Patel AB. Aneurysm embolization treatment efficiency: comparing the Penumbra Coil 400 system to conventional coils (abstract 347). Presented at the Congress of Neurological Surgeons Annual Meeting; Chicago, IL, USA. October 6-10, 2012.

[34]   Cruz JP, Chow M, O'Kelly C, *et al.* Delayed ipsilateral parenchymal hemorrhage following flow diversion for the treatment of anterior circulation aneurysms. AJNR Am J Neuroradiol 2012; 33: 603-8.

[35]   Ding YH, Lewis DA, Kadirvel R, Dai D, Kallmes DF. The Woven EndoBridge: a new aneurysm occlusion device. AJNR Am J Neuroradiol 2011; 32: 607-11.

[36]   Kwon SC, Ding YH, Dai D, Kadirvel R, Lewis DA, Kallmes DF. Preliminary results of the luna aneurysm embolization system in a rabbit model: a new intrasaccular aneurysm occlusion device. AJNR Am J Neuroradiol 2011; 32: 602-6.

[37]   Agostoni P, Foley D, Lesiak M, *et al.* A prospective multicentre registry, evaluating real-world usage of the Tryton side branch stent: results of the E-Tryton 150/Benelux registry. EuroIntervention 2012; 7: 1293-300.

[38]   Gil RJ, Vassilev D, Michalek A, *et al.* Dedicated paclitaxel-eluting bifurcation stent BiOSS(R) (bifurcation optimisation stent system): 12-month results from a prospective registry of consecutive all-comers population. EuroIntervention 2012; 8: 316-24.

[39]   Latib A, Colombo A, Sangiorgi GM. Bifurcation stenting: current strategies and new devices. Heart 2009; 95: 495-504.

[40]   Turk A, Turner RD, Tateshima S, *et al.* Novel aneurysm neck reconstruction device: initial experience in an experimental preclinical bifurcation aneurysm model. J Neurointerv Surg 2013; 5: 346-50.

Frontiers in Neurosurgery, Vol. 1, 2015, 121-138

CHAPTER 5

Spinal Vascular Pathology

E. Orrù[2], G. Guarnieri[1,*], J. Gabrieli[2], M. Muto[1] and F. Causin[2]

[1]*Neuroradiology Service, AO Cardarelli Hospital, Naples, Italy;* [2]*Neuroradiology Service, University Hospital of Padua, Padua, Italy*

Abstract: Spinal cord vascular malformations are vessel disorders involving, directly or indirectly, the spinal cord tissue. Their management and treatment remain complex and require a deep knowledge of the "lesional" and regional anatomy. The object of this chapter is to explain the vascular embryology, the anatomy of the spinal cord and the treatment of vascular malformations such as arteriovenous malformations, dural arteriovenous fistulas and aneurysms.

Keywords: Dural spinal AVM, endovascular treatment, intramedullary, malformation, perimedullary, Spinal AVM, spinal arteriovenous, spinal arteriovenous fistula.

SPINAL CORD ANATOMY

The spinal cord is constituted of neural tissue (gray matter, neural pathways and glial cells) extending from the foramen magnum up to conus medullaris at L1-L2 level, where it continues as the cauda equina. It terminates with the filum terminalis, anchoring to the coccyx. The spinal cord is covered by the meninges: the dura mater, the arachnoid and the pia mater, delimiting three compartments. Between the dura mater and the bone of the vertebrae there is the epidural space, filled with adipose tissue and containing vascular structures. The interface between the dura mater and the arachnoid is the subdural space (a virtual space). The space between the arachnoid and the pia mater is the subarachnoid space containing the cerebrospinal fluid, a pial arterial network formed by the longitudinal arteries (the anterior spinal artery [ASA] and the two posterior spinal arteries [PSAs]) and coronal arteries supplying the spinal cord and the medullary veins.

SPINAL CORD VASCULATURE

Appropriate knowing of the spinal vascular system is essential element in order to understand the different types of vascular malformations.

---

*Corresponding author G. Guarnieri: Neuroradiology Service, AO Cardarelli Hospital, Naples, Italy; Tel: 081 7473838; Fax: 081 7473125; E-mail: gianluigiguarnieri@hotmail.it

Simone Peschillo (Ed.)

Embryology: The Constitution of the Anterior and Posterior Spinal Arteries

Like for the brain, the spinal cord vessels development has different phases: (i) vasculogenesis - de novo formation of blood vessels from precursors of endothelial cells (angioblasts) derived from the mesoderm; (ii) luminogenesis - when neighboring angioblasts group to form a vascular lumen; and (iii) angiogenesis - the remodeling and development of the primitive vascular network thanks to sprouting phenomena [1]. Vessel genesis involves different phenomena such as fusion, unfusion and regression of the primary arteries, all of which take place with blood circulating at arterial pressure [1]. During the third week of intra-uterine growth, embryonic structures of the chordates located on both sides of the neural tube form from the mesoderm of 31 somites. They are composed of consecutive units all along the antero-posterior axis of the embryo. Each somite receives bilateral arteries from the dorsal aorta: 31 couples of segmental arteries (8 cervical, 12 thoracic, 5 lumbar, 5 sacral, 1 coccygeal) that distribute to the developing bones, muscles and nervous structures. The spinal cord receives its vascularization from a dorso-medial branch of each ipsilateral segmental artery. The central portion of the developing nerve brings the corresponding artery towards the neural tube. Thus, the vascular supply to the neural tube is provided by paired, symmetrical segmental arteries. At this stage, a thin vessel network is developed all around the neural tube [1].

During the fourth to sixth weeks of intra-uterine life there is progressive constitution of the classical adult arrangement. The two anterior longitudinal vascular axes of the neural tube migrate toward the midline fusing into a single ventral longitudinal vessel: the ASA. Sometimes in the event of a misfusion this process can be incomplete, resulting in a fenestrated ASA. An unfused ventral spinal artery is usually associated with bilateral (most often symmetrical) persistence of the segmental radiculo-medullary arteries [1].

At the dorsal aspect of the neural tube two long, separate and less developed longitudinal para-median vascular axes persist, with dominant longitudinal flow: these are the future posterior-lateral arteries or PSAs (the two names are often used synonymously in the literature; in this chapter the vessel is referred to as the PSA).

The arterial supply to this vascular network is initially brought by segmental arteries at each level. During the development of the embryo these vessels progressively involute through summation and desegmentation processes, eventually resulting in the regression of most of these radicular contributions to the anterior and posterior spinal cord axes. When the development finishes, only about four to eight anterior radicular arteries and ten to twenty posterior radicular arteries will persist. The remnants of the other segmental arteries to the neural derivates will maintain supply to the spinal nerve dura and bony structures [1].

Within the first month of intra-uterine life, the sulcal arteries appear at the dorsal aspect of each paired ventral axis. They remain lateralized when the fusion occurred. The pial network develops secondarily and vascularizes the spinal cord funiculi *via* the perforating arteries [1].

Spinal Vascular Anatomy

At the end of vasculogenesis, vascular supply and drainage of the spinal cord is provided by arterial and venous vessels variable in both nature and number.

This vascular organization can be distinguished into extrinsic vascularization and intrinsic vascularization. The extrinsic vascularization of the spinal cord and nerve roots is formed by radicular arteries, radiculo-pial arteries, and radiculo-medullary arteries with the pial arterial network (longitudinal and axial).

As minimal contribution of the embryonic segmental system to neural crest derivatives, a radicular artery can be found at each vertebral level. The radiculo-pial arteries follow and vascularize the nerve root, reach the surface of the cord and participate in the constitution of the spinal cord pial network, which has longitudinal and axial systems [1]. The radiculo-medullary arteries terminate in the ASA. They initially follow the anterior nerve roots, then abandon the anterior pial arteries and reach the anterior sulcus eventually dividing into a dominant ascending branch and a smaller descending one [1].

The spinal cord pial (superficial) network has longitudinal and axial systems. The longitudinal one is formed by the ASA and both PSAs with a pial anastomotic network, while the axial system is formed by radially penetrating branches (*vasa corona*) that can be divided into a *dorsal plexus* (close to the midline with perforating arteries for the posterior funiculi), two *lateral plexuses* (between anterior and posterior roots) and a *ventral plexus* (small pial branches of radiculo-pial arteries, the radiculo-medullary artery and the sulco-commissural artery) [1].

The ASA descends in front of the medulla oblongata and along the anterior medial fissure of the spinal cord (medulla spinalis) to supply the anterior two thirds of the cord. It is reinforced by a succession of a few inconstant radiculo-medullary branches joining the vertebral canal through the intervertebral foramina and pierce the dura following the nerve roots [1]. The biggest anterior radiculo-medullary artery is the artery of Adamkiewicz, or artery of the lumbar enlargement arising between T9 and T12 in 75% of cases, frequently left-sided; if the artery is found above T8 or below L2 then an other major contributor is expected [1].

The cervical segment and the upper thoracic segment are fed by segmental arteries arising from the vertebral arteries, from the ascending and deep cervical arteries and from the pharyngo-occipital system. A large feeder of the ASA in the cervical tract can be seen and is known as the artery of the cervical enlargement or, less frequently, as the artery of Lazorthes. Below the cervical region the blood supply comes from paired intercostal and lumbar radicular arteries that provide major anastomoses and join the spinal cord alongside the dorsal and ventral nerve roots [1].

The PSAs, two vessels along the back surface of the cord on each side, supply the posterior third of the cord. They can be better described as a discontinuous longitudinal system on the dorsal aspect of the spinal cord that is reinforced by radiculo-pial branches which usually supply no more than a few levels.

The common origin of both anterior and posterior radiculo-medullary arteries at the same segmental level is known as the "configuration of Lazorthes".

Inferiorly, the anterior and posterior systems are anastomosed around the conus medullaris in the so-called arterial "basket". The continuity of the ASA below the basket gives the artery of the filum terminalis [1].

The intrinsic vascularization of the spinal cord is formed by sulcal arteries, radial perforating arteries, with intrinsic anastomoses.

The sulcal arteries arise from the ASA, perforate the ventral sulcus, anastomose with each other (without anastomoses on the midline) within the sulcus on the same side and then penetrate the cord supplying the gray matter (centrifugal system).

The radial perforating arteries arise from the pial/coronal network to penetrate into the white matter (centripetal system) vascularizing mainly the funiculi. They divide into axial and longitudinal branches. The perforating arteries anastomose inside the spinal cord with branches of the sulco-commissural arteries dorsolaterally, ventrolaterally, and ventrally. At each vertebral level, radial arteries form short extramedullary anastomotic branches connecting adjacent levels, however, in the case of arterial occlusion they may not provide adequate blood supply considering their small size. The dorsolateral pial network is considered primarily as an axial system of arterial supply [1]. "The venous drainage of the cord is guaranteed by radially symmetric intrinsic spinal cord veins and small superficial pial veins that open into the superficial longitudinal median anterior and posterior spinal cord veins" [2-5].

By transmedullary anastomoses, a venous network with anterior and posterior veins is created. Transdural emissary bridging veins do not follow the nerve roots; they pierce the dura through a separate ostium going into epidural plexus and extra-spinal veins, with a mechanism preventing reflux within the dura mater. At the upper cervical level, bridging veins running through the occipital foramen connect the vertebral plexus to the inferior dural sinuses. Venous drainage is guaranteed by the internal and external venous vertebral plexuses, anastomosed to the azygos and hemiazygos venous systems.

CLINICAL AND IMAGING DATA

Spinal symptoms secondary to a vascular pathology depend on the type of lesion and its location (paraspinal, epidural, dural, intradural, and intramedullary). Symptoms include myelopathy (sensory and/or motor deficits, bowel and/or bladder dysfunction), radicular pain and back pain [6]. Spinal cord hemorrhage, venous hypertension, arterial steal and a mass effect are the most frequently detected causative events.

Hemorrhage can happen into the cord or into the subarachnoid space, in both cases presenting with an acute onset of symptoms or with a sudden worsening of already present neurological deficits. The risk of hemorrhage depends on the type of vascular lesion. Generally, it is greater in spinal cord arteriovenous malformations (AVMs) than in other lesions. Large and giant spinal cord dural arteriovenous fistulas (DAVFs) and cervical or intracranial DAVFs with perimedullary venous congestion have a lower bleeding risk. Small spinal cord DAVFs and thoracic and lumbar DAVFs are the lesions that are less likely to bleed [7, 8]. If a spinal artery is involved or there are intranidal aneurysms, the risk of hemorrhage is higher.

Venous hypertension is typically associated with arteriovenous (AV) malformations with perimedullary venous drainage. This phenomenon can occur also with spinal DAVFs, or pial AVFs of the spinal cord or intracranial DAVFs that have perimedullary venous drainage. Arterial steal phenomenon is typically due to high-flow AV shunts [9]. Rarely, myelopathy results from a mass effect. Large low-related aneurysms or large dilated vein may compress the spinal cord or nerve roots leading to myelopathy, radicular pain or a neurological deficit. Spinal MRI study is used when a vascular malformation and should is suspected and it can be carried out with the following protocol: sagittal T1WI, T2WI, T2WI with fat saturation, T1WI with contrast. The accuracy of magnetic resonance angiography with contrast injection is debated [10]. Magnetic resonance angiography performed with more advanced 3T machines, or computed tomography angiography performed with new multidetector scanners, can indicate the site of the lesion, in order to reduce both the extent and duration of catheter angiography.

Selective spinal digital subtraction angiography is the gold standard in imaging to evaluate the feeder origin and to examine the angioarchitecture of all vascular malformations with optimal detection of normal vasculature of the examined territories, from arterial to venous phase, and proper visualization of spinal cord veins, vessels in pathological territories, planning the diagnosis and treatment, and visualizing associated lesions.

The examination is performed *via* a femoral access using a 5 French catheter, studying the deep cervical, ascending cervical arteries and all the intercostal and lumbar arteries bilaterally down to the median sacral artery and the hypogastric, ileolumbar and lateral sacral arteries. Different catheter shapes may be necessary in order to obtain a precise selective injection of all possible pedicules.

If an AV shunt or malformation is not identified, all the cerebral vessels should be studied selectively, including both vertebral arteries, internal carotid arteries (with special regard to the meningohypophyseal trunk) and external carotid branches, such as the ascending pharyngeal artery, middle meningeal artery and occipital artery, in order to exclude an intracranial DAVF with spinal venous drainage (Cognard type 5). An essential part of the examination is always to identify the ASA, the PSAs and the radiculo-medullary arteries, in particular the artery of Adamkiewicz.

The aim of this multimodality imaging approach is to detect:

- *Parenchymal conditions*: hemorrhage, venous congestion, atrophy, syringomyelia and enhancement pattern;

- *Abnormal vessels*;

- *AV shunts*: nidus/fistula; size; location (epidural/dural/ perimedullary/ intramedullary/radicular/filum);

- *Arteries*: feeders, aneurysms, normal cord supply;

- *Draining veins*: location, direction, thrombosis, venous pouches, normal cord drainage;

- *Multiple lesions*: metameric/somatic/extension;

Before performing any endovascular treatment, it is essential to have the most precise understanding of the lesional and regional vascular anatomy.

CLASSIFICATIONS OF ARTERIOVENOUS LESIONS

Different classifications exist in order to clarify the angioarchitecture of each spinal AV lesion (AVM or DAVF) and their treatment indication or planning. The Bicetre group [11, 12] classified spinal cord AV lesions into three main groups:

1) Genetic hereditary lesions that are caused by a genetic disorder affecting the vascular germinal cells, such as malformations associated with hereditary hemorrhagic telangiectasia;

2) Genetic nonhereditary lesions, such as the Cobb syndrome (or spinal AV metameric syndrome), the Klippel-Trenaunay and the Parkes-Weber syndromes. Patients with these conditions have multiple shunts of the spinal cord and nerve root, bone, paraspinal, subcutaneous and skin tissue;

3) Single lesions that may reflect the incomplete expression of one of the previously mentioned situations and include the spinal cord, nerve roots, and filum terminale AV lesions.

The majority of the spinal vascular malformations with both pial and dural AV shunts, are included in the third group.

Krings *et al.* [13] presented a classification based on vascular anatomy and hemodynamic criteria with an overview of the anatomy and the physiopathology of each spinal AV shunt, used as a reference for the indication, contraindication, and technique of endovascular treatment. Two different types with multiple subgroups were proposed:

A. AVMs with the presence of a nidus between artery and vein:

1. Intramedullary (also known as type II or glomus-type AVM)

2. Pial

3. Epidural

4. Intra- and extramedullary (also known as type III, intradural-extradural, juvenile AVM, or metameric AVM)

B. AV fistulas (AVFs) with a direct shunt between artery and vein:

1. Pial AVFs (also known as type IV, spinal cord AVFs, ventral intradural AVF, or perimedullary AVFs)

   a. Small

   b. Large

   c. Giant

2. DAVFs (also known as type I or dorsal intradural AVFs)

3. Epidural AVFs (also known as extradural AVFs)

At the date, the following classification, created between 1991 and 1998 by different authors [14-16], is the most accepted and widely used.

Type I: DAVFs

Type II: intradural glomus-type AVMs

Type III: juvenile or combined AVMs

Type IV: intradural perimedullary AVFs.

Type I: Dural Arteriovenous Fistulas

DAVFs are the most common type of spinal cord AVM, representing 70% of all spinal AVMs, with a male predominance (80%) in late adulthood (age 40-60 years) [17]. With regards to cerebral dural fistulas a strong association with cerebral venous thrombosis [18], factor V Leiden and protein C deficiency [19, 20], infection [21] or trauma has been demonstrated but without clear predominance [22-24]. A typical presentation is radiculo-myelopathy, followed by progressive neurological defict. Subarachnoid hemorrhage is very uncommon as is an acute deterioration in neurological function. The majority of fistulas are solitary lesions at thoraco-lumbar level. The fistula is located inside the dura where a radiculo-meningeal artery enters the corresponding radicular vein, close to the spinal nerve root. The progressive clinical worsening is caused by increasing pressure in the venous system that leads to venous congestion and decreased normal venous drainage. The increased venous pressure causes chronic spinal cord ischemia and atrophy [25, 26]. The essential diagnostic tools are magnetic resonance imaging and selective catheter angiography. On MRI, the typical patterns are cord edema, perimedullary arterialized dilated veins, and cord enhancement. Magnetic resonance angiography gives information about the level of the AV. Some authors have described that multidetector computed tomography is effective for finding the site of a fistula [27-29]. Catheter angiography is still the gold standard for spinal DAVFs diagnosis.

Treatment

The vascular structure of the fistula must be carefully investigated to establish if the arterial feeder is a dural branch or a radiculo-medullary artery. In the latter case the feeder contributes to the spinal cord vasculature (ASA or PSAs). This condition excludes endovascular treatment, to avoid damage to the spinal cord. In rare cases the high flow of the fistula could hide a segmental medullary branch, even when selectively injected.

The goal of treatment is identification and isolation of the feeder and subsequent disconnection of the fistulous point with interruption of the AV shunting, thus normalizing the venous pressure.

Two treatment options are available: (i) embolization of the feeders with injection of glue or another liquid embolic agent, positioning the microcatheter very distally and close to the fistula; and (ii) direct surgical exeresis, through laminectomy and opening of the dura with direct exposure of the fistula. Surgical resection or embolization of arterialized veins is not necessary and should be avoided.

Embolization can be a safe and effective therapy for DAVFs. Direct surgical exposure should be preferred in those cases in which glue migration in the draining veins could be predicted or in cases in which the feeder is a segmental medullary artery.

Type II: Intramedullary Glomus Arteriovenous Malformations

These are true intramedullary AVMs of the spinal cord. They can run along the whole spinal cord axis and located inside the parenchyma (intramedullary), at the surface of the spinal cord (pial AVMs), in the epidural space (epidural AVMs), or they can have both intramedullary and extramedullary components. The AVMs located in the conus medullaris constitute a distinct type and can extend to the cauda equina and along the filum terminalis. The "glomus type" are the most commonly encountered intramedullary vascular malformations, accounting for about 20% of all spinal vascular malformations. These malformations are formed by a compact intramedullary nidus that occupies a short segment of the spinal cord, with multiple feeders from the anterior or posterior spinal arteries, or both, and venous drainage into coronal venous plexus [9, 30]. Like brain AVMs, intramedullary glomus AVMs is a focal network of AV shunts draining into the spinal veins often associated with an intra-nidal flow-related aneurysm [31]. Intramedullary AVMs occur with an equal incidence in men and women, and generally in earlier age. Typical symptoms are progressive and fluctuating myelopathy, paraplegia and pain, overlaid by periods of acute neurological deficit due to hemorrhage within the AVM. Sudden and severe neurological impairment and possible transverse myelopathy, are commons. Subarachnoid and intramedullary hemorrhage often occurs in these lesions. The mortality rate related to type II malformations was reported to be 17.6%. After the first hemorrhage, the risk of re-bleeding is estimated to be about 10% within the first month and 40% within the first year [31].

Treatment

Despite the high risk carried by any treatment modality, there is a general consensus among the scientific community about the importance to treat intramedullary AVMs, in order to modify its the natural history of the disease and decreasing the risk of rupture, especially after a first bleed has occurred. The prognosis of non-treated spinal cord AVMs is poor. It was found that 36% of patients younger than 40 years developed severe impairment after 3 years of natural, unmodified evolution of the condition [8, 32, 33]. The therapeutic strategy includes: embolization, surgery or a combination of the two approaches. Surgical treatment has an high intraoperative risk of neurological injury, especially for lesions in the anterior spinal cord. Posterior superficial lesions are more amenable to surgical resection, which is safer for these lesions [34]. Partial or complete embolization has an important role in the management of intramedullary AVMs and can modify the patient's natural history. It is performed using liquid embolic agents in order to reduce arterial steal and to improve cord perfusion. Recanalization, however, occurs over time, with a continued risk of hemorrhage. Liquid agents, such as N-butyl cyanoacrylate (NBCA) glue and Onyx, combine a more permanent occlusion with the a very low recanalization rate [9,35]. An alternative treatment option is CyberKnife radiosurgery [36] resulting in a delayed obliteration effect.

Conus medullaris AVMs: these particular type II malformations are characterized by the presence of anterior and dorsal intradural AV shunts with multiple feeders and an intramedullary AVM. They are more complex lesions with multiple arterial feeders, difficult to treat by embolization alone. Combined treatment with embolization followed by surgical resection might be preferred.

Type III: Juvenile (Diffuse-Type) Arteriovenous Malformations

Juvenile spinal AVMs are extremely rare high flow lesions, characterized by an intramedullary nidus with or without extramedullary or extraspinal paraspinous extension. Juvenile AVMs are large and complex lesions, with multiple feeding arteries often arising from different levels of the spinal cord [9, 13]. Peri-nidal Flow-related aneurysm are common associated. Cardiac output requirements may be significantly increased and a bruit is commonly noted. These AVMs occur most commonly in children and young adults with different clinical onset. Symptoms and treatment are similar to those of type II AVMs. Acute onset is secondary to subarachnoid hemorrhage, while a vascular steal phenomenon, venous hypertension or a mass effect on the spinal cord and/or nerve roots are often associated with progressive motor and sensory deficit with sphincter disturbance. Subarachnoid hemorrhage usually occurs from rupture of a venous or arterial aneurysm. Hematomyelia has also been observed after rupture of subpial spinal veins. Asymmetric neurological deficits are highly suggestive of a mass effect on the cord and/or nerve roots. Selective spinal angiography reveals scattered vessels in the spinal cord matter, direct AVM feeders from the ventral or dorsal spinal arteries, and sometimes from the radiculo-pial arteries. The AVM drains into dilated perimedullary veins. Intramedullary AVMs are typically a conglomeration of vessels extending on the surface of the spinal cord.

Treatment

Considering the size and vascular complexity of these lesions and their natural history, the prognosis after any kind of treatment should be considered very poor. A multidisciplinary approach is mandatorily tailored on each lesion's extension, location and angioarchitectural features. The options are surgery or embolization alone or in combination. It is very difficult to obtain a definitive, curative therapy for these lesions without increased morbidity. Palliative treatment could be considered with an endovascular or surgical approach and could be performed in order to relieve symptoms due to hemorrhage, arterial steal, venous hypertension, or a direct mass effect.

Type IV: Perimedullary Arteriovenous Fistulas

These lesions are AVFs. The fistulous connection is intradural but extramedullary, sited on the ventral or on the dorsal surface of the spinal cord, arising from the ASA with dilated vein without an interposed vascular network. The clinical onset occurs during the third to sixth decade [9] with subarachnoid hemorrhage or acute neurological deficit. A chronic and progressive neurological deficit is common. Intradural spinalAVFs have been divided in 3 subgroup:

- Type IVa fistulas feature a single feeding artery, often the artery of Adamkiewicz, with low flow through the AV shunt and moderate venous enlargement. Because of small size of the feeders, surgical treatment is preferred while an endovascular approach is more difficult.

- Type IVb fistulas are intermediately sized, often with multiple feeders, and venous enlargement. Venous dilatation can be developed at the shunt point. Thanks to the larger size of the feeding arteries, embolization is possible. If there is incomplete shunt obliteration, direct surgical excision may be recommended.

- Type IVc are large multi-pedunculated fistulas, with high blood flow, and enlarged, tortuous draining veins. Vascular steal can cause spinal ischemia. Due to size of these lesions, direct surgery is technically difficult. The best treatment option is to perform flow-reduction by an endovascular approach and follow this with surgical excision.

Spinal Aneurysms

Spinal aneurysms, not related to the increased flow of a vascular malformation, are rare. They seldom occur at branching points, rather than developing along the course of an artery [37]. Spinal aneurysms lack a clear neck and usually appear as fusiform dilations. The fusiform nature of these lesions makes clipping difficult and favors sacrifice of the parent artery. Endovascular techniques can also be considered.

New Classification Schemes for Spinal Arteriovenous Lesions

Recently, in order to clarify indications for treatment, new classifications of spinal AV lesions based on hemodynamic, topographic and anatomical criteria have been developed [38, 39].

Spetzler *et al.* [39, 40] and Zozulya *et al.* [38] performed new classifications of spinal vascular pathological entities based on anatomical, pathophysiological or angioarchitectural features. Krings [9] defined a classification based on hemodynamic criteria.

Geibprasert *et al.* [41] published a new classification that combines the spectrum of cranial and spinal DAVFs in a single classification. They redefined DAVFs into three groups according to the embryologic development of the venous drainage of the surrounding structures: the ventral, dorsal, and lateral epidural groups.

1) "The ventral epidural group represents a group of shunts into those veins that normally drain structures developed from the notochord (*i.e.*, the vertebral body at the spinal level). They are the basivertebral venous plexus, which subsequently drains into the anterior internal vertebral venous plexus, located in the ventral epidural space of the spinal canal, which cranially joins the basilar venous plexus and the cavernous sinus. The previously called "epidural," "posteodural," or "paravertebral" AV shunts can be categorized into this group. Because the draining veins of these shunts do not drain the spine but the bone, these shunts do not become symptomatic due to venous congestion of the cord. They can be

symptomatic due to compression of the spinal cord or nerve roots by the enlarged epidural venous pouches. Only a few cases are reported describing associated perimedullary reflux causing congestive myelopathy. A hypothesis about a possible defective valve-like mechanism normally impeding retrograde flow from the epidural plexus to perimedullary veins has been put forward to explain this finding. However, it may also discussed that the reflux is due to an extensive thrombosis of the normal epidural outlets that leads to secondary retrograde drainage into the perimedullary veins" [7].

2) "The dorsal epidural group of AV shunts is related to veins that normally drain the spinous process and lamina at the spinal level. Although they are due to the major dural venous sinuses (superior sagittal sinus, torcular and transverse sinuses) at the cranial level, the corresponding veins at the spinal level are poorly developed and consist of a pair of longitudinal channels (*i.e.*, the posterior internal venous plexus). Patients affected by dural AV shunts within this space present with spontaneous epidural hematomas. These shunts are extremely rare".

3) "The most common "classic" types of spinal DAVFs are the lateral epidural DAVFs. These AV shunts develop in the lateral epidural space at the junction of the bridging (or radicular) veins that connect the spinal cord drainage to the epidural venous system. Outflow stenosis of its adjacent venous outlet, either due to thrombosis or fibrosis related to aging, will then lead to immediate drainage into the perimedullary veins. As a result, patients present with aggressive clinical symptoms and at an older age. A strong male predominance is also observed, which is similar to that in the cranially located lateral epidural DAVFs, such as those in the foramen magnum (medulla bridging vein) and tentorium (petrosal bridging vein)" [7].

MANAGEMENT

The indication for treatment, whether surgical, endovascular or a combination, for patients affected by spinal AVMs should be derived from a careful consideration of the possible benefits versus the risks. The natural history of these pathologies remains uncertain and not well-classified. However, not treating could potentially result in significant damage and hemorrhage, leading to serious neurological deficits or death. To date, there are no algorithms or protocols to help determine the indication for treatment. Probably the best strategy is to evaluate the circumstances case-by-case. Different options for treating AVMs and DAVFs can be considered: microsurgery, endovascular embolization, and radiosurgery. The choice of treatment depends largely on the symptoms, location and angioarchitectural features (size, arterial feeders and venous drainage) of the malformation and at the date best option is the combined treatment [42].

To simplify these extremely complex anatomo-pathological entities we can postulate that in spinal DAVFs, the fistula is superficial or subpial; in spinal AVMs, the nidus can be superficial, subpial, subarachnoid or intramedullary, usually superficial to the cord when small and embedded into the cord when large. This description needs to be integrated with symptoms and information from all possible imaging techniques in order to understand the lesional and regional anatomy and to choose an appropriate treatment strategy.

In type I DAVFs symptoms increase over the time with progressive weakness of the legs and concurrent bowel or bladder difficulties. Surgical or endovascular treatment is essential in these patients, and it is imperative to occlude the shunt as soon as possible in order to interrupt the spinal cord damage [43]. In 2008, Narvid *et al.* [44] described a 20-year experience with both surgical and endovascular approaches treating 39 patients by endovascular embolization obtaining complete obliteration of the fistulas in 69% patients compared to 83% in 24 patients who were treated successfully with a surgical approach alone. However, the results of endovascular therapy for spinal DAVFs has growth significantly over the last years. The majority of recent studies published report success rates of 70-90% with NBCA or other liquid embolic agents. Surgery is useful in the case of failed embolization and recurrence or for lesions not able to embolization. Clinical outcomes are similar to surgical treatment when the fistula and draining vein remain persistently occluded. Improving in gait and motor function are considered as successful treatment, whereas urinary improvements less frequently occur.

In cases of intradural AVMs/AVFs (types 2 and 4) the patients' preoperative neurological status is an important consideration before the treatment. Patients typically suffer acute intraparenchymal or subarachnoid hemorrhage. Rarely, patients present because of a vascular steal phenomenon or chronic myelopathy, in which oxygenated arterial blood shunted through the AVM causes vascular hypoperfusion surrounding normal parenchyma or high flow fistulas cause venous engorgement. Lastly, patients affected by intradural lesions can suffer from a mass effect caused by the growth of feeders and draining veins of the AVM. The enlarged vascular malformation compresses the surrounding neural tissue, impairing neurological function. Treatment planning depends on the hemodynamic aspects of the lesion, its site and its angioarchitecture. Embolization is the first treatment option for many spinal vascular malformations. However, surgery continues to have a important role, and a multidisciplinary approach is essential.

Good results can be obtained if the treatment is performed early before severe clinical deterioration.

Bleeding due to a spinal AV shunt is a good indication for treatment in order to prevent re-bleeding [45]. In 2004, Rodesch *et al.* [12] described their experience in 155 patients affected by symptomatic high flow spinal cord AV shunts showing improvement in more than 70% of patients.

Endovascular treatment has an important role in the management of dural and intramedullary spinal AVMs using embolic agents or associated with surgery. NBCA and Onyx achieve a more permanent occlusion with a very low recurrence rate [9,35]. The liquid agent should be delivered within or as close to the shunt as possible in order to control the injection better and to ensure complete occlusion with maximum safety. Coils are not used in lesions located in the spinal cord, because they achieve only proximal arterial occlusion, leading to the development of collateral flow to the shunts. Distal occlusion of the vein in large AV shunt by the embolic agent can carry an increased risk of bleeding. As mentioned above, too proximal an occlusion of feeding artery gives poor result because other arterial anastomoses will be developed subsequently to supplying the shunt. The targets of treatment are the fistulous point for AV shunts and the nidus for spinal AVMs.

ACKNOWLEDGEMENTS

Declared none.

CONFLICTS OF INTEREST

The authors confirm that this chapter contents have no conflict of interest.

REFERENCES

[1]   Lasjaunias PL, Berenstein A, Ter Brugge KG. Surgical Neuroangiography, Vol. 1: Clinical Vascular Anatomy and Variations. Springer Verlag, Heidelberg, 2001.
[2]   Santillan A, Nacarino V, Greenberg E, Riina HA, Gobin YP, Patsalides A. Vascular anatomy of the spinal cord. J NeuroIntervent Surg 2012; 4: 67-74.

[3]   Krings T, Geibprasert S, Thron A. Spinal vascular anatomy. In: Naidich T, ed. Neuroradiology of the Brain and Spine. New York: Elsevier; 2009.

[4]   Thron AK. Vascular Anatomy of the Spinal Cord. Neuroradiological Anatomy and Clinical Syndromes. Springer Verlag, Vienna. 1988

[5]   Gillilan LA. Veins of the spinal cord. Anatomic details; suggested clinical applications. Neurology 1970; 20: 860-8.

[6]   Jellema K, Tijssen CC, van Gijn J. Spinal dural arteriovenous fistulas: a congestive myelopathy that initially mimics a peripheral nerve disorder. Brain 2006; 129: 3150-64.

[7]   Krings T, Geibprasert S. Spinal dural arteriovenous fistulas. AJNR Am J Neuroradiol 2009; 30: 639-48.

[8]   Hurth M, Houdart R, Djindjian R, *et al*. Arteriovenous malformations of the spinal cord: clinical, anatomical and therapeutic consideration: a series of 150 cases. Progr Neurol Surg 1978; 9: 238-66.

[9]   Patsalides A, Knopman J, A. Santillan A, Tsiouris AJ, Riina H, Gobin YP. Endovascular treatment of spinal arteriovenous lesions: beyond the dural fistula. AJNR Am J Neuroradiol 2011; 32: 798-808.

[10]   Backes WH, Nijenhuis RJ. Advances in spinal cord MR angiography. AJNR Am J Neuroradiol 2008; 29: 619-31.

[11]   Rodesch G, Hurth M, Alvarez H, *et al*. Classification of spinal cord arteriovenous shunts: proposal for a reappraisal - the Bicetre experience with 155 consecutive patients treated between 1981 and 1999. Neurosurgery 2002; 51: 374-9.

[12]   Rodesch G, Hurth M, Alvarez H, *et al*. Angio-architecture of spinal cord arteriovenous shunts at presentation: clinical correlations in adults and children - the Bicetre experience on 155 consecutive patients seen between 1981–1999. Acta Neurochir (Wien) 2004; 146: 217-26.

[13]   Krings T, Mull M, Gilsbach JM, *et al*. Spinal vascular malformations. Eur Radiol 2005; 15: 267-78.

[14]   Bao YH, Ling F. Classification and therapeutic modalities of spinal vascular malformations in 80 patients. Neurosurgery 1997; 40: 75-81.

[15]   Barrow DL, Awad IA (eds): Conceptual overview and management strategies. In: Spinal Vascular Malformations. Park Ridge, IL: The American Association of Neurological Surgeons, 1999; 169-80.

[16]   Berenstein A, Lasjaunias P. Spinal dural arteriovenous fistulas. In: Surgical Neuroangiography: Endovascular Treatment of Spine and Spinal Cord Lesions. Springer, Berlin Heidelberg New York Tokyo. 1992.

[17]   Koch C. Spinal dural arteriovenous fistula. Curr Opin Neurol 2006; 19: 69-75.

[18]   Tsai LK, Jeng JS, Liu HM, Wang HJ, Yip PK. Intracranial dural arteriovenous fistulas with or without cerebral sinus thrombosis: analysis of 69 patients. Neurol Neurosurg Psychiatry 2004; 75: 1639-41.

[19]   Kraus JA, Stuper BK, Berlit P. Association of resistance to activated protein C and dural arteriovenous fistulas. J Neurol 1998; 245: 731-3.

[20]   Kraus JA, Stuper BK, Nahser HC, Klockgether T, Berlit P. Significantly increased prevalence of factor V Leiden in patients with dural arteriovenous fistulas. J Neurol 2000; 247: 521-3.

[21]   Foix CH, Alajouanine T. [La myelite necrotique subaigue.] Rev Neurol 1926; 46: 1-42.

[22]   Jellema K, Tijssen CC, Fijnheer R, de Groot PG, Koudstaal PJ, van Gijk J. Spinal dural arteriovenous fistulas are not associated with prothrombotic factors. Stroke 2004; 35: 2069-71.

[23]   Gerlach R, Boehm-Weigert M, Berkefeld J, *et al*. Thrombophilic risk factors in patients with cranial and spinal dural arteriovenous fistulae. Neurosurgery 2008; 63: 693-98; discussion 698-9.

[24]   Jellema K, Tijssen CC, Sluzewski M, van Asbeck FW, Koudstaal PJ, van Gijn J. Spinal dural arteriovenous fistulas - an underdiagnosed disease. A review of patients admitted to the spinal unit of a rehabilitation center. J Neurol 2006; 253: 159-62.

[25]   Merland JJ, Riche MC, Chiras J. Intraspinal extramedullary arteriovenous fistulae draining into the medullary veins. J Neuroradiol 1980; 7: 271-320.

[26]   Thron A. [Spinal dural arteriovenous fistulas.] [In German] Radiologe 2001; 41: 955-60.

[27]   Mull M, Nijenhuis RJ, Backes WH, *et al*. Value and limitations of contrast-enhanced MR angiography in spinal arteriovenous malformations and dural arteriovenous fistulas. AJNR Am J Neuroradiol 2007; 28: 1249-58.

[28]   Yamaguchi S, Eguchi K, Kiura Y, *et al*. Multi-detector-row CT angiography as a preoperative evaluation for spinal arteriovenous fistulae. Neurosurg Rev 2007; 30: 321-6.

[29]   Hetts SW, Moftakhar P, English JD, *et al.* Spinal dural arteriovenous fistulas and intrathecal venous drainage: correlation between digital subtraction angiography, magnetic resonance imaging, and clinical findings. J Neurosurg Spine 2012; 16: 433-40.

[30]   Berenstein A, Ter Brugge K, Lasjaunias P. Surgical Neuroangiography. Vol. 2: Clinical and endovascular treatment aspects in adults. Second edition. Springer. 2004.

[31]   Biondi A, Merland JJ, Hodes JE, Pruvo JP, Reizine D. Aneurysms of spinal arteries associated with intramedullary arteriovenous malformations. I. Angiographic and clinical aspects. AJNR Am J Neuroradiol 1992; 13: 913-22.

[32]   Aminoff MJ, Logue V. The prognosis of patients with spinal vascular malformations. Brain 1974; 97: 211-8.

[33]   Bostrom A, Krings T, Hans FJ, *et al.* Spinal glomus-type arteriovenous malformations: microsurgical treatment in 20 cases. J Neurosurg Spine 2009; 10: 423-9.

[34]   Connolly ES Jr, Zubay GP, McCormick PC, *et al.* The posterior approach to a series of glomus (type II) intramedullary spinal cord arteriovenous malformations. Neurosurgery 1998; 42: 774-85, discussion 785-6.

[35]   Corkill RA, Mitsos AP, Molyneux AJ. Embolization of spinal intramedullary arteriovenous malformations using the liquid embolic agent, Onyx: a single center experience in a series of 17 patients. J Neurosurg Spine 2007; 7: 478-85.

[36]   Sinclair J, Chang SD, Gibbs IC, Adler JR Jr. Multisession CyberKnife radiosurgery for intramedullary spinal cord arteriovenous malformations. Neurosurgery 2006; 58: 1081-9.

[37]   Gonzalez LF, Zabramski JM, Tabrizi P, Wallace RC, Massand MG, Spetzler RF. Spontaneous spinal subarachnoid hemorrhage secondary to spinal aneurysms: diagnosis and treatment paradigm. Neurosurgery 2005; 57: 1127-31.

[38]   Zozulya YP, Slin'ko EI, Al-Qashqish II. Spinal arteriovenous malformations: new classification and surgical treatment. Neurosurg Focus 2006; 20: E7.

[39]   Kim LJ, Spetzler RF. Classification and surgical management of spinal arteriovenous lesions: arteriovenous fistulae and arteriovenous malformations. Neurosurgery 2006; 59: S195-201.

[40]   Spetzler RF, Detwiler PW, Riina HA, Porter RW. Modified classification of spinal cord vascular lesions. J Neurosurg 2002; 96: 145-56.

[41]   Geibprasert S, Pereira V, Krings T, *et al.* Dural arteriovenous shunts: a new classification of craniospinal epidural venous anatomical bases and clinical correlations. Stroke 2008; 39: 2783-94.

[42]   Krings T, Thron AK, Geibprasert S, *et al.* Endovascular management of spinal vascular malformations. Neurosurg Rev 2010; 33: 1-9.

[43]   Cenzato M, Versari P, Righi C, *et al.* Spinal dural arteriovenous fistulae: analysis of outcome in relation to pretreatment indicators. Neurosurgery 2004; 55: 815-22.

[44]   Narvid J, Hetts SW, Larsen D, *et al.* Spinal dural arteriovenous fistulae: clinical features and long-term results. Neurosurgery 2008; 62: 159-66.

[45]   Konan AV, Raymond J, Roy D. Transarterial embolization of aneurysms associated with spinal cord arteriovenous malformations: report of four cases. J Neurosurg 1999; 90: 148-54.

Frontiers in Neurosurgery, Vol. 1, 2015, 139-153   139

CHAPTER 6

Endovascular Reperfusion Management for Acute Ischemic Stroke

Paolo Machi[1,*], Kiriakos Lobotesis[2] and Alain Bonafé[1]

[1]*Centre Hospitalier Universitaire Gui de Chauliac, Montpellier, France;* [2]*Imperial College Healthcare NHS, London, United Kingdom*

Abstract: Early recanalization of a thrombosed cerebral artery in a patient with acute ischemic stroke is related to better outcome and reduced mortality. Intravenous administration of rt-PA within 4.5 hours from stroke onset is the recommended therapy for acute ischemic stroke. However, several studies demonstrated improvements, in terms of anatomical and clinical results when intravenous therapy is associated with intra-arterial approach. Although improvement in outcome of patients treated by mechanical approach reported in various case series, three recent randomized controlled failed to demonstrate the superiority of mechanical thrombectomy over intravenous fibrinolysis. In the first part of this chapter we report the results of these randomized trials and discuss their biases and limitations. We then describe stentriever thrombectomy techniques and the mechanical approach to tandem occlusions.

Keywords: Embolectomy, endovascular treatment, intracranial revascularization, intravenous fibrinolysis, ischemic stroke, mechanical treatment, tandem occlusions, thrombectomy, stentrievers.

INTRODUCTION

Intravenous fibrinolysis (IVF) is the treatment of choice for acute ischemic stroke even though in a number of retrospective series it was found that the results, in terms of rate of vessel recanalization, were better when an intra-arterial approach (IAA) was used. To date there are no prospective, randomized trials demonstrating the superiority of this latter treatment, compared to IVF. In 2013 three articles were published in The New England Journal of Medicine comparing the efficacy of IAA versus IVF. These randomized controlled trials, which we analyze below, have not swayed the neurovascular community, mainly because of weaknesses in the studies' design. None of these studies compared IVF

---

*Corresponding author Paolo Machi: Centre Hospitalier Universitaire Gui de Chauliac, Montpellier, France; Tel/Fax: 0033467337888; E-mail: paolo.machi@gmail.com

Simone Peschillo (Ed.)

with mechanical thrombectomy performed with stent retrievers which is, as reported below, the current treatment of reference used worldwide for IAA.

The Synthesis Trial

This trial [1] compared the clinical outcome at three months of two groups of patients with acute ischemic stroke presenting within 4.5 hours who were treated by IVF or IAA. One hundred eighty-one patients were assigned to the IVF arm and received (rt-PA) intravenously a median of 2.75 hours after the onset of symptoms. The same number of patients (181) was assigned to the IAA arm and by a median of 3.75 hours after the onset of symptoms were treated with intra-arterial thrombolysis, mechanical clot disruption or retrieval or a combination of these approaches. The three-month assessment showed a better clinical outcome for patients assigned to the IVF arm. Sixty-three patients (of 181; 34.8%) in the IVF arm were alive without disability, with a modified Rankin scale (mRS) score <2, compared to 55 patients (of 181; 30.4%) in the IAA arm. The authors concluded that the results of this trial indicate that endovascular therapy is not superior to standard treatment with intravenous t-PA for patients with acute ischemic stroke. One major drawback of this study is the fact that patients assigned to the IAA arm were treated in different ways, giving the study a very low level of reproducibility. In 109 patients endovascular treatment was not performed with thrombectomy devices. This group of patients was given intra-arterial injections of t-PA administered through a microcatheter that had been navigated into the thrombus; in some cases operators additionally performed manual clot fragmentation using a microwire. These thrombectomy techniques were only available in the early phase of the trial (early 2008). These mechanical approaches are now considered ineffective. In the other 56 patients of this cohort an appropriate thrombectomy device was used: Solitaire FR (EV3, Covidien) Merci retriever (Concentric, Medical), Penumbra System (Penumbra) or Treevo (Stryker). Only in 23 patients (out of 163 who underwent IAA treatment) was the device of choice a stent retriever. Furthermore, patients assigned to IAA did not receive intravenous t-PA while awaiting endovascular treatment.

This approach differs from current combined intravenous/intra-arterial strategies in which t-PA is administered intravenously to patients waiting for mechanical thrombectomy. Although it has not been demonstrated, intravenous t-PA may facilitate mechanical fragmentation or retrieval of the clot. Another major drawback of this study was the type of imaging used to select patients. The only neuroradiological study performed for patient selection was non-contrast-enhanced computed tomography of the brain. This investigation is of limited value for the assessment of the infarct core and does not enable evaluation of the presence of vessel occlusion or thrombus location. Potentially, this could have led to inclusion of patients without any vessel occlusion or a penumbra.

Interventional Management of Stroke III Trial

In this international, phase 3, randomized, open-label clinical trial [2], with blinded outcomes, stroke patients were randomized to be treated within three hours of the onset of symptoms either by IVF alone or by IVF and an additional IAA, in a 2:1 ratio. As for the Synthesis trial the primary endpoint of this study was the clinical outcome at three months evaluated using the mRS. This study was stopped early because of futility after 656 patients had been recruited, with 434 patients assigned to the IVF arm and 222 to the IVF plus IAA arm. The proportion of patients presenting with a mRS score=2 at the three-month follow-up examinations did not differ significantly according to the type of treatment received. The percentage of patients with a mRS score =2 at three months was 40.8% for the IVF plus IAA arm and 38.7% for the IVF arm. As for the Synthesis trial, the authors concluded that there is no significant difference in functional independence following treatment with IAA after IVF as compared with IVF alone. Again in this trial, the major drawback was that patients treated with the endovascular approach underwent different types of treatment. In this trial, patients assigned to the combined IVF/IAA arm underwent thrombectomy performed with a Merci retriever (Concentric, Medical), a Penumbra System (Penumbra) or Solitaire FR (EV3, Covidien) or endovascular administration of t-PA delivered by Micro Sonic SV infusion (EKOS) or by a standard microcathater. Only four patients out of the 434 in this trial were treated with a stent retriever, Solitaire FR. Imaging criteria used for patient selection in this trial, as for the Synthesis trial, constituted another important bias of the study since, at least in the early phase, no neurovascular imaging was performed before randomization. Another bias of this study was the delay between stroke onset and the interventional procedures. Overall patients received IVF within 3 hours of symptom onset. Randomization was required within 40 minutes after the initiation of the infusion. Patients assigned to the IAA arm had to be treated as soon as possible, either in the hospital that initiated the treatment or in another participating hospital; the angiographic procedure had to be initiated within 5 hours and completed within 7 hours of the onset of symptoms. This could be a cause of late and futile recanalization. In fact, as reported even by the authors of the study, the clinical outcome of stroke patients is related to arterial recanalization but also to the timing of the recanalization. The earlier the artery is reopened, the higher the probability that the patient will have a good clinical outcome.

MR Rescue Trial

This phase 2b, randomized, controlled, open-label (blinded outcome), multicenter trial [3] was designed to evaluate the three-month outcome of stroke patients treated with either IVF or IVF and IAA within 8 hours after stroke onset. In this study computed tomography or magnetic resonance imaging of the "penumbral" or "non-penumbral" pattern permitted stratification during randomization into favorable versus non- favorable imaging patterns. Patients assigned to the IAA arm underwent embolectomy performed with a Merci retriever (Concentric, Medical) or Penumbra System (Penumbra Inc.) or with intra-arterial injection of t-PA. One hundred twenty-seven patients were randomized: 70 were assigned to undergo embolectomy and 57 to receive standard care. Among the 118 eligible patients in this study, 58% had a favorable penumbral pattern. Revascularization was achieved in 67% of the patients in the embolectomy group. The three-month mortality rate was 21%, and the rate of symptomatic intracranial hemorrhage was 4%; neither rate differed between the treatment groups. The mean mRS scores did not differ between patients treated with embolectomy or standard care (3.9 versus 3.9; P=0.99). Embolectomy was not superior to standard care in patients with either a favorable penumbral pattern (mean score, 3.9 versus 3.4; P=0.23) or anon-favorable pattern (mean score, 4.0 versus 4.4; P=0.32). In the primary analysis of mRS scores at 90 days, there was no interaction between the pre-treatment imaging pattern and treatment assignment (P=0.14). The authors concluded that a favorable penumbral pattern on neuroimaging did not identify patients who would benefit differentially from endovascular therapy for acute ischemic stroke, nor was embolectomy shown to be superior to standard care. Nevertheless, in the discussion section, the authors offered an interesting possible explanation of the neutral results obtained in the comparison of the IAA and IVF groups. The lack of a better 90-day outcome for patients in the embolectomy group was probably related to the low rate of recanalization obtained with old-generation embolectomy devices. The authors suggested that it is possible that new-generation stent retrievers would have a treatment benefit and a benefit in patients with a favorable penumbral pattern because of both higher recanalization rates and lower complication rates.

Need for Further Investigations of the Treatment of Acute Ischemic Stroke

As reported above, three international, prospective, randomized, controlled trials published in 2013 in The New England Journal of Medicine failed to demonstrate a superior three-month clinical outcome from IAA for the treatment of acute ischemic stroke in comparison to the standard IVF. Nevertheless, these trials had several weaknesses. As described above and as also discussed by the authors of the trials, one of the major weaknesses of all these studies was that patients assigned to the IAA arms were not treated with the same approach and only a small number of patients assigned to IAA were treated with stent retrievers. Another important issue was the lack of homogeneity in the participating centers regarding imaging criteria for the selection of patients. Moreover, the delay in treatment for patients assigned to the IAA arms (up to 8 hours) seems to be too long according to the results of several stroke studies demonstrating that clinical outcome is directly related to prompt vessel recanalization. This chapter is not intended to describe how to design a clinical trial on stroke therapy. Nevertheless, it seems to us that the ideal study comparing IAA versus IVF should be a randomized trial in which patients assigned to the IAA arm are treated with the same procedure and the same device (a stent retriever) in experienced centers in which there is a high volume of thrombectomy procedures performed for strokes. Moreover, the same imaging selection criteria (using dedicated computed tomography or magnetic resonance stroke selection software) should be applied to all patients and the delay in the thrombectomy procedure should not go beyond 4.5 hours from symptom onset.

ENDOVASCULAR REVASCULARIZATION TECHNIQUES

Mechanical Thrombectomy and Stent Retrievers

Intravenous administration of fibrinolytic drugs (recombinant-PA) within 4.5 hours of the onset of the stroke is the most common therapy for acute ischemic stroke worldwide. In spite of the encouraging results reported after with mechanical thrombectomy with different thrombectomy systems, none of them is accepted worldwide as a standard tool for recanalization procedures. Furthermore, mechanical treatment is not recognized as a more suitable treatment for patients amenable to IVF.

Stentrievers

Stentrievers are stent-based thrombectomy systems with an open or closed-cell design with or without a split section. These devices are advanced and delivered within the thrombus *via* a standard microcatheter (inner lumen diameter of 0.021" or 0.027"). The stent-based design provides dual functionality: first they act as temporary intracranial by-passes, immediately restoring flow through the thrombus, and secondly they act as clot retrievers, trapping the thrombus in their cells, enabling the clot to be removed.

Several intrarterial tools and techniques have been reported so far. Thrombectomy devices have been subdivided into proximal and distal devices depending on where they apply force to the thrombus [4-6]. Moreover, various types of devices have been used, off-label, as recanalization instruments, e.g. angioplasty balloons, self-expanding stents and balloon-mounted coronary stents [6, 7]. There are extensive reports on the clinical experience with the MERCI® retriever device (Concentric Medical, Mountain View, CA, USA) [6].

In the Multi-MERCI trial a revascularization rate of 69.5% (91/131 patients) was reported for cases in which the mechanical thrombectomy was associated with intra-arterial rt-PA. Intracerebral hemorrhage was recorded in 9.8% of the patients (16/131 patients) and intra-procedural adverse events were reported in 5.5% of the cases (9/131 patients). The number of device passes per intervention was on average 2.9. Comparison of results of this study with those of studies in which patients were treated with a Solitaire FR stentriever, showed an inferior rate of target arterial recanalization (65.5% versus 89.2%), a higher number of passes performed per procedure (2.9 versus 2), and higher rates of significant peri-operative intraprocedural complications and symptomatic hemorrhagic complications. Although the MERCI® retriever device has been approved by the Food and Drug Administration, the relatively long learning curve required for its use has probably not encouraged worldwide acceptance of this device. Furthermore, in 2011 Concentric Medical launched Treevo®, another stentriever, on the European market. The investigators from the Penumbra Pivotal Stroke Trial [7] reported on 125 acute stroke patients treated with the Penumbra System. In this series 81.6% of the target vessels were revascularized to TIMI grade 2 to 3. Eighteen procedural events in 16 patients (12.8%) were reported. The all-cause mortality rate was 32.8% and a total of 35 patients (28%) were found to have intracranial hemorrhage on the 24-hour computed tomography evaluation, with the hemorrhage being symptomatic in 14 (11.2%) cases. At 90 days 25% of the patients had achieved a mRS score of = 2. In contrast to the lower estimated incidence of traumatic events caused by a proximal device, such as the Penumbra System, in comparison to a distal thrombectomy device, the rate of intracranial hemorrhages seems to be high compared with results reported in the literature for Solitaire FR. Nevertheless the 90-day follow-up of the Penumbra Trial cohort (25% of patients with a mRS score=2) does not seem to correlate well with the incidence of artery recanalization (81.6%), probably because the TIMI score, used to measure the degree of recanalization of the target artery is not correlated with the degree of the parenchymal reperfusion. Hence, a TIMI score of 3 is not necessarily correlated with brain parenchymal and clinical recovery. Penumbra Inc. also started to produce a stentriever in 2012. Intracranial self-expanding stents have been successfully employed as temporary or permanent endovascular bypasses in the invasive management of acute ischemic stroke [7-10]. In this technique the stent is deployed at the point of vessel occlusion and expands, displacing the thrombus circumferentially and restoring blood flow. The re-establishment of flow through the occlusion site promotes immediate dissipation of prothrombotic factors. At the same time the restored arterial flow allows thrombolytic medications to come into contact with the thrombotic material trapped within the mesh of the stent and against the arterial wall [11]. Levy *et al.* [11] reported on a series of 18 patients with 19 acute phase arterial thrombotic occlusions treated with permanent stent placement in combination with other mechanical maneuvers and pharmacological therapy. Complete recanalization (TIMI 3) was achieved in six out of the 19 cases (31.5%) but stent placement was associated with angioplasty (before or after stent placement), clot-retrieval (MERCI® retriever), thrombolytic drugs (recombinant t-PA and abciximab) and antiplatelet medications (aspirin, clopidogrel). The overall incidence of intracranial hemorrhage was 36.8% (7 out of 19 cases). This high incidence was probably related to the combination of thrombolytic medication with antiplatelet therapy required when a stent is placed permanently. Such a multimodal approach results in consumption of time and resources and requires a very experienced neurointerventionist team. Kelly *et al.* [12] described a technique in which the Enterprise® stent (Cordis, Miami Lake, FL, USA), a reconstrainable self-expanding microstent, was used successfully as a temporary endovascular by-pass to recanalize a middle cerebral artery refractory to pharmacological thrombolysis. In this case the stent was partially deployed (two- thirds) across the site of the arterial occlusion. The radial expansion of the stent displaced and disrupted the occlusive thrombus. After flow restoration, abciximab was administered. Twenty minutes after deployment, the stent was reconstrained and retrieved and an additional intra-arterial dose of abciximab and recombinant t-PA was administered. Temporary stent deployment has the advantages described for permanent stent placement without the risks of complications related to antiplatelet therapy, which is mandatory in the case of permanent stent deployment. Whether stent opening is sufficient to re-establish flow in any type of thrombus remains a matter of debate. Since 2010 several groups worldwide have published data on their experience using the Solitaire FR in stroke patients [13];

the overall results of these studies confirm the superiority of this device, in terms of high rate of vessel recanalization and low rates of peri- and post-procedural complications, in comparison with the "no-stentriever" thrombectomy devices. Furthermore, these studies showed a better long-term (three months) clinical outcome, as determined by a mRS score of =2, for patients treated with Solitaire FR.

From a technical point of view, stentrievers are easily navigated to the occlusion point and the deployment across the thrombus is also simple. Since the learning-curve for the use of these devices is very short, the efficacy of stentrievers seems to be less operator-dependent than that of more complex devices. The simplicity of their deployment and retrieval enables consistent results to be achieved throughout the entire neurointervention team. One could imagine that retrieval of a fully deployed stent might be dangerous in terms of vessel damage.

However, no cases of vessel dissection have been reported, so far, in the literature. On the other hand, there are reports of episodes of vasospasm, after stent retrieval, with these resolving after intra-arterial injection of nimodipine. Furthermore, the occluding balloon guide catheter plays an important role in thrombus removal. In fact, sometimes the thrombus is found in the 50 cc syringe after manual aspiration performed during the device retrieval.

In these cases the stent probably just displaced the clot, which would have remained in the vasculature if the blood had not been aspirated.

Description of the Procedure

Thrombectomy procedures are performed *via* a femoral artery access under general or local anesthesia. For the anterior circulation, a 6, 8 or 9 French guide catheter (with or without an occlusion balloon) is introduced through a femoral sheath into the concerned carotid artery. For the posterior circulation, a 6 French guidecatheter is navigated into the dominant vertebral artery. A 0. 21" internal diameter microcatheter is advanced distal to the clot over a steerable microwire and an angiographic run is done through the microcatheter in order to control the downstream vasculature and the distal edge of the thrombus. The microwire is then exchanged with the stentriever which is released within the thrombus.

Upon stentriever placement, a new angiographic control is done to evaluate the opening of the stent. There after the device is maintained in place for 3-7 minutes in order to allow the optimal expansion of the nitinol struts. Hence, the stentriever is gently retrieved within the guide catheter. During the retrieval, for cases in which a balloon guide catheter is used, the balloon guide catheter is inflated and manual aspiration (e.g. with a 50 cc syringe) is performed in order to reduce the risk of thromboembolic complications. Using the same device, or a second one, up to five passes can be made into the occluded vessel, if necessary. In the case of tortuous vessels a co-axial system could be used in order to help navigation and manipulation of the delivery stentriever microcatheter. In this setting two or three guide catheters are navigated co-axially above the vessel tortuosity.

Selection of Patients for Endovascular Treatment

Patients must be examined on admission by a senior stroke neurologist in order to assess the severity of the neurological deficit using the National Institutes of Health Stroke Scale (NIHSS) [14]. Clinical outcome must then be re-evaluated at 24 hours, and every day during the hospitalization and at discharge using the NIHSS and the mRS. Patients should be evaluated in the acute phase with magnetic resonance imaging or computed tomography-perfusion studies in order to evaluate the extent of the ischemic lesion. Computed tomography or magnetic resonance angiography is used to locate the site of occlusion and, in cases in which patients are studied by magnetic resonance T2 and FLAIR weighted imaging, to determine the timing of the ischemic lesions. Perfusion imaging, in both computed tomography and magnetic resonance studies, is used to evaluate the contribution of the collateral supply to the ischemic zone. For patients presenting with MCA stroke, the Alberta Stroke Program Early Computed Tomography (ASPECT) score, calculated on diffusion weighted images or on perfusion computed tomography, could be used to determine the ischemic core. Patients with an ASPECT score inferior or equal to 5 are good candidates for thrombectomy. According to the literature patients presenting within 4.5 hours of the onset of stroke symptoms due to occlusion of a carotid "T" or common carotid artery associated with an intracranial occlusion (tandem occlusion) are good candidates for the combined approach of intravenous fibrinolysis together with mechanical thrombectomy. The rationale of this dual approach is the very low rate of vessel recanalization obtained by fibrinolysis alone. Patients presenting with isolated M1 occlusions are good candidates for intravenous fibrinolysis alone. Nevertheless, this subgroup of patients can take advantage from mechanical thrombectomy as a rescue therapy if clinical improvement (increase in NIHSS score of at least 4 points) is not obtained within 60 minutes of the intravenous injection (rescue therapy). Furthermore, several studies have demonstrated the superiority of a combined approach in comparison with an intravenous approach alone.

While intravenous treatment is easily reproducible, the endovascular treatment is variable depending on institutional protocols and operator choices.

Mechanical Recanalization Strategy for Tandem Occlusions Using Stentrievers

The optimal treatment in the acute phase of occlusion of the cervical internal carotid artery (ICA) associated with carotid bifurcation (carotid "T") or middle cerebral artery occlusion is not established looking at the literature a relatively small number of patients with "tandem obstruction" achieve full recanalization and have an improvement in clinical outcome after intravenous treatment [14, 24]. Consequently, more aggressive treatments, such as intra-arterial fibrinolysis or mechanical thrombectomy have been proposed in association with conventional intravenous treatment. The SAME authors of THIS chapter reported on the efficacy and safety of endovascular approach to tandem occlusions.

They reported about a tapered technique of such challenging occlusions for which the proximal extracranial internal carotid thrombosis is treated firstly with aspiration or angioplasty in order to permit the advancement of the guide catheter and subsequently the intracranial thrombectomy. The aim of this technique is to obtain the intracranial revascularization as soon as possible since it is directly related with the clinical outcome. After intracranial revascularization achievement, further treatment is addressed to the extracranial thrombosis and the underlying stenosis, eventually. Cervical carotid stenting is performed only in cases for which standing-alone angioplasty is not sufficient in obtaining adequate blood flow within the artery. The rational of this "tapered" technique is to reduce the need of antiplatelet medications which increases the risk of bleeding in acute stroke patients. Endovascular procedures for tandem occlusions of the anterior circulation Endovascular treatments are performed with the patient on general or local anesthesia depending on different institutional protocols. An 8 or 9 French normal or balloon guide catheter is navigated into the common carotid artery *via* a femoral artery approach and an initial angiographic study of the proximal occlusion is performed. Thereafter the guide catheter is advanced within the thrombus over the guide wire and manual thrombus aspiration is performed meanwhile. The technique differs when the proximal occlusion is the consequence of a dissection of the cervical carotid, in this setting the guide catheter is advanced over a microcatheter within the dissected artery. The use of the microcatheter, instead of a standard guide wire, allows a more accurate navigation through the true lumen of the dissection. Once the guide catheter, or the coaxial guide catheter, is placed above the dissection, the intracranial thrombus is retrieved as previously described. After intracranial revascularization the guide catheter is retrieved in the cervical carotid below the level of the proximal occlusion. Thereafter, a new angiographic evaluation of the proximal stenosis is carried out. In cases of significant residual stenosis (>70%) or unstable plaque, additional angioplasty and the stenting of the carotid eventually can be performed. 250 mg of aspirin are administered intravenously in cases of stent placement. In cases of tandem occlusion due to cervical internal carotid dissection, the stenting of the artery is performed only when collateral blood supply to the concerned hemisphere through the communicating arteries is not present or adequate.

Rationale for a Mechanical Approach to Tandem Occlusions

Intravenous fibrinolysis is less effective in obtaining intracranial recanalization for cases of tandem occlusion in comparison with cases of isolated m1 occlusion [15, 16]. Tandem occlusion is a recognized independent risk factor for poor clinical outcome in stroke patients treated with intravenous fibrinolysis [17]. Furthermore, fibrinolysis is less effective in cases of internal carotid terminus occlusion [18]. Nevertheless, in cases of tandem occlusion, early recanalization of the intracranial occlusion leads to better clinical outcome regardless of persistent proximal cervical occlusion [19]. This is the rational of the strategy we reported above, which first addresses distal clot removal and flow re-establishment and then treats the causative proximal occlusion. Several publications present in literature have shown that distal occlusion can be treated by intra-arterial injection of rt-pa previous stenting of the cervical carotid artery. This procedure delays the intracranial recanalization because the time needed for both carotid stenting and intracranial thrombus dissolution. This "time-wasting" may lead to poor clinical outcome in spite of complete recanalization.

Ozdemir *et al.* [20] treated 8 patients presenting with tandem occlusions with "*in situ*" intra-arterial or combined intravenous "*in situ*" intra-arterial injection of rt-pa performed with a microcather navigated *via* the communicating arteries system to the intracranial clot. The proximal cervical occlusion in patients of this series was not treated. Only 2 out of 8 patients showed intracranial recanalization, nevertheless 3 months outcome was favorable for overall patients. The described technique is practicable only in patients in which communicating arteries are present. Moreover in cases of cervical carotid occlusion associated with terminal carotid occlusion the access to the distal thrombus seems to be precluded. Finally, the permanence of the cervical thrombus, source for potential emboli, is an independent risk factor for early re-occlusion after rt-pa [21]. Lavalée *et al.* [21] reported on ten cases of tandem occlusions due to cervical carotid dissection treated within three hours from stroke onset. Four out of 10 patients received only intravenous rt-pa while in the remaining 6 cases intra-arterial treatment of the distal thrombus was performed by mechanical means (5 cases) or "*in situ*" rt-pa injection (1 case). Intracranial recanalization was noted in all patients treated intrarterially. In the conclusion section author state that intra-arterial treatment seems to be more effective than the intra-venous approach. Whether intra-arterial treatment is also effective in cases of tandem occlusions associated with cervical carotid atherosclerotic plaques rests a matter of debate.

Malik *et al.* [22] treated 27 patients presenting with tandem occlusions. Patients received intra-arterial treatment of the distal clot previous cervical carotid stenting. The intracranial clot was addressed with either mechanical means or "*in situ*" rt-pa, or both. Mechanical thrombectomy was performed with merci clot retriever device (Concentric medical, mountain view, Ca, USA), or penumbra system (Penumbra inc, alameda, Ca, USA), or with intracranial angioplasty followed or not by stenting. During the procedure patients received intravenous heparin in order to obtain an activated clotting time double from the baseline. Moreover, in the early phase of the study patients received an intravenous bolus of eptifibatide after stent placement and clopidogrel and aspirin thereafter. Later in the study, antiplatelets (clopidogrel and aspirin) were administered to patients only *via* the nasogastric tube after stent placement. The rate of complete proximal and distal recanalization of this series was 75.3%, the hemorrhagic complication rate was 10.4%, thromboembolic complication rate was 3.9%. The mortality rate was 24.6%. Favorable outcome was recorded in 41.6% of patients. Authors state that the reopening of the cervical carotid allows immediate intracranial revascularization and consents a stable placement of the guide catheter. Furthermore, the stent placed within the cervical carotid upon the proximal thrombus decreases the risk of distal embolization. However, authors admit that this approach could require prolonged time for stent placement and that the dual antiplatelet therapy is dangerous in patient with large stroke extension especially in patients for which intracranial thrombectomy was not effective. Authors suggest that rate of hemorrhagic complications could decrease by treating the proximal cervical occlusion uniquely with angioplasty even if this treatment is less durable than stenting. Recanalization rate for each technique used for intracranial thrombectomy is not available. Nevertheless, given the assortment of tools and techniques used, results of this study seem poorly reproducible. Srinivasan *et al.* [23] treated 7 patients presenting with tandem occlusion. In this series the proximal occlusion was due to: atherothrombosis in five cases, to dissection in one case and to consequences of endoartherectomy in one case. Six patients presented with associated m1 occlusion. M1 recanalization was obtained in all cases by intra-arterial rt-pa injected *via* a microcatheter navigated within the cervical occlusion. Thereafter the cervical occlusion treatment was tapered depending on the type of underlying cause. In cases of atherothrombotic plaque (four cases) the cervical carotid was treated by stenting and angiolplasty. In the case of dissection two covered stent were deployed along the dissected segment. Four patients out of six had good clinical evolution at one month. Authors claim that in tandem occlusion stroke the intracranial occlusion should be addressed first since it is the cause of the neurological symptoms. We agree with this attitude since in our opinion the aim of the endovascular treatment of tandem occlusions should be the prompt recanalization of the intracranial artery [24-27]. Initial approach to the cervical carotid is performed to obtain placement of the guide catheter above the proximal occlusion. Thereafter intracranial clot removal is performed with stentrievers. The cervical carotid is subsequently treated with angioplasty or stenting or medical management depending on the etiology and the status of the artery. Stenting is performed in cases of dissection (without collateral supply) and atherothrombotic occlusive plaque. Aspirin (250 mg) is administered intravenously after stent placement. Stand-alone angioplasty should be performed in cases of non occlusive thrombus. The carotid stenting could be scheduled after the acute phase. This staged treatment reduce the rate of infarcted zone hemorrhagic transformation and allows for better antiplatelet preparation of the patient.

ACKNOWLEDGEMENTS

Declared none.

CONFLICT OF INTEREST

The authors confirm that this chapter contents have no conflict of interest.

REFERENCES

[1]   Ciccone A, Valvassori L, Nichelatti M, *et al*. Endovascular treatment for acute ischemic stroke N Engl J Med 2013; 368: 904-13.
[2]   Broderick J, Palesch Y, Demchuk A, *et al*. Endovascular therapy after intravenous t-PA versus t-PA alone for Stroke. N Engl J Med 2013; 368: 893-903.

[3]   Kidwell C, Jahan R, Gornbein J, *et al.* A trial of imaging selection and endovascular treatment for ischemic stroke. N Engl J Med 2013; 368: 914-23.

[4]   Higashida RT, Furlan AJ, Roberts H, *et al.* Trial design and reporting standards for intra-arterial cerebral thrombolysis for acute ischemic stroke. Stroke 2003; 34: e109-37.

[5]   The IMS II Trial Investigators. The Interventional Management of Stroke (IMS) II study. Stroke 2007; 38: 2127-35.

[6]   Smith WS, Sung G, Saver J, *et al.* Mechanical thrombectomy for acute ischemic stroke: final results of the Multi MERCI trial. Stroke 2008; 39: 1205-12.

[7]   Penumbra Pivotal Stroke Trial Investigators. The Penumbra Pivotal Stroke trial: safety and effectiveness of a new generation of mechanical devices for clot removal in intracranial large vessel occlusive disease. Stroke 2009; 40: 2761-8.

[8]   Mazighi M, Serfaty JM, Labreuche J, *et al.* Comparison of intravenous alteplase with a combined intravenous –endovascular approach in patients with stroke and confirmed arterial occlusion (RECANALISE study): a prospective cohort study. Lancet Neurol 2009; 8: 802-9.

[9]   Gralla J, Schroth G, Remonda L, *et al.* Mechanical thrombectomy for acute ischemic stroke: thrombus-device interaction, efficiency, and complications *in vivo*. Stroke 2006; 37: 3019-24.

[10]   Hussain MS, Kelly ME, Moskowitz SI, *et al.* Mechanical thrombectomy for acute stroke with the alligator retrieval device. Stroke 2009; 40: 3784-8.

[11]   Levy EI, Ecker RD, Horowitz MB, *et al* Stent-assisted intracranial recanalization for acute stroke: early results. Neurosurgery 2006; 58: 458-63.

[12]   Kelly ME, Furlan AJ, Fiorella D, *et al.* Recanalization of an acute middle cerebral artery occlusion using a self-expanding, reconstrainable, intracranial microstent as a temporary endovascular bypass. Stroke 2008; 39: 1770-3.

[13]   Machi P, Costalat V, Lobotesis K, *et al.* Solitaire FR thrombectomy system. immediate results in 56 consecutive acute ischemic stroke patients. J Neurointerv Surg 2012; 4: 62-6.

[14]   Costalat V, Machi P, Lobotesis K, *et al.* Rescue, combined, and stand-alone thrombectomy in the management of large vessel occlusion stroke using the Solitaire device: a prospective 50-patient single-center study: timing, safety, and efficacy. Stroke 2011; 42: 1929-35.

[15]   Kim K, Garami Z, Mikulik R, *et al.* Early recanalization rates and clinical outcomes in patients with tandem internal carotid artery/middle cerebral artery occlusion and isolated middle cerebral artery occlusion. Stroke 2005; 36: 869-71.

[16]   Linfante I, Llinas R.H, Selim M, *et al.* Clinical and vascular outcome in internal carotid artery versus middle cerebral artery occlusions after intravenous tissue plasminogen activator. Stroke 2002; 33: 2066-71.

[17]   The National Institute of Neurological Disorders and Stroke rtPA Stroke Study Group. Tissue plasminogen activator for acute ischemic stroke. N Engl J Med 1995; 333: 1581-7.

[18]   Christou I, Feldeberg RA, Demchuk AM, *et al.* Intravenous tissue plasminogen activator and improvement in acute ischemic stroke patients with internal carotid artery occlusion. J Neuroimaging 2002; 12: 119-23.

[19]   Mourand I, Brunel H, Vendrell JF, *et al.* Endovascular stent-assisted thrombolysis in acute occlusive carotid artery dissection. Neuroradiology 2010; 52: 135-40.

[20]   Ozdemir O, Bussiere M, Leung A, *et al.* Intra-arterial thrombolysis of occluded middle cerebral artery by use of collateral pathways in patients with tandem cervical carotid artery/ middle cerebral artery occlusion AJNR Am J Neuroradiol 2008; 29: 1596-600.

[21]   Lavallée PC, Mickaël M, Saint-Maurice JP, *et al.* Stent-assisted endovascular thrombolysis versus intravenous thrombolysis in internal carotid artery dissection with tandem cerebral artery occlusion. Stroke 2007; 38; 2270-4.

[22]   Malik AM, Nirav AV, Ridwan L *et al.* Endovascular treatment of extracranial/intracranial anterior circulation occlusion. Stroke 2011; 42: 1653-7.

[23]   Srinivasan A, Goyal M, Stys P, Sharma M, Lum C. Microcatheter navigation and thrombolysis in acute symptomatic cervical internal carotid occlusion. AJNR Am J Neuroradiol 2006; 27: 774-9.

[24]   Rubiera M, Ribo M, Delgado-Mederos R. *et al.* Tandem internal carotid artery/middle cerebral artery occlusion: an independent predictor of poor outcome after systemic thrombolysis. Stroke 2006; 37: 2301-5.

[25]   Zaidat OO, Suarez JI, Sunshine JL, *et al*. Thrombolytic therapy of acute ischemic stroke: correlation of angiographic recanalization with clinical outcome. AJNR Am J Neuroradiol 2005: 26: 880-4.

[26]   Kimura K, Iguchi Y, Shibazaki K, *et al*. Large ischemic lesions on diffusion-weighted imaging done before intravenous tissue plasminogen activator thrombolysis predicts a poor outcome in patients with acute stroke. Stroke 2008; 39: 2388-91.

[27]   Malgorzata M, Michels P, Jensen AM, *et al*. Endovascular treatment in proximal and intracranial carotid occlusion 9 hours after symptom onset. Neuroradiology 2008; 50: 599-604.

CHAPTER 7

State-of-the-Art and Future Perspective of Devices for Neuroendovascular Treatment

Arani Bose[1,2,*], John Lockhart[2], Dave Barry[2] and Sophia S. Kuo[2]

[1]*Interventional Neuroradiologist, New York, USA;* [2]*Penumbra Inc., Alameda, California, USA*

Abstract: In this chapter, we discuss the history of devices developed for neuro-endovascular therapy, culminating with the state-of-the-art devices in each category. Innovative tools for intracranial access including guide catheters, intermediate catheters, microcatheters, and guidewires which were critical to the development of neuro-interventional procedures are addressed first. With the introduction of coil embolization, aneurysms became amenable to minimally invasive treatment. Stents brought the strategy of parent vessel reconstruction to assist coiling of wide neck aneurysms, while disruption of flow at the aneurysm neck to enhance stagnation of blood in the sac enabled treatment of previously untreatable aneurysms, without sacrificing the parent vessel. For revascularization in acute ischemic stroke, mechanical thrombectomy devices were developed for clot removal. Subsequently, advances in polymer and materials technology and engineering breakthroughs in catheter design made it possible to deliver 5 French and 6 French catheters safely and reliably to the middle cerebral artery, thus allowing the promise of simple aspiration thrombectomy to be realized. The future of stent design and the exciting promise of neurointervention are also considered.

Keywords: Aneurysm coiling, coil embolization, flow diverter, intracranial access, mechanical thrombectomy, microcatheter, reperfusion catheter, stent retriever, thrombus revascularization.

OVERVIEW

It is a true privilege to have witnessed the blossoming of our field from a cottage industry to a global, multinational, multidisciplinary brand. In the late 1980s there were only a handful of centers worldwide that were training neurointerventionalists. Devices were hand-crafted in the angio suite, and the international working group of practitioners in the field could fit into a moderate sized conference room.

*Corresponding author Arani Bose:** Penumbra Inc., 1351 Harbor Bay Parkway, Alameda, California, USA 94502; Tel: 510-748-3200, 510-814-8305; E-mail: arani.bose@penumbrainc.com

Simone Peschillo (Ed.)

We started out treating a few thousand patients worldwide with esoteric brain and spinal vascular malformations. We then progressed to treating tens of thousands of patients with brain aneurysms. And now we have fast, effective tools to treat the hundreds of thousands of patients with acute ischemic stroke.

We are just beginning to develop therapeutic neurointerventional strategies to address the unmet clinical needs in hemorrhagic stroke, tissue regeneration, movement disorders, and epilepsy, among others. It is our challenge and responsibility to our young specialty, as physicians and industry, to continue to innovate and open new horizons and expand the field for the next generation.

ACCESS

Introduction

Procedure development and device development in neurointervention have been at least a quarter of a century behind similar developments in cardiac intervention. One important reason for this time lag is that the coronary ostia are relatively easy to access with large bore catheters and therefore large profile devices. In addition, the coronary vasculature is far less fragile than intracranial vessels and is encased in cardiac muscle. However, by necessity of evolution the intracranial vessels must course through the neck and enter the cranial vault with a great deal of redundancy. This enables the many degrees of freedom of rotation, tilt, and swivel of the cervical spine that allow tracking of prey without fear of cutting off the blood supply to the brain.

Intracranial access through the skull base and around the ophthalmic genu has been the bane of endovascular neurosurgeons for the entire history of the field. This problem has become more pronounced in the past decade as the devices we strive to bring up to the intracranial vasculature are larger, stiffer, and more complex. This advancement in therapeutic devices drove the need for innovation in access devices.

Guide Catheters

A decade ago, before the introduction of the Neuron catheter, guide catheters would sit low in the cervical internal carotid artery (ICA). Devices would be introduced *via* a microcatheter through the guide catheter. As the ICA traversed through the skull base, the microcatheter would meet tortuosity and resistance. The operator, in order to overcome this resistance, would apply more force to the microcatheter where it entered the groin. This force could often not be transmitted to the tip of the microcatheter and would be transmitted back to the guide catheter, causing the guide to back out of the ICA, sometimes all the way into the aortic arch, necessitating repositioning of the entire guide catheter/microcatheter system. This was not only time-consuming and inconvenient but often made the entire interventional procedure impossible.

This problem was essentially solved by developing a guide catheter designed specifically for neurointerventional procedures, called Neuron. Neuron is a variable stiffness guide catheter, designed to be positioned much higher than standard guides. The Neuron family of guide catheters is meant to be positioned around the right angles of the skull base (Fig. **1**) [1]. In this manner, when the force delivered through the micro-catheter is transmitted back to the Neuron, instead of backing out, the Neuron locks in place taking advantage of the right-angled bends of the skull base. In this way Neuron turns the disadvantage of tortuous skull base anatomy into an advantage conferring added stability, thereby allowing a variety of neuroendovascular procedures that would have otherwise been impossible.

Intermediate Catheters

As more complex therapeutic devices (flow diverters and clot retrieval devices) evolved so did the need for more distal support. These intermediate catheters (DAC®, Concentric Medical and ReFlex, Reverse Medical) had lumens large enough to deliver microcatheters, yet had distal flexibility profiles soft enough to be placed even higher in the anatomy. Two limiting factors of these intermediate catheters were their limited proximal support and lower quality angiograms due to lower contrast injection rates. To overcome the lack of proximal support, physicians would rely on long sheaths (Shuttle, Cook Medical and Neuron Max, Penumbra Inc) for proximal support. To address the lower quality angiograms, a new line of intermediate catheters (5MAX DDC, Penumbra Inc) used a tapered inner diameter. By having a larger proximal lumen (0.064 inch) for most of the length, then tapering to 0.054 inch, these catheters retained the contrast flow rate equivalent to a 0.062 inch catheter, while still having the highly flexible 5 French distal tip that can be placed high in the anatomy.

Microcatheters

The original Tracker microcatheter developed by Target Therapeutics in the late 1980s opened the door for endovascular treatment of neurovascular lesions. These highly flexible microcatheters enabled access for treatment, but significant manipulation was required to place them. To address this limitation, the addition of hydrophilic coats on the FasTracker catheter lubricated the surface, thereby reducing the friction and manipulation of placing the microcatheter.

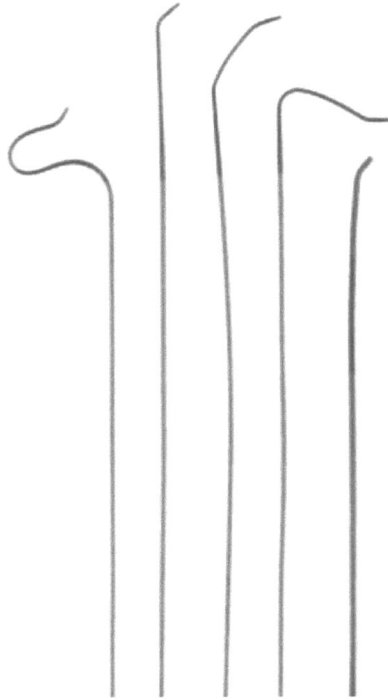

Figure 1: The Neuron family of guide catheters.

The Tracker catheters still had one major limitation. These catheters had liners made from polyethylene and lacked reinforcement. The polyethylene liners were fairly lubricious, but were not durable. This resulted in the liner being scored as coils passed through the lumen. This lumen scoring resulted in increased friction that eventually resulted in the inability to pass additional coils through the catheter. This usually happened after five to ten coils, and the catheter would need to be replaced. The second limitation was that these catheters had no proximal or distal reinforcement. When advancing through tortuous anatomy, this could result in ovalization or kinking of the distal end. When ovalization occurred, the friction and scoring of the liner during coil insertion was significantly increased, whereas a kinked catheter resulted in catheter replacement and the potential inability to treat if additional catheters could not be placed without kinking. The proximal end of these catheters relied only on stiff polymers. This limited the pushability and torqueability of these catheters.

In the mid 1990s the limitations of the Tracker catheters were addressed by the Transit and Rapid Transit (Cordis Corporation) microcatheters. These microcatheters featured a durable, lubricious polytetrafluoroethylene (PTFE) liner that would not score during coil insertion. They also had a distal platinum coil to decrease ovalization and increase kink resistance. The proximal end of the catheter used a stainless steel braid to maximize pushability and torqueability. As PTFE-lined and reinforced catheters gained acceptance, further improvements occurred in distal tip flexibility (Prowler, Cordis Corporation, and SL-10, Boston Scientific) using softer polymers and optimizing the distal reinforcement.

Guidewires

Like microcatheters, guidewires have undergone significant evolution. Due to the limitations of the original Tracker catheters, placing the catheter required three different guidewires. Physicians would start with a Taper (Target Therapeutics) wire. Once initial tortuosity was encountered, the Taper wire was replaced with a Seeker (Target Therapeutics). Once past the initial level of tortuosity, the Seeker was replaced with a Dasher (Target Therapeutics) wire. These wires all used stainless steel cores. The Dasher wire allowed the physician access to the lesion. The first guidewire innovation beyond these initial wires was the creation of the Instinct wire (Cordis Corporation). This wire had a lubricious PTFE coating and used a nitinol core wire. By using nitinol, the shape setting that was seen in the earlier stainless steel wires was eliminated. Next came the introduction of the FasDasher wire (Target Therapeutics). The FasDasher used both a hydrophilic coating and more advanced heat treatment to the stainless steel core. With the addition of the Instinct and FasDasher wires, physicians were generally then able to bring the microcatheter to the lesion with one wire. The FasDasher was still limited in torqueability due to its tendency to shape-set, while the nitinol core of the Instinct limited physicians to preshaped tips.

With the acquisition of Target Therapeutics by Boston Scientific, the guidewire design and processing knowledge gained from coronary interventions was applied to the neurovasculature. The addition of the Transcend (Boston Scientific) resulted in a hydrophilic wire that was shapeable by the physician with a high level of torque response. The next innovation in guidewires (Synchro, Precision

Vascular) was to replace the distal over-coil of the wire with a micro-machined hypo-tube. This advance allowed for a wire that provided one-to-one torque control even in tight anatomies.

Embolization

Coils

Aneurysm therapy can arguably be credited with ushering in the modern age of neurointervention. Prior to the advent of coiling, the means existed to perform minimally invasive surgery in the brain, namely femoral puncture and neuroendovascular access with flexible microcatheters. However, only rare and complex procedures were being performed, such as embolization of arteriovenous malformations (AVMs) with cyanoacrylate glue or polyvinyl alcohol (PVA) particles. With the advent of coiling, a major disease state, intracranial aneurysms, became amenable to minimally invasive treatment.

Historically, spherical balloons filled with various biocompatible substances were expanded in irregularly shaped aneurysms, often with disastrous results [2-4]. In the early 1990s, the introduction of the Gugliemi detachable coil (GDC) enabled safer, more controlled endovascular treatment of intracranial aneurysms (Fig. **2**) [5, 6]. Detachability was a crucial innovation in delicate brain aneurysms because it allowed the operating physician to have confidence in the safety and appropriate placement of the embolic material prior to releasing it in the aneurysm. The original GDC coil (Target Therapeutics) was a 0.015 inch diameter platinum coil that was pushed through microcatheters with 0.018-0.019 inch inner diameters. Hence, the coils were categorized as "18" system coils in reference to the size of the microcatheter that delivered them. These coils were relatively stiff due to the thick platinum filament that was necessary to prevent the coil from unraveling upon withdrawal. Thus these early coils were limited in their ability to pack the aneurysm sac densely. The polymer technology behind the 18-microcatheters of the time also contributed to relatively stiff microcatheter tips and thus limited control within the aneurysm sac.

The next phase of innovation in aneurysm coiling was miniaturization. Smaller microcatheters were developed with inner diameters of 0.015 inches (i.e. Prowler-10, Cordis Neurovascular) and 0.0165 inches (i.e. SL-10, Boston Scientific Neurovascular). These microcatheters were made with softer polymers and navigated to aneurysms and controlled within the aneurysms to a degree not possible with the older, larger catheters. Coils with 0.010 inch diameters were developed that were compatible with these microcatheters; however the nomenclature changed, and these coils were called "10" system coils, referring now to the coil's outer diameter, not the delivery microcatheter.

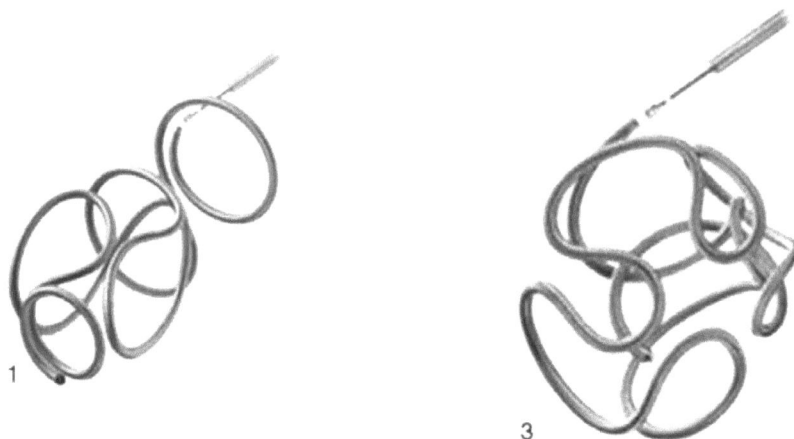

Figure 2: The bare platinum GDC 360° coil and GDC 10 3D coil which are available in 0.010-inch and 0.018-inch wire thickness or 0.010-inch wire thickness, respectively [54].

It is interesting to note that the physics of coils requires bending stiffness to be directly proportional to the filament size but inversely proportional to the outer diameter of the coil [7]. Thus, the smaller 0.010 inch "10" system coils, all other things being equal, would be stiffer in bending than the old 0.015 inch coils. To compensate for this increase in bending stiffness, the new 0.010 inch coils employed much thinner platinum filaments than had previously been used. As a predictable consequence, the "10" coils were weak in tension and prone to unravel during withdrawal. "Stretching," or unraveling of a coil during an intervention was not uncommon in the early days of "10" coils and could lead to serious consequences during the procedure including embolization of the downstream artery and the need for further intervention to retrieve the coil. The engineering response to this problem was the advent of the "stretch-resistant" feature in 0.010 inch coils. This innovation involved passing a suture of various materials, but commonly polypropylene, down the center lumen of the coil during the manufacturing process and securing it at both ends. Thus, tension could be placed on the coil during withdrawal and rather than that tension being resisted by the platinum coil loops, the inner tension member held the coil together. Stretch resistance ushered in the ability to develop extremely soft coils despite their small

0.010 inch diameter by using extremely fine platinum filament. The GDC Ultrasoft (Boston Scientific Neurovascular) was one of the first of this new generation of coils allowing for denser packing of aneurysms than previously achievable. In addition, these very soft coils, dubbed "finishing" coils, spawned a progressive coiling technique in which stiffer coils would be used initially to "frame" the aneurysm. Coils of medium softness were used to "fill" the aneurysm and finally the stretch-resistance-enabled "finishing" coils were used last resulting in a denser, more complete overall occlusion.

As 0.010 inch platinum coil technology was beginning to mature, a series of modifications to the bare metal coils were introduced. These modifications included hydrogel materials designed to swell in the presence of blood and progressively occlude the aneurysm. Bioabsorbable suture material was also introduced in various configurations, designed to dissolve over time and by virtue of elution of that material, induce a more aggressive healing cascade ideally concluding with the growth of new endothelial tissue across the aneurysm neck and thus cure of the aneurysm (Fig. **3**) [8].

Around the end of the first decade of the 21st century a series of randomized studies looking at the various modifications had all produced disappointing results [9-12]. Whether by increasing filling or by inducing a bioactive healing cascade, these technologies failed to satisfy the hope of improved, long-term durability of treatment. Other bare platinum coils introduced during the same period reversed the trend in coil diameter reduction. The Orbit coil (Cordis Neurovascular) was a 0.012 inch diameter coil deliverable through the same "10"-system microcatheters already on the market. The Orbit coil took advantage of the greater volume filling and softness inherent in larger diameters. This trend reversal found its ultimate conclusion for "10" system coils in the Cashmere coil (Micrus Endovascular). The Cashmere was 0.014 inches in diameter and, using stretch resistance to maintain coil integrity, combined the benefits of a very fine platinum filament and larger diameter to create a particularly soft and supple coil resulting in dense aneurysm packing.

A further innovation in aneurysm coiling was introduced in the years following the failed trials of modified coils. The Penumbra Coil 400 (Penumbra, Inc.) is a 0.020 inch diameter coil, breaking the trend of coil size limited by "10" size delivery microcatheters (Fig. **4**). The Penumbra Coil 400 introduced several innovations at once [13]. A specialized, compatible microcatheter with an 0.025 inch inner diameter, the PX Slim (Penumbra, Inc.) was developed using the latest polymer materials and reinforcement design enabling tip softness equivalent to that of the smaller "10" size microcatheters despite its larger size. The Penumbra Coil also made use of a nitinol stretch resistance tension element instead of suture which enabled various softness levels and further carried the overall helical or spherical shape of the coil. Finally, this nitinol stretch-resistance wire, combined with another nitinol coil mounted inside the platinum coil, holds the promise of resisting coil mass compaction and thus aneurysm recurrence by virtue of its super-elastic, shape memory property. The Penumbra Coil, due to the combination of large volume, very soft bending resistance and nitinol inner elements promises more efficient aneurysm occlusion due to higher packing densities and lower recanalization rates, with dramatically fewer coils and shorter procedure times at reduced cost [14].

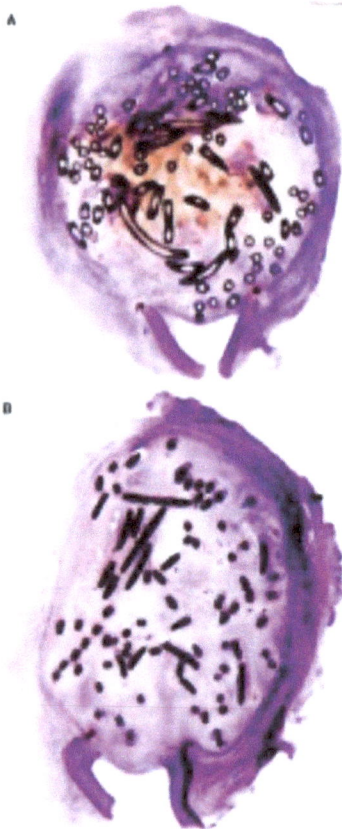

Figure 3: Growth of new endothelial tissue across the aneurysm neck shown in hematoxylin and eosin-stained light microscopic images of the aneurysm 14 days after embolization with GDC coils (A) or Matrix coils (B) [8].

In recent years, non-coil intrasaccular solutions for aneurysm occlusion have been introduced. Web (Sequent Medical) is a multi-layer, nitinol, cylindrical, closed-end mesh which is collapsed for microcatheter delivery and expands radially when deployed in the aneurysm [15-17]. Another device with similar technology is the Luna device (NFocus Medical) which is a spherical nitinol basket designed to match the inner surface of the aneurysm sac (Fig. **5**) [18, 19]. Studies of these products in multicenter experiences continue.

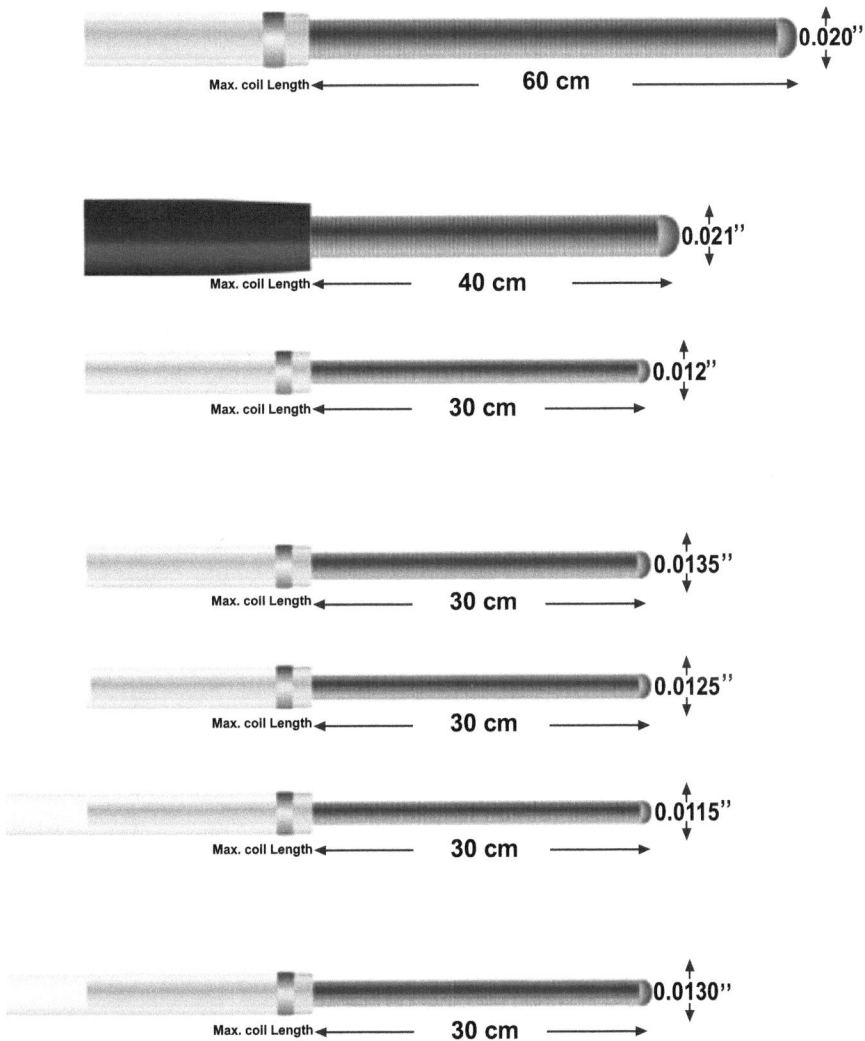

Figure 4: Penumbra 0.020 inch platinum PC 400 coil platform.

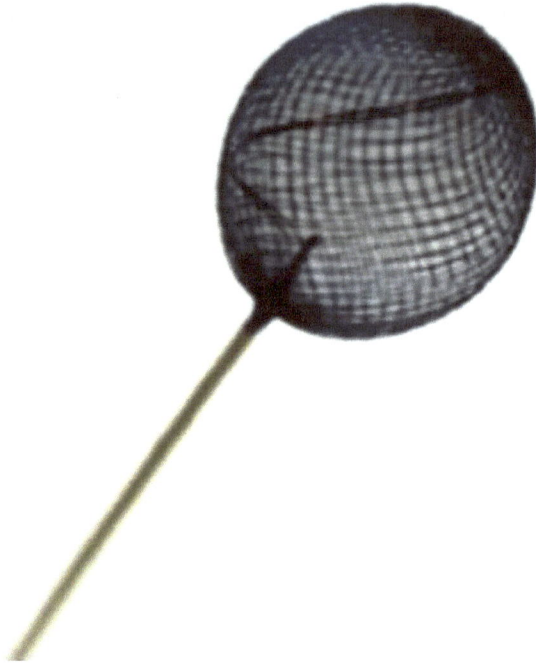

Figure 5: Luna AES, "a self-expanding ovoid ball-like implant" [19].

Stents

In the late 1990s, while several companies were pursuing various modifications of the shape and surface of platinum coils, one start-up company, Smart Therapeutics, was pursuing parent vessel reconstruction *via* the Neuroform stent. Neuroform was the first self-expanding, microcatheter-deliverable stent designed specifically for delivery and implantation in the neurovasculature (Fig. **6**) [20-22]. The pursuit of parent vessel reconstruction was informed by the belief that the central problem in aneurysm pathophysiology was not the dome but rather the neck of the aneurysm. Addressing the aneurysm neck would not only improve coil retention within the aneurysm but also modify flow. An early indication of this potential was noted serendipitously during the Neuroform trial. A blister aneurysm of the middle cerebral artery was covered by a Neuroform stent during stent-assisted coil treatment of the index aneurysm in the ICA. At the six-month follow up, not only was the ICA aneurysm well healed, but the middle cerebral artery blister aneurysm was also healed despite placement of a Neuroform stent with only 7% surface coverage and no coils.

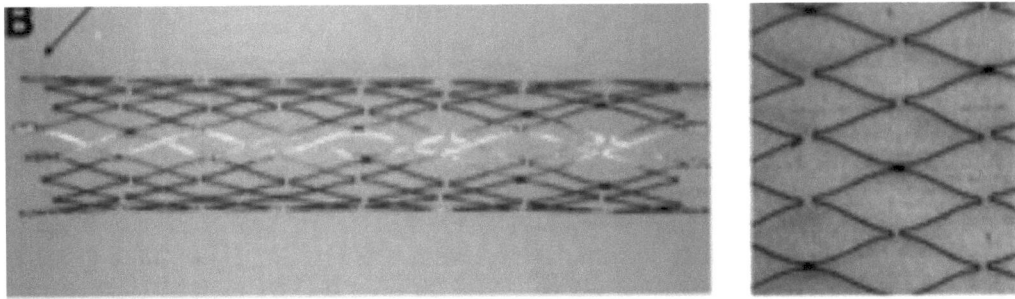

Neuroform - Semi-open Cell Design

Figure 6: The Neuroform stent was the first intracranial stent for aneurysm treatment and featured a semi-open cell design [55].

The Neuroform stent, cleared by the Food and Drug Administration in 2002, ushered in the era of parent vessel reconstruction and stent-assisted coiling of wide neck aneurysms. The strut width of the Neuroform was 75 microns, which coincided with three concurrent facts. First, literature on neuroanatomy indicated that important perforating arteries had a cross-sectional diameter of 150 microns. Second, laws of fluid dynamics indicated that half the cross-sectional diameter of a vessel could be obstructed without significantly compromising flow within that vessel. And third, chemical etching and electro-polishing techniques had recently been invented that allowed nitinol to be worked with at a thickness of 75 microns without compromising its super-elastic and shape memory properties.

Neuroform became the standard tool for stent-assisted coiling and was later joined by the Enterprise stent (Cordis Neurovascular) [23]. The Enterprise stent was also manufactured from laser cut, nitinol hypo-tube but was differentiated from Neuroform by its closed-cell design, which allowed its central advantage of being able to be re-sheathed (Fig. **7**). The advantages of conformability that Neuroform's open-cell design offered were offset by the possible opening of a strut segment into a wide aneurysm neck when positioned on the outside of a curve (see Fig. **8A**). Similarly, the resheathability offered by the closed-cell design of the Enterprise stent was offset by the lack of conformability and easy kinking when placed within bends (Fig. **8B**).

In the decade since the Food and Drug Aministration's clearance of the Neuroform stent, much advancements have occurred in nitinol processing. While continuing to push the envelope of technology, the Liberty stent (Penumbra, Inc.) now has struts of 20 micron thickness which enable supple microcatheters to insinuate themselves across the high mesh density plane and enter the aneurysm neck for the placement of coils. The novel design of the stent allows much greater surface coverage as compared to Neuroform or Enterprise, a completely conformable yet fully resheathable device that does not kink on a curve, and a stent with excellent wall opposition (Fig. **9**). This device is currently undergoing an international clinical study for regulatory approval as a next-generation, stent-assisted coiling implant [24].

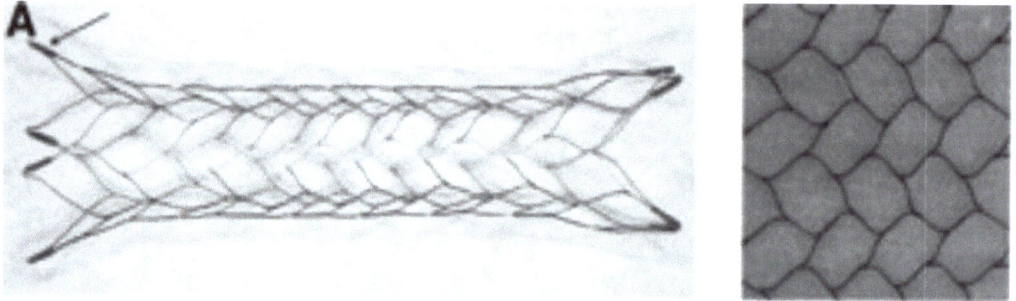

Enterprise - Closed Cell Design

Figure 7: The Enterprise stent was also a laser cut, nitinol hypo-tube but was differentiated from Neuroform by its closed cell design [55].

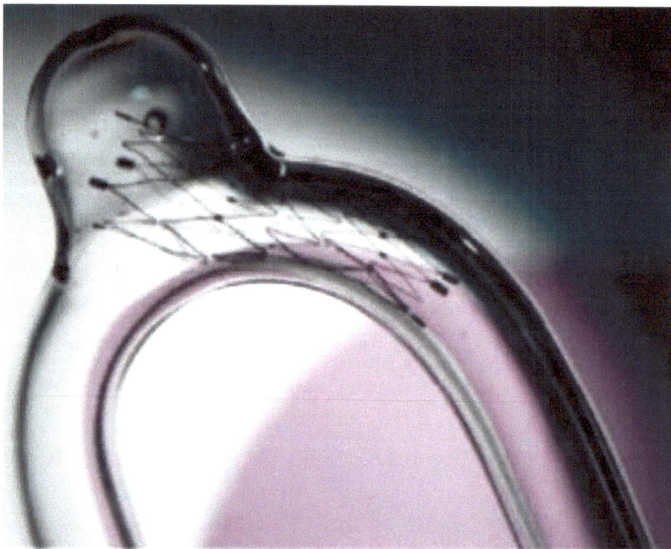

Figure 8A: The advantages of conformability that Neuroform's open cell design offered were offset by a possible displacement of the end of the stent into a wide aneurysm neck shown in an aneurysm model [56].

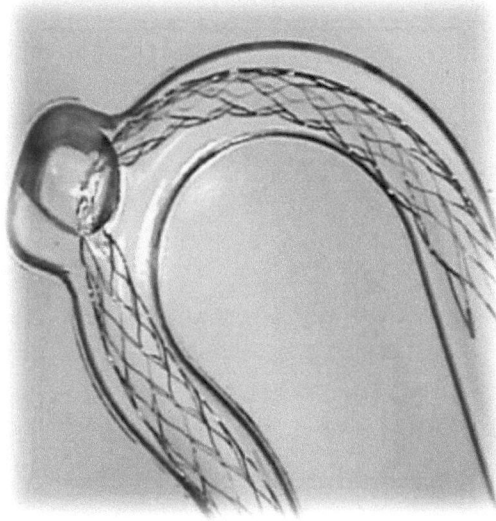

Figure 8B: Resheathability offered by the closed cell design of the Enterprise stent was offset by the lack of conformability and easy kinking when placed within bends.

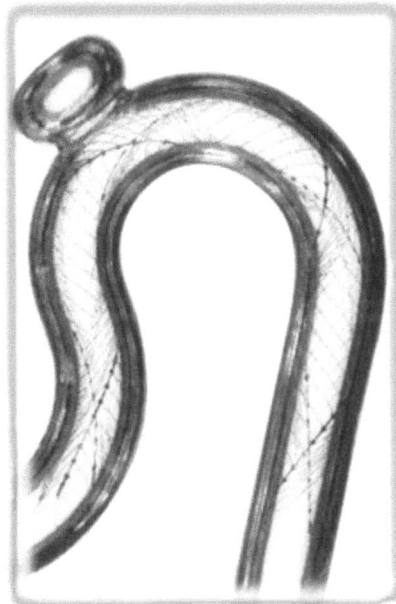

Figure 9: The novel design of the Liberty stent, including advanced nitinol technology, provides robust radial force, while its hybrid cell structure and helical twist confer conformability to vessel curvature. A Liberty device within a glass aneurysm model shows optimized coverage of the aneurysm neck, minimal foreshortening and excellent wall apposition.

Another class of devices, dubbed flow diverters, has been added to the neurointerventional toolkit in recent years: these devices include Silk (Balt) [25], Pipeline (Covidien) [26-29], and Surpass (Stryker) [30] (Figs. **10** and **11**). These densely woven wire-based devices disrupt flow at the aneurysm neck in an attempt to enhance stagnation of blood in the sac and thus trigger the thrombosis-based healing cascade without the use of intrasaccular embolic material. There were some stunning successes in otherwise untreatable giant and fusiform ICA aneurysms in the early experience with these devices (Fig. **12**) [31, 32]. As their use broadened globally to smaller, posterior, and more distal anterior aneurysms, the results became more mixed. Delayed rupture of some previously asymptomatic unruptured aneurysms caused concern, as did unexplained distal parenchymal hemorrhages in the territory of the stent placement [33-36]. As a reaction to these complications, many operators began placing embolic coils behind the flow diverter, especially for larger intradural aneurysms, to enhance the immediate occlusion of the aneurysm sac and, it was hoped, to prevent complications. Many questions about the indications, acute, and long-term outcomes of flow diverters remain, and studies of the various products are ongoing.

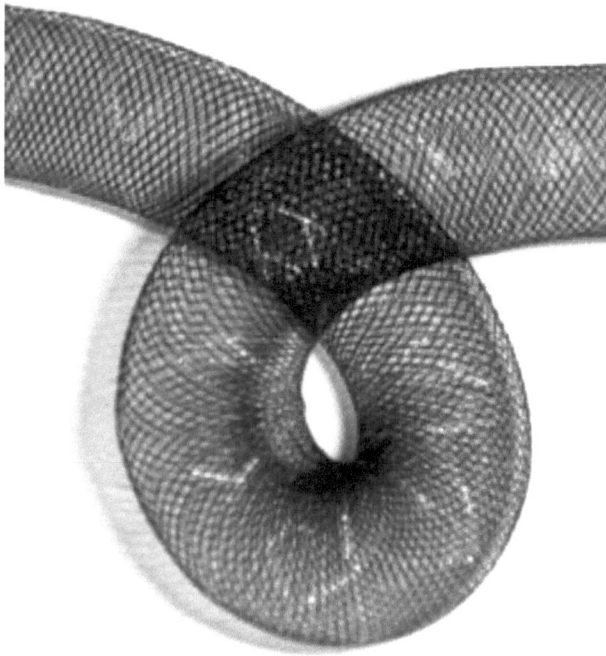

Figure 10: Silk flow diverter [25].

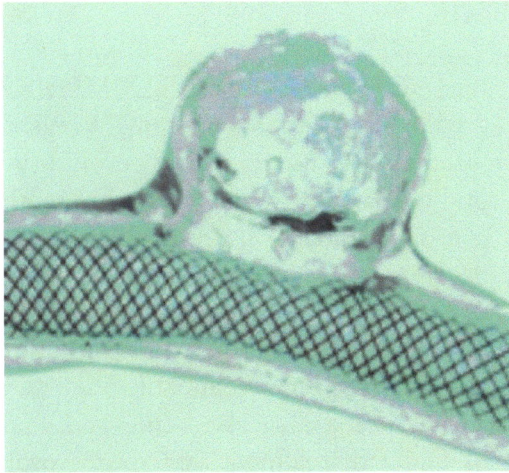

Figure 11: Pipeline flow diverter which aims to disrupt flow at the aneurysm neck [57].

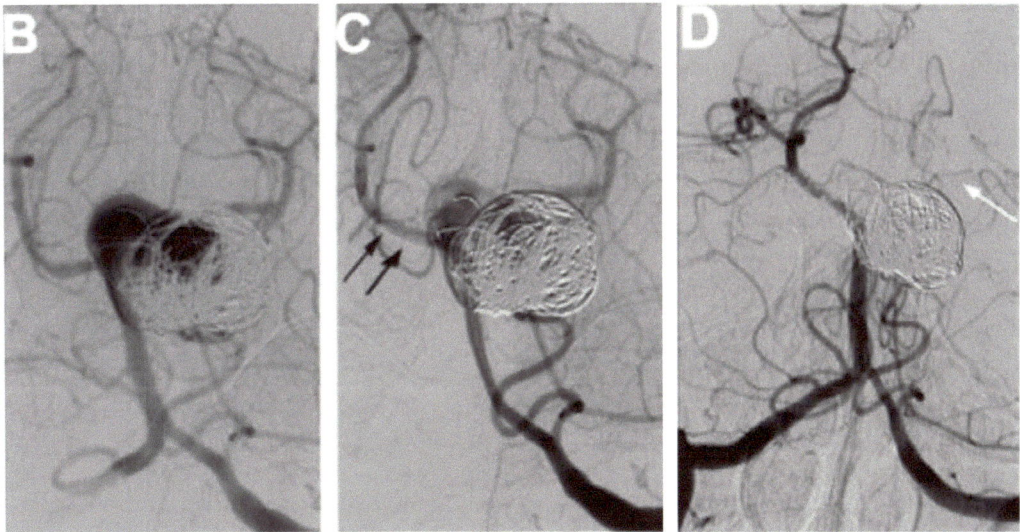

Figure 12: Angiogram showing the left vertebral artery demonstrates partial coil occlusion of the dome of a giant, distal basilar aneurysm incorporating the left P1 segment (B). Angiogram immediately following placement of a single Pipeline embolization device (PED) from the mid-basilar to the right posterior cerebral artery (PCA) (arrows) showing a slight decrease in intra-aneurysmal flow, as evidenced by diminished contrast density within the aneurysm cavity (C). Angiogram several minutes following PED placement showing occlusion in the aneurysm cavity and the left PCA (arrow), along with thrombus formation within the PED in the right PCA (D) [32].

REVASCULARIZATION

There has now been one randomized trial, SAMMPRIS, demonstrating that angioplasty and stenting with a self-expanding stent, Wingspan (Boston Scientific Neurovascular) is not effective in reducing the morbidity and mortality from intracranial atherosclerotic disease [37]. The results of another randomized trial, VISSIT, which was a phase III study of the Pharos Vitesse Neurovascular Stent System (Codman Neurovascular) compared to best medical therapy for the treatment of intracranial atherosclerotic disease, were recently presented. This trial reached the same conclusion with the use of a balloon expandable stent [38]. It is interesting to note that the balloon expandable stent fared much worse than the self-expanding stent in these trials. The Wingspan stenting procedure was based on the premise of targeted treatment of the atherosclerotic segment with Wingspan, after pre-dilatation to 80% of the parent vessel diameter with the Gateway balloon, and no post-dilatation [39, 40]. The Wingspan stent was moderately oversized to allow for adequate wall apposition and the potential for ongoing positive remodeling force on the atherosclerotic lesion (Fig. **13**).

Since the development of the Wingspan system for the treatment of intracranial atherosclerotic disease, there have been many pharmacological advances in the treatment of this disease. With the advent of aspirin and clopidogrel as antiplatelet agents, the commonplace use of statins, and tighter control of hypertension and diabetes, modern medical management has dramatically reduced the need for device-based revascularization for intracranial atherosclerotic disease since the time of the Warfarin-Aspirin Symptomatic Intracranial Disease (WASID) study [41].

Thrombectomy

If aneurysm coiling ushered in the modern era of neurointervention, then acute stroke thrombectomy is ushering in its future. Only 3-5% of strokes are caused by bleeding in the subarachnoid space due to aneurysm rupture. Approximately 87% of strokes are ischemic in nature due to extracranial embolus, *in-situ* thrombosis, or other causes. Although neurointerventional treatment of strokes is limited today to substantial clot burden located within the large vessels of the Circle of Willis, and treated within eight hours of symptom onset, this subset still represents at least *ten-fold* more patients than the whole of the treated aneurysm population. Ischemic stroke thrombectomy remains by far the largest opportunity for expansion of the neuroendovascular profession, as well as for having a positive impact on patients' lives.

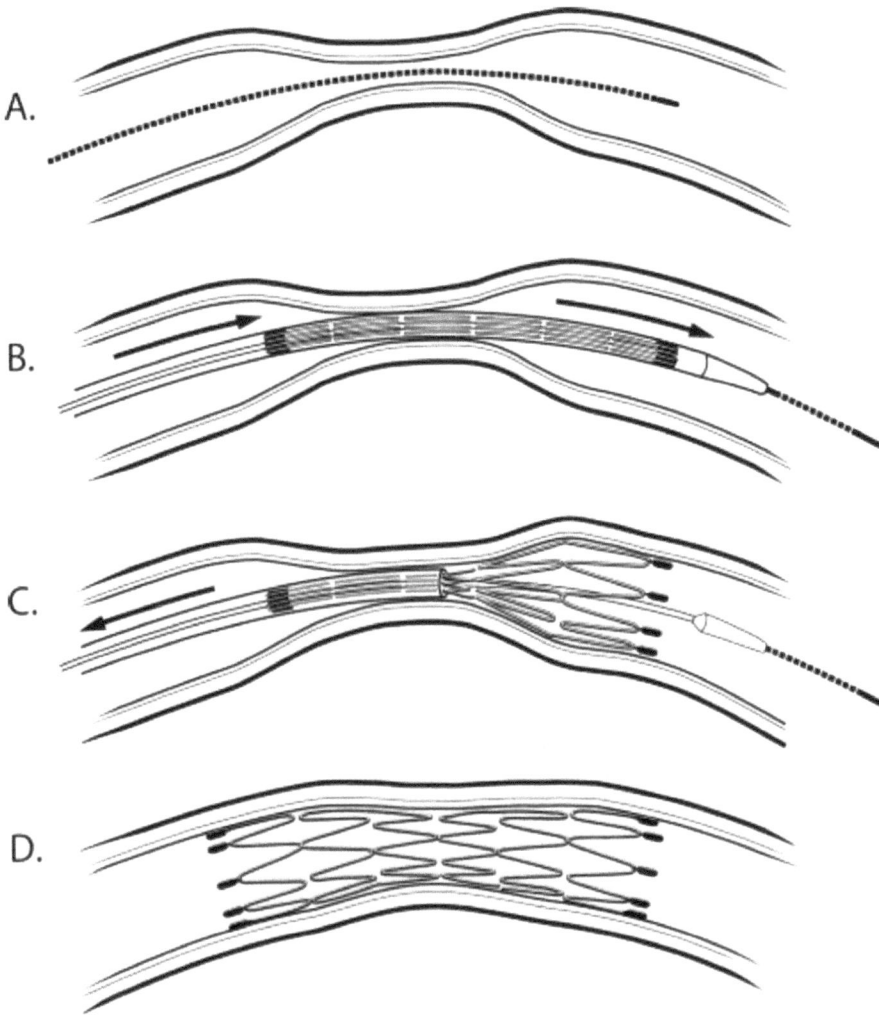

Figure 13: The self-expanding Wingspan stent designed for targeted treatment of the atherosclerotic segment in patients with intracranial atherosclerotic disease [40].

Thrombectomy of clots causing an ischemic event has been a legitimate procedure since catheters were first placed in the neurovasculature. Gerhard Schroth first described catheter-based suction thrombectomy as early as the late 1980s. Basic aspiration would remain central to neurointerventional thrombectomy since that time. In 2004, the first product specifically designed for thrombectomy in acute stroke patients, called the Merci Retriever (Concentric Medical), was launched after clearance from the Food and Drug Administration. The first generation 'X' devices resembled a wire in the shape of a corkscrew, which was deployed inside the clot in an effort to engage and grab the clot, enabling it to be pulled out of the body. A balloon-tipped guide catheter would be placed in the ICA and inflated prior to removing the Merci completely. Aspiration was then placed on the balloon guide to capture residual emboli and thrombus not retained by the Merci. Later generations, including the "L" and "K-mini" devices, varied the shape of the grabber wire, also adding suture strands to help engage the clot. The Merci device was only moderately successful in the marketplace being somewhat difficult to use with consistent success. Complete or mostly complete revascularization of the brain (TICI 2A-3 or TIMI 2/3) was achieved in only 48% of cases in a major study [42].

Four years later, in January 2008, the Penumbra System (Penumbra, Inc.) became available in the United States. The Penumbra System used aspiration as its primary mode of operation. A flexible, large-bore microcatheter was delivered to the site of occlusion and aspiration placed directly on the lesion itself. However, the early Penumbra System catheters, the largest of which was 0.041 inches in internal diameter, were not quite big enough to avoid becoming clogged by clot burden and so another component, a Separator, was introduced and moved back and forth at the tip of the microcatheter to continually break up and macerate the clot once ingested under aspiration. Without the Separator, the early microcatheters would clog, necessitating removal and clearance, a tedious process. Thus the Separator allowed continuous thrombectomy under constant aspiration supplied by an external vacuum pump. This system improved the rate of successful revascularization to 81.6% in the Pivotal trial for Food and Drug Administration approval [43], which further increased to 87% in the real-world POST trial [44].

Further innovation in the Penumbra System line included the Reperfusion Catheter 054, a larger bore version of the 041, including a mid-shaft inner diameter taper that increased to 0.064 inches, which further increased the flow rate over the distal tip enlargement alone [45]. Next came a refinement of the whole line of Penumbra System catheters called MAX. This technology consisted of softer polymers, enhanced nitinol reinforcement, and a greater number of stiffness transitions to make navigation to the site of occlusion much easier [46].

In this same time frame, a variety of stent retrievers were introduced including the Solitaire FR (Covidien) and the Trevo (Concentric Medical). Stent retrievers built on the mode of action of the MERCI Retriever, as far as utilizing a distal grabber to engage the clot and a proximal balloon guide to aspirate through, as the retriever was withdrawn. The grabber devices in this case are cylindrical constructs in the shape of a non-implantable stent, which are deployed within the clot. These devices fared better than their older predecessor, the MERCI Retriever, successfully removing the clot in 68.5% of cases when the Solitaire was used [47] and in 86% of cases when the Trevo was used [48].

As the concept of distal grabbers combined with proximal aspiration experienced a renaissance following the days of the MERCI Retriever, a new concept was elaborated by Turk *et al.* called ADAPT: A Direct Aspiration first Pass Technique [49]. ADAPT is a systematic approach to treating large vessel occlusion in the brain whereby a large-bore aspiration catheter, usually the 5MAX (Penumbra, Inc.) is introduced to the site of occlusion and the clot is suctioned with no adjunctive product usage, including the Penumbra Separator. The clot is usually engaged deep into the catheter *en bloc*, retaining the clot's integrity and allowing complete removal without distal emboli by fully withdrawing the catheter from the body. In fact, the authors reported a 97% rate of successful revascularization (TICI 2B-3) and a never-before-seen rate of complete revascularization, solely TICI 3, of 65%. This quest for perfect revascularization, TICI 3, became the new standard. The outcome numbers reported earlier, and used historically in the field to represent "successful" revascularization, included TICI 2A or TIMI 2. This means that one half of the middle cerebral artery area could remain occluded and yet the revascularization would still be counted as "successful". This standard may have been considered useful for the purposes of clinical trials, but the patient would not have found the outcome satisfactory. Tools and techniques were then available which allowed fast, easy, and complete clot removal to become commonplace.

Within a few months of publication of the ADAPT technique, another significant innovation was released, the ACE catheter (Penumbra, Inc.). ACE revolutionized acute stroke thrombectomy. Now with an 0.060 inch distal internal diameter, and building upon all the polymer and reinforcement technology improvements of the MAX line, the ACE catheter could easily reach the territory of the middle cerebral artery over a mere microcatheter, and had the aspiration capacity to often fully ingest and remove the clot from the body without further manipulation or withdrawal of the catheter (Fig. **14**). This means that a large lumen catheter is still available at the clot site to deliver any back-up or adjunctive products needed should ACE alone fail to work. As reported at the ABC-WIN conference in Val d'Isere, France in 2014, ACE achieved TICI 2B/3 (not including TICI 2A) in 96% of cases, while the incidence of perfect revascularization, TICI 3, remains very high at 66% [50-52].

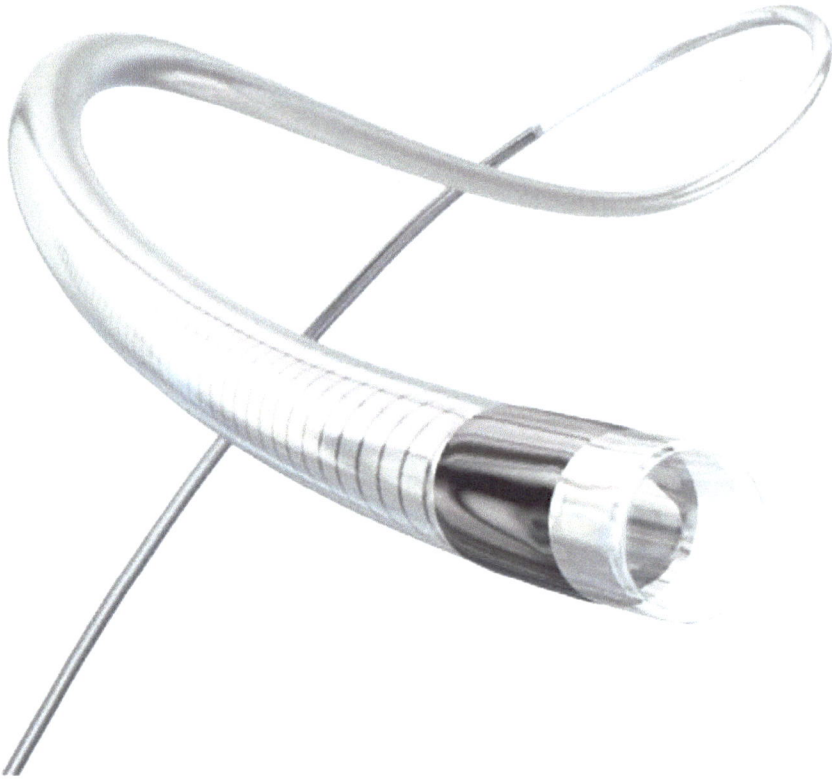

Figure 14: The novel ACE™ catheter which has the aspiration capacity to frequently fully ingest and remove intracranial thrombus without further manipulation or withdrawal of the catheter.

We have reached an age in which the question is no longer "Can we remove the clot?", but is "How well can we remove the clot?" There is now a wide variety of modalities and devices that can be used to remove a clot causing an acute ischemic stroke [53]. The number of untreated stroke patients who languish, dying or disabled, in hospitals and rehabilitation facilities today is in the hundreds of thousands in the United States alone, and many times that around the world. Treating these patients - completely removing the clot causing their stroke - and giving them better than a fifty-fifty chance of continuing their life without severe disability, is now an imperative in our society. We have a moral mandate as neurointerventional physicians to use the tools at our disposal, which are simple, safe, and highly effective, to save patients from death and disability in numbers an order of magnitude higher than those suffering from ruptured intracranial aneurysms. This will be the future and the dominant calling of the neurointerventional profession from now on.

ACKNOWLEDGEMENTS

The preparation of this chapter was funded by Penumbra Inc.

CONFLICT OF INTEREST

JL, DB, and SK are full-time employees of Penumbra Inc. AB is the chairman, founder, and chief medical officer of Penumbra Inc.

REFERENCES

[1]   Turk A, Manzoor MU, Nyberg EM, Turner RD, Chaudry I. Initial experience with distal guide catheter placement in the treatment of cerebrovascular disease: clinical safety and efficacy. J Neurointerv Surg 2013; 5: 247-52.

[2]   Serbinenko FA. Balloon catheterization and occlusion of major cerebral vessels. J Neurosurg 1974; 41: 125-45.

[3]   Monsein LH, Debrun GM, Chazaly JR. Hydroxyethyl methylacrylate and latex balloons. AJNR Am J Neuroradiol 1990; 11: 663-4.

[4]   Yang X, Wu Z, Li Y, *et al*. Re-evaluation of cellulose acetate polymer: angiographic findings and histological studies. Surg Neurol 2001; 55: 116-22.

[5]   Guglielmi G, Viñuela F, Sepetka I, Macellari V. Electrothrombosis of saccular aneurysms *via* endovascular approach. Part 1: Electrochemical basis, technique, and experimental results. J Neurosurg 1991; 75: 1-7.

[6]   Guglielmi G, Viñuela F, Dion J, Duckwiler G. Electrothrombosis of saccular aneurysms *via* endovascular approach. Part 2: Preliminary clinical experience. J Neurosurg 1991; 75: 8-14.

[7]   White JB, Ken CG, Cloft HJ, Kallmes DF. Coils in a nutshell: a review of coil physical properties. AJNR Am J Neuroradiol 2008; 29: 1242-6.

[8]   Murayama Y, Tateshima S, Gonzalez NR, Vinuela F. Matrix and bioabsorbable polymeric coils accelerate healing of intracranial aneurysms: long-term experimental study. Stroke 2003; 34: 2031-7.

[9]   Molyneux AJ, Clarke A, Sneade M, *et al*. Cerecyte coil trial: angiographic outcomes of a prospective randomized trial comparing endovascular coiling of cerebral aneurysms with either cerecyte or bare platinum coils. Stroke 2012; 43: 2544-50.

[10]   Coley S, Sneade M, Clarke A, *et al*. Cerecyte coil trial: procedural safety and clinical outcomes in patients with ruptured and unruptured intracranial aneurysms. AJNR Am J Neuroradiol 2012; 33: 474-80.

[11]   White PM, Lewis SC, Gholkar A, *et al*.; HELPS trial collaborators. Hydrogel-coated coils versus bare platinum coils for the endovascular treatment of intracranial aneurysms (HELPS): a randomised controlled trial. Lancet 2011; 377: 1655-62.

[12]   White PM, Lewis SC, Nahser H, Sellar RJ, Goddard T, Gholkar A; HELPS Trial Collaboration. HydroCoil Endovascular Aneurysm Occlusion and Packing Study (HELPS trial): procedural safety and operator-assessed efficacy results. AJNR Am J Neuroradiol 2008; 29: 217-23.

[13]   Mascitelli JR, Polykarpou MF, Patel AA, Kamath AA, Moyle H, Patel AB. Initial experience with Penumbra Coil 400 versus standard coils in embolization of cerebral aneurysms: a retrospective review. J Neurointerv Surg 2013; 5: 573-6.

[14]   Milburn J, Pansara AL, Vidal G, Martinez RC. Initial experience using the Penumbra coil 400: comparison of aneurysm packing, cost effectiveness, and coil efficiency. J Neurointerv Surg 2014; 6: 121-4.

[15]   Lubicz B, Klisch J, Gauvrit JY, *et al*. WEB-DL endovascular treatment of wide-neck bifurcation aneurysms: short- and midterm results in a European study. AJNR Am J Neuroradiol 2014; 35: 432-8.

[16]   Pierot L, Klisch J, Cognard C, *et al*. Endovascular WEB flow disruption in middle cerebral artery aneurysms: preliminary feasibility, clinical, and anatomical results in a multicenter study. Neurosurgery 2013; 73: 27-34; discussion 34-5.

[17]   Lubicz B, Mine B, Collignon L, Brisbois D, Duckwiler G, Strother C. WEB device for endovascular treatment of wide-neck bifurcation aneurysms. AJNR Am J Neuroradiol 2013; 34: 1209-14.

[18]   Turk AS, Turner RD, Chaudry MI. Evaluation of the Nfocus LUNA, a new parent vessel occlusion device: a comparative study in a canine model. Neurosurgery 2011; 69(1 Suppl Operative): ons20-6.

[19]   Kwon SC, Ding YH, Dai D, Kadirvel R, Lewis DA, Kallmes DF. Preliminary results of the luna aneurysm embolization system in a rabbit model: a new intrasaccular aneurysm occlusion device. AJNR Am J Neuroradiol 2011; 32: 602-6.

[20]   Biondi A, Janardhan V, Katz JM, Salvaggio K, Riina HA, Gobin YP. Neuroform stent-assisted coil embolization of wide-neck intracranial aneurysms: strategies in stent deployment and midterm follow-up. Neurosurgery 2007; 61: 460-8.

[21]   Lylyk P, Ferrario A, Pasbón B, Miranda C, Doroszuk G. Buenos Aires experience with the Neuroform self-expanding stent for the treatment of intracranial aneurysms. J Neurosurg 2005; 102: 235-41.

[22]   Brisman JL, Song JK, Niimi Y, Berenstein A. Treatment options for wide-necked intracranial aneurysms using a self-expanding hydrophilic coil and a self-expandable stent combination. AJNR Am J Neuroradiol 2005; 26: 1237-40.

[23]   Higashida RT, Halbach VV, Dowd CF, Juravsky L, Meagher S. Initial clinical experience with a new self-expanding nitinol stent for the treatment of intracranial cerebral aneurysms: the Cordis Enterprise stent. AJNR Am J Neuroradiol 2005; 26: 1751-6.

[24]   Lopes D, Woo H, Barraza L, Sit S, Bose A for the Penumbra Liberty trial investigators. The Penumbra Liberty trial: safety and effectiveness in the treatment of wide-neck intracranial aneurysms. Presented at the AANS Meeting, New Orleans, LA, April 2013.

[25]   Kulcsár Z, Ernemann U, Wetzel SG, *et al*. High-profile flow diverter (silk) implantation in the basilar artery: efficacy in the treatment of aneurysms and the role of the perforators. Stroke 2010; 41: 1690-6.

[26]   Becske T, Kallmes DF, Saatci I, *et al*. Pipeline for uncoilable or failed aneurysms: results from a multicenter clinical trial. Radiology 2013; 267: 858-68.

[27]   Nelson PK, Lylyk P, Szikora I, Wetzel SG, Wanke I, Fiorella D. The pipeline embolization device for the intracranial treatment of aneurysms trial. AJNR Am J Neuroradiol 2011; 32: 34-40.

[28]   McAuliffe W, Wycoco V, Rice H, Phatouros C, Singh TJ, Wenderoth J. Immediate and midterm results following treatment of unruptured intracranial aneurysms with the pipeline embolization device. AJNR Am J Neuroradiol 2012; 33: 164-70.

[29]   Phillips TJ, Wenderoth JD, Phatouros CC, *et al*. Safety of the pipeline embolization device in treatment of posterior circulation aneurysms. AJNR Am J Neuroradiol 2012; 33: 1225-31.

[30]   De Vries J, Boogaarts J, Van Norden A, Wakhloo AK. New generation of flow diverter (surpass) for unruptured intracranial aneurysms: a prospective single-center study in 37 patients. Stroke 2013; 44: 1567-77.

[31]   Sise AB, Osher JM, Kolsky MP, Stemer A, Bank WO, Garfinkel RA. Pipeline embolization device: a new source for embolic retinal vascular occlusion. J Neuroophthalmol 2013; 33: 373-6.

[32]   Lall RR, Crobeddu E, Lanzino G, Cloft HJ, Kallmes DF. Acute branch occlusion after Pipeline embolization of intracranial aneurysms. J Clin Neurosci 2014; 21: 668-72.

[33]   Turowski B, Macht S, Kulcsár Z, Hänggi D, Stummer W. Early fatal hemorrhage after endovascular cerebral aneurysm treatment with a flow diverter (SILK-Stent): do we need to rethink our concepts? Neuroradiology 2011; 53: 37-41.

[34]   Fargen KM, Velat GJ, Lawson MF, Mocco J, Hoh BL. Review of reported complications associated with the Pipeline Embolization Device. World Neurosurg 2012; 77: 403-4.

[35]   Cruz JP, Chow M, O'Kelly C, *et al*. Delayed ipsilateral parenchymal hemorrhage following flow diversion for the treatment of anterior circulation aneurysms. AJNR Am J Neuroradiol 2012; 33: 603-8.

[36]   Siddiqui AH, Abla AA, Kan P, *et al*. Panacea or problem: flow diverters in the treatment of symptomatic large or giant fusiform vertebrobasilar aneurysms. J Neurosurg 2012; 116: 1258-66.

[37]   Derdeyn CP, Chimowitz MI, Lynn MJ, *et al*; Stenting and Aggressive Medical Management for Preventing Recurrent Stroke in Intracranial Stenosis Trial Investigators. Aggressive medical treatment with or without stenting in high-risk patients with intracranial artery stenosis (SAMMPRIS): the final results of a randomised trial. Lancet 2014; 383: 333-41.

[38]   Zaidat OO, Castonguay AC, Fitzsimmons BF, *et al*; VISSIT Trial Investigators. Design of the Vitesse Intracranial Stent Study for Ischemic Therapy (VISSIT) trial in symptomatic intracranial stenosis. J Stroke Cerebrovasc Dis 2013; 22: 1131-9.

[39]   Henkes H, Miloslavski E, Lowens S, Reinartz J, Liebig T, Kühne D. Treatment of intracranial atherosclerotic stenoses with balloon dilatation and self-expanding stent deployment (WingSpan). Neuroradiology 2005; 47: 222-8.

[40]   Fiorella D, Levy EI, Turk AS, *et al*. US multicenter experience with the wingspan stent system for the treatment of intracranial atheromatous disease: periprocedural results. Stroke 2007; 38: 881-7.

[41]   Chimowitz MI, Kokkinos J, Strong J, *et al*. The Warfarin-Aspirin Symptomatic Intracranial Disease Study. Neurology 1995; 45: 1488-93.

[42]   Smith WS, Sung G, Starkman S, *et al*; MERCI Trial Investigators. Safety and efficacy of mechanical embolectomy in acute ischemic stroke: results of the MERCI trial. Stroke 2005; 36: 1432-8.

[43]   Penumbra Pivotal Stroke Trial Investigators. The Penumbra Pivotal stroke trial: safety and effectiveness of a new generation of mechanical devices for clot removal in intracranial large vessel occlusive disease. Stroke 2009; 40: 2761-8.

[44]   Tarr R, Hsu D, Kulcsar Z, *et al*. The POST trial: initial post-market experience of the Penumbra system. Revascularization of large vessel occlusion in acute ischemic stroke in the United States and Europe. J Neurointerv Surg 2010; 2: 341-4.

[45]   Frei D, Gerber J, Turk A, *et al*. The SPEED study: initial clinical evaluation of the Penumbra novel 054 Reperfusion Catheter. J Neurointerv Surg 2013; 5 (Suppl 1): i74-6.

[46]   Farkas J, Arcot KM, Walzman DE, *et al*. Initial clinical experience with the Penumbra 4MAX and 3MAX reperfusion catheters for acute stroke intervention. Presented at the SVIN Meeting, Miami, FL, October 2012.

[47]   Saver JL, Jahan R, Levy EI, *et al*; SWIFT Trialists. Solitaire flow restoration device versus the Merci Retriever in patients with acute ischaemic stroke (SWIFT): a randomised, parallel-group, non-inferiority trial. Lancet 2012; 380: 1241-9.

[48]   Nogueira RG, Lutsep HL, Gupta R, *et al*; TREVO 2 Trialists. Trevo versus Merci retrievers for thrombectomy revascularisation of large vessel occlusions in acute ischaemic stroke (TREVO 2): a randomised trial. Lancet 2012; 380: 1231-40. Erratum in: Lancet 2012; 380(9849): 1230.

[49]   Turk AS, Spiotta A, Frei D, *et al*. Initial clinical experience with the ADAPT technique: a direct aspiration first pass technique for stroke thrombectomy. J Neurointerv Surg 2014; 6: 231-7.

[50]   Turk A. The US multi-center ADAPT technique experience. Paper presented at: ABC-WIN Seminar, January 19-24, 2014; Val d'Isère, France.

[51]   Frei D. Prospective stroke thrombectomy experience in a busy US stroke center in 100 consecutive patients in 2013. Paper presented at: ABC-WIN Seminar, January 19-24, 2014; Val d'Isère, France.

[52]   Farkas J, Arcot K, Azhar S, Janjua S. Initial clinical experience of the Penumbra ACE Reperfusion Catheter in acute ischemic stroke therapy. Paper presented at: ABC-WIN Seminar, January 19-24, 2014; Val d'Isère, France.

[53]   Spiotta AM, Chaudry MI, Hui FK, Turner RD, Kellogg RT, Turk AS. Evolution of thrombectomy approaches and devices for acute stroke: a technical review. J Neurointerv Surg 2014; Jan 2 [Epub ahead of print].

[54]   van Rooij WJ, Sluzewski M. Packing performance of GDC 360 degrees coils in intracranial aneurysms: a comparison with complex orbit coils and helical GDC 10 coils. AJNR Am J Neuroradiol 2007; 28: 368-70.

[55]   Wakhloo AK, Deleo MJ 3rd, Brown MM. Advances in interventional neuroradiology. Stroke 2009; 40: e305-12.

[56]   Broadbent LP, Moran CJ, Cross DT 3rd, Derdeyn CP. Management of neuroform stent dislodgement and misplacement. AJNR Am J Neuroradiol 2003; 24: 1819-22.

[57]   Kallmes DF, Ding YH, Dai D, Kadirvel R, Lewis DA, Cloft HJ. A new endoluminal, flow-disrupting device for treatment of saccular aneurysms. Stroke 2007; 38: 2346-52.

CHAPTER 8

Endovascular Management of Brain Tumors: What's in the Future?

A. Caporlingua[1], F. Caporlingua[1] and S. Peschillo[2,*]

[1]*Department of Neurology and Psychiatry, Neurosurgery, "Sapienza" University of Rome, Rome, Italy;* [2]*Department of Neurology and Psychiatry, Endovascular Neurosurgery/Interventional Neuroradiology, "Sapienza" University of Rome, Rome, Italy*

Abstract: Neuroendovascular techniques have evolved rapidly during the last decades extending the range of treatment options available for neuroendovascular surgeons and creating new applications other than those in the field of cerebrovascular diseases. Endovascular approaches for the management of head and neck tumors date back to the 1970s when the French surgeon Manelfe described the first pre-surgical embolization for an intracranial meningioma. Thereafter, indications for such treatment widened to other intracranial hypervascular tumors such as hemangiopericytomas and hemangioblastomas or extra/intracranial neoplasms including paragangliomas and juvenile nasopharyngeal angiofibromas. Moreover, the possibility of reaching specific regions of the brain *via* the endovascular route made intra-arterial chemotherapy for brain tumors feasible, mitigating complications related to systemic exposure to toxic drugs. The indications, outcomes and complications of these relatively new techniques are discussed in depth.

Keywords: Dangerous anastomoses, embolization, endovascular, head and neck tumors, hemangioblastomas, hemangiopericytomas, intracranial meningiomas, juvenile nasopharyngeal angiofibromas, paragangliomas.

INTRODUCTION

Pre-Surgical Embolization of Brain Tumors

At the beginning of the 20th century, in his book entitled "The treatment of certain malignant growths by excision" published precisely in 1903, Dawbarn described an endovascular approach to the management of neoplasms occurring in the territory of the external carotid artery (ECA). The so-called "starvation operation" entailed ligation of the ECA and subsequent intra-arterial injection of paraffin,

*Corresponding author S. Peschillo: Department of Neurology and Psychiatry, Endovascular Neurosurgery/ Interventional Neuroradiology, "Sapienza" University of Rome, Rome, Italy; Tel/Fax: +390649979185; E-mail: simone.peschillo@gmail.com

an embolic agent. For this purpose the paraffin had to be maintained in its liquid form and thus kept at very high temperatures. Using a boiled syringe with adequate short tubing and cannula the operation had to be performed rapidly in order both to preserve the operators' hands from burn wounds and to keep the paraffin in the liquid state which gave it its penetration potential. Observing how clotting tended to occur when blood came into contact with the hot solution, thus jeopardizing distal distribution of the embolic agent, Dawbarn proposed injecting a warm salt solution to distend and flush out the vessels and their branches distal to the ligature just before the paraffin injection. Well aware of the vascular anatomy in the ECA territory he tried to embolize vessels supplying the lesion, leaving the arterial blood supply for normal tissue needs as unaltered as possible [1, 2].

With the introduction of cerebral angiography, thanks to the efforts of the Portuguese Egas Moniz, endovascular surgery techniques evolved while, at the same time, providing a diagnostic and therapeutic approach to cerebrovascular diseases. Building on that, during the 1970s, the French Djindjian foresaw how angiography would aid neurosurgeons dealing with brain or spinal hypervascular tumors with pre-operative embolization of the major arterial pedicles supplying the neoplasm and developed a technique which allowed superselective catheterization of arterial vessels using a finely tapered microcatheter. However, embolic materials were still primitive and consisted of small pieces of Gelfoam or autologous muscle, as the more advanced "pellets" (silastic spheroids) would not enter the microcatheter given its small diameter [3, 4]. A co-national of Djindjian, Manelfe, is credited with the first pre-surgical embolization of an intracranial meningioma in 1973 [5]. Soon after, others reported their experience, including Hekster who described the embolization of a left superficial parietal brain tumor in a 39-year old woman whose blood group was very rare so blood loss during surgery had to be minimal. Injecting emboli (small pieces of Spongostan, also known as Gelfoam) into the ipsilateral ECA *via* the transfemoral route he supposed that the emboli would be "sucked" from the tumor vascularization. The patient tolerated the procedure and blood loss during the following surgical resection was minimal [6]. The use of pre-surgical embolization has now broadened not only to intracranial neoplasms such as meningiomas, but also to hemangioblastomas, hemangiopericytomas and to extracranial tumors including paragangliomas and juvenile nasopharyngeal angiofibromas which often extend intracranially. Furthermore embolization may be used as a stand-alone approach to inoperable tumors or when surgery is contraindicated because of a patient's comorbidities. However, the indications for pre-surgical or palliative embolization are still controversial and vary greatly depending on operators' preferences and experience, availability of equipment and habits within an institution. Given the great variability in outcomes, benefits and risks, this technique struggles to be included in the standard of care for brain tumors; nonetheless, it is invaluable in selected cases of hypervascular neoplasms whose vasculature cannot be reached in the early stages of surgery.

Intra-Arterial Chemotherapy for Brain Tumors

Since the discovery and description of the blood-brain barrier in the 1950s, oncologists have tried to limit the collateral effects of chemotherapy agents by delivering the drugs directly to the tumor while minimizing exposure of systemic tissues [7]. The goal of intra-arterial chemotherapy is to produce a high concentration of the drug in the arterial blood stream which supplies the tumor, thereby increasing uptake of the drug into malignant cells and, consequently, increasing these cells' death. Since 1991 when the coils of Guglielmi were introduced into clinical practice, there has been a considerable evolution of endovascular techniques [8]. Subsequently, the treatment of cerebral aneurysms shifted from open surgery to a multimodal approach. More selective catheterization started being a common neuroendovascular practice and was found to be useful as an alternative route for delivering drugs to brain tumors. Super-selective intra-arterial cerebral infusion (SIACI) held the hope of minimizing the neurotoxicity of chemotherapeutic agents while concomitantly increasing their efficacy.

PRE-SURGICAL EMBOLIZATION FOR BRAIN TUMORS

Goals and Benefits Versus Risks and Complications

The main purpose of embolization is devascularization of a neoplasm prior to its surgical resection. The benefits of the procedure include reduction of intraoperative blood loss which, in turn, increases both the tolerability of the procedure and the quality of the resection because vision during tissue dissection is far less impeded by blood in the surgical field. Furthermore, deprivation of the arterial supply triggers a series of reactions which result in a reduction in the consistency and volume of tumor tissues. As a natural consequence, better resection reduces recurrence rates. When used as a palliative measure, embolization is intended to achieve the best reduction or containment of tumor growth rate.

Fever and localized pain are the most frequent transient complications following embolization procedures [9]. Local complications include puncture site hematomas, which may be divided into mild or severe depending on whether they do not or do need surgical correction. Endovascular navigation itself is not without any risk; in particular vessel wall perforation or damage due, respectively, to wires and hemodynamic changes resulting from the embolization [10] may lead to thromboembolic accidents whose severity varies depending on the vascular region affected. Accidental distal dissemination of embolic particles is the main embolization-specific complication. The mechanisms underlying this complication are variable: pure distal dissemination, reflux, passage of embolisates in the anastomotic circulation (see "Tumor vascularization: anatomy and pitfalls"), and patency of the foramen ovale, which may lead to paradoxical embolic accidents [11]. Intracranial embolization is burdened with a 3-6% risk of stroke and intracerebral hemorrhage [12, 13]. In 2000, Gruber *et al.* published results from a series of 128 endovascular embolization procedures for intracranial meningiomas (n = 41), juvenile nasopharyngeal angiofibromas (n = 7) and temporal paragangliomas (n = 18) collected between 1982 and 1998; they reported only three complications of which two were embolic strokes and one was a cerebellar infarction (2.3% complication rate). Moreover they outlined how all these complications occurred in the early period of the study and that there were absolutely no complications, such as distal dissemination through unexpected anastomoses or vasa nervorum damage [14-17], during the end of the period studied, advocating that dramatic improvements in both expertise and equipment had been decisive factors in this achievement [18].

Tumor necrosis following embolization may produce an increase in peritumoral edema and tissue swelling, ultimately leading to abrupt neurological and clinical deterioration requiring either steroid therapy or an emergency surgical resection [18-21]. Embolization of ECA branches may lead to scalp necrosis and impair the process of wound healing if cutaneous branches of the ECA are improperly occluded [20, 22]. Moreover surgical resection of embolized tumors may further jeopardize the arterial supply of the scalp, especially when the design of the cutaneous flap is poor [23]. Cranial nerve palsies may be exacerbated by disruption of the microscopic vasa nervorum whose patency can be compromised when using ultra-small particles in certain branches of the ECA [24, 25]. Tumor-specific complications are described in depth in each dedicated section.

Tumor Vascularization: Anatomy and Pitfalls

Head and neck tumors may have a single or double vascularization arising from the internal carotid artery (ICA), the ECA or both. Typically embolization is far more beneficial and safe for tumors supplied exclusively or predominantly by the ECA. Indeed superselective catheterization of ICA branches is more complex because of their tortuous anatomy and consequently higher risk of arterial wall perforation and thromboembolic accidents that can produce transient or permanent neurological morbidity. Thorough knowledge of normal and pathological cerebrovascular anatomy is essential in order to avoid potentially disastrous complications.

External Carotid Artery

In the case of the ECA, several branches contribute to the arterial supply of cranial nerves *via* the microscopic vasa nervorum, while other branches are or may be connected to the ICA circulation thus potentially enabling unwanted dissemination of an embolic agent into the intracranial circulation. The most commonly encountered "dangerous" anastomoses that should always be identified before any embolization is performed are: (i) the distal internal maxillary artery (IMA) connected to the ICA *via*, respectively, the middle meningeal artery (MMA) and the posterolateral branch of the inferolateral trunk (ILT); (ii) the accessory meningeal artery (AMA) and the posteromedial branch of the ILT; and (iii) the artery of the foramen rotundum and the anterolateral branch of the ILT [26-28]. The ascending pharyngeal artery at the odontoid arterial arch, the occipital arteries at the C1-C2 interspace and branches of the posterior auricular artery may communicate with the vertebral artery (VA). Exploration of the MMA should always look for a meningolacrimal branch which runs into the territory of the ophthalmic artery supplying the retina.

Post-embolization cranial nerve palsies are often caused by smaller embolic particles with great penetration potential which enables the particles to occlude vasa nervorum supplying the nerves. The neuromeningeal trunk arising from the ascending pharyngeal artery or posterior auricular arteries supplies the lower cranial nerves: the glossopharyngeal (IX), the vagus (X) and the accessory (XI) nerves. The petrous branches of the MMA may supply the VIIth cranial nerve (the facial nerve). In an effort to minimize the incidence of such complications, pre-embolization diagnostic tests have been developed. As Kerber and Horton pointed out [29], intra-arterial injection of lidocaine may be useful for early identification of branches of the ECA supplying cranial nerves. Positivity of this provocative test might motivate the use of larger particles to reduce the risks of vasa nervorum embolization. However, the test may further increase the overall risks related to embolization procedures as intra-arterial injection of lidocaine itself is not free from risk; for instance, reflux of lidocaine into the intracranial or systemic circulation may result in seizures and cardiorespiratory arrest, respectively. Deveikis *et al.* described sequential injection of barbiturates (sodium amytal), normally used for identification of the dominant hemisphere during the Wada test, and then lidocaine. Amobarbital injections can rule out the presence of anastomoses between the ECA and ICA, identified through continuous neurological monitoring of the patient maintained under local anesthesia for the duration of the procedure; when such anastomoses have been excluded, lidocaine can help to exclude a contribution of the vasa nervorum of the cranial nerves [30]. Despite this, the use of provocative tests use is not widespread mainly because of the additional costs, risks and, above all, the high incidence of false positive and false negative results [27]. As an alternative, intraoperative somatosensory evoked potentials may increase safety by early identification of ischemia during embolization [31].

Internal Carotid Artery

Embolization of tumor vessels arising from the ICA may be required, especially when the vessels are surgically inaccessible, for instance in the case of skull base or ICA-encasing lesions. Despite being challenging, embolization of ICA branches has been described in the literature. Using hydrophilic microcatheters of various stiffness, cavernous ICA branches have been catheterized [27]. In 1986 Theron *et al.* [32] described a technique, which he used in six patients, for embolizing cavernous ICA branches in cases of brain arteriovenous malformations and intracranial tumors. By inflating a balloon in the ICA distally to the selected branches, polyvinyl alcohol (PVA) was injected safely and embolization successfully achieved. Jungreis *et al.* [33] described the use of ethanol as the embolic agent for this technique. The balloon was deflated only after proper flushing of the ICA with a heparinized solution to remove PVA remnants in the lumen of the artery. Although quite ingenious, this technique carries some risks and may have complications such as balloon displacement or failed balloon deflation leading to distal dissemination of embolic agents [34]: furthermore, it depends entirely on the presence of a completely developed circle of Willis which would compensate for the temporary occlusion of the ICA or VA [32].

For ophthalmic lesions or anterior skull base tumors supplied by the ophthalmic artery *via* the ethmoidal arteries, embolization is often contraindicated in an effort to avoid complications endangering vision; nevertheless, embolization of branches of the ophthalmic artery is feasible and has been reported for cases in which surgery did not provide direct access to these branches or when surgery itself was not an option. Visualization of the choroidal blush is of the utmost importance as it confirms the anatomy of the central retinal artery. Provocative tests with sodium amobarbital may be used to rule out any risk of blindness with embolization of the selected vessels prompting either the suspension of the embolization or the use of larger embolic materials (coils or particle >400 μm) to reduce the risk of retinal ischemia. Lefkowitz *et al.* reported on a series of 12 patients with ophthalmic vascular lesions or tumors requiring embolization [35]. Interestingly, when dealing with ophthalmic lesions that have already caused monocular blindness, caution must be used as ischemic necrosis of the affected retina may trigger an antibody reaction capable of endangering the contralateral, functioning retina as a result of release of segregated antigens [36]. Embolization of pial vessels should be avoided as this carries a higher risk of thromboembolic accidents given the fragility of these vessels.

When dealing with lesions involving or encasing the ICA, it is essential to perform an occlusion test in order to evaluate the feasibility of sacrificing the ICA during surgery. Sekhar described various possible ways of making this evaluation. One approach is to perform angiography with the affected ICA manually compressed while injecting the contrast agent in the contralateral ICA: observing the venous phase on an anteroposterior view is the most reliable proof as delayed venous filling and emptying corroborate the presence of a poor collateral circulation. The more widely adopted balloon occlusion test may be performed with ICA occlusion for 30 minutes, with the patient awake and under clinical monitoring looking for neurological deficits. This test must be performed under systemic heparinization and a single dose of 325 mg of aspirin must be given the day before the scheduled procedure [29, 30]. The occlusion test may be coupled with a transcranial Doppler: a 30% drop in middle cerebral artery velocities indicates borderline collateralization; a drop of 40% indicates insufficient collateral flow, inadequate to support cerebral perfusion. The ILT may be connected to the ophthalmic artery by a deep recurrent branch of the latter, hence there is an associated risk of blindness when this vessel is catheterized; moreover it supplies the IIIrd, IVth and VIth cranial nerves as well as the Gasserian ganglion [37].

Embolic Materials

Polyvinyl Alcohol

Shaved into precisely sized particles from an original block, polyvinyl alcohol (PVA) is the most common particulate used for embolization of all tumors. The size of these particles varies from 50 to 150 μm to 500 to 1200 μm. Preparation of the emboli is important as PVA particles tend to clump together and so the overall diameter of a particle may differ as a function of the level of aggregation. Penetration potential is inversely proportional to particle diameter: in other words, the bigger a particle, the less its penetration. Penetration potential may be described as a double-edged weapon as it provides better results in terms of devascularization, but also increases the risk of unwanted distal embolization leading to either thromboembolic accidents or cranial nerve palsies depending on the vascular region affected. PVA particles are inert and hydrophobic; their tendency to expand after injection enables the occlusion of vessels whose diameter is superior to that of the catheter. Furthermore PVA triggers inflammatory responses involving polymorphonuclear cells (2 weeks) and giant cells (3 months) leading to a partially calcified thrombus (9 months) [38-40]. The main limitations of the use of PVA include particulate degradation and subsequent thrombus absorption by endogenous lytic agents within several weeks to months, leading to the risk of recanalization of the embolized vessel within this period. The poor long-term devascularization results are the reason why PVA is better suited for pre-surgical embolization [38, 39, 41]. PVA may provoke catheter occlusion given its high friction coefficient. Furthermore during the mixing process, PVA particles tend to fragment into smaller sized particles, contaminating the final mixture with "dangerous" emboli with excessive penetration and dissemination potential.

Tissue Adhesive Embolisates: n-butyl Cyanoacrylate Glue

N-butyl cyanoacrylate (NBCA) is a stable, non-absorbable, liquid polymerizing agent. It is commonly used for the treatment of cerebrovascular diseases such as brain arteriovenous malformations or fistulas, but rarely for tumors. It is mixed with an oil-based contrast agent (ethiodol). The glue polymerizes when in contact with ionic solutions and, given its liquid form, can reach both proximal and distal arterial feeders. Considering its outstanding and, at the same time, poorly controllable penetration potential, it is clear why its use is far more limited than that of PVA when dealing with tumors, since the risks of unwanted dissemination are too high to be safely manageable.

Cellulose Beads and Trisacryl Gelatin Microspheres

Kai *et al.* tested cellulose porous beads (200-μm diameter) in 141 consecutive patients with intracranial meningiomas [42]. Produced starting from frozen and then fixed liquid cellulose microscopic droplets, cellulose porous beads have a uniform size, globoid shape with many micropores, and a specific gravity similar to that of whole blood [43]. Differently from PVA, superficial positive charges prevent clumping of the particles and, more importantly, cellulose porous beads are not susceptible to reabsorption with subsequent thrombus degradation resulting in recanalization. These features enable them to reach the vascular bed of the tumor without occluding pre-capillaries, thus providing better results in terms of devascularization and tumor tissue softening, especially when surgical resection is delayed for more than 7 days.

Trisacryl gelatin microspheres, also known as Embospheres, are hydrophilic, non-absorbable, collagen-coated, deformable embolic agents which do not have a tendency to aggregate [44]. Bendszus *et al.* [45] published a comparative prospective study of 30 consecutive patients treated with Embospheres and 30 with PVA. Blinded to the patients' treatment, the authors found that Embospheres could penetrate more deeply in the tumor vascular bed with resulting better devascularization and greater reduction of intraoperative blood loss.

Ethanol

Ethanol is a powerful sclerotic and cytotoxic agent which causes anoxic cell damage, protein precipitation, and fibrinoid necrosis of the intimal lining [46] resulting in the obliteration of small caliber arterial feeders. Its great penetration potential is nonetheless associated with a higher risk of complications such as cranial nerve palsies and distal embolization [33, 47]. Ethanol induces a robust inflammatory response that obliterates tissue planes, which may not be beneficial during a delayed surgical resection. Horowitz *et al.* [48] described the use of alcohol in patients with a carotid body tumor. In an effort to prevent distal penetration of the liquid agent they used a balloon-assisted technique and limited the dose to prevent excessive tissue damage. Surgical resection was performed 24 hours later. Lonser *et al.* [49] described intratumoral ethanol injection into three pial epidural masses and one hemangiobalstoma, reporting "visible blanching of the tumor". Ethanol is not widely used because of its excessive aggressiveness and poor reliability which are not compatible with the currently widely adopted "complication avoidance strategy" when planning pre-surgical embolization.

Gelatin Foam (Gelfoam)

Widely known and used in the operating room for its hemostatic properties, Gelfoam is commonly used for the endovascular management of brain arteriovenous malformations and fistulas. The high penetration potential of Gelfoam is due to the small size of its pieces, ranging from 40 to 60 μm. Despite being easy to use and to deliver, endogenous lytic agents rapidly degrade Gelfoam. Its main limitations are a high risk of distal embolization and rapid absorption by the body.

Coils

Commonly used in combination with other embolic agents, coils prevent recanalization better when used on proximal arterial feeders after embolization of distal feeders. Coils are indicated when angiography shows the presence of anastomoses between the ECA and ICA circulations and in the case of positivity of provocative tests. Indeed in these particular circumstances using smaller particulates may be unacceptably risky for the patients and coils or other larger embolic agents are valid alternatives in order to minimize complications.

Fibrin Glue

Richling first described the indications for the use of fibrin glue in endovascular procedures in 1982 [43, 44]. Fibrin glue is a two-component adhesive agent originating from the combination of homologous fibrinogen and thrombin and has several surgical, particularly neurosurgical, applications such as tissue gluing and hemostasis. Probst *et al.* reported on its use [50] in a series of 80 patients of whom two developed permanent neurological complications. They advocated that the main advantages of fibrin glue are the possibility of conducting continuous radiological monitoring given the radio-opaque nature of the mixture and the substantial shortening of procedure duration in comparison with embolization performed using small diameter PVA particles with comparable results in terms of distal embolization of the vascular bed of the tumor. The limitations include a risk of allergic reaction, infection (minimized since donors are tested meticulously for viral markers) and recanalization due to endogenous thrombolytic agents. Because of this last limitation, fibrin glue embolization cannot be used as a stand-alone procedure.

Miscellaneous

Microfibrillar collagen is derived from purified bovine collagen and is commonly used during surgery for hemostatic purposes. It induces platelet aggregation and is effective even in the case of heparinization and underlying coagulopathies. Kumar *et al.* tested its use for embolization and reported better results than with PVA [51].

Phenytoin is rarely used, but Kasuya *et al.* [52] described its properties when administered *via* a microcatheter at a dose of 250-500 mg, reporting ischemic and hemorrhagic necrosis with resulting devascularization of meningiomas.

Hydroxyapatite ceramic microparticles are made of calcium phosphate, have a microporous structure, and range in size from 100 to 250 μm. These microparticles were originally intended for prosthetic grafts in orthopedic surgery, plastic and reconstructive surgery, spinal surgery, cranial reconstruction, and oral surgery. However, in 2003 Kubo *et al.* investigated their use as embolic agents [53]. Subsequently he described his clinical experience in 13 patients with intracranial meningiomas, reporting excellent results in terms of devascularization, biocompatibility and visibility of the hydroxyapatite microspheres [54].

Delay in Surgical Resection after Embolization

The time between embolization and surgical resection varies and a standard has still not been officially established [24, 27, 50, 55]. When tumor tissues are deprived of their arterial supply a series of reactions is triggered. Anoxic damage induces necrosis which, in turn, causes the tumor to shrink, to soften and to be less prone to hemorrhage which are the most appealing effects for neurosurgeons entrusted with the subsequent surgical resection. Unfortunately, the effect of embolization may not be permanent: a collateral circulation may develop after a certain period of time or the embolic material may dissolve or be degraded by endogenous lytic agents [56]. In the literature the reported timing of surgery ranges from 24 hours after embolization [12, 57], to three to five days [17, 55, 58] and to one to three weeks [24, 59, 60]. Precocious resection (within 24 hours) is to be considered contraindicated as devascularization effects have not yet occurred and, according to Chun *et al.* [19], there may be greater intraoperative blood loss. Histological specimens of embolized paragangliomas collected by Pauw *et al.* [61] showed peculiar features, such as thrombosis and a multinucleated giant cell reaction, within seven days of embolization. After a week these changes regressed due to partial or complete revascularization which was more likely to occur in the 30% of embolized vessels, suggesting better surgical outcomes when resection is performed within one week of embolization. Comparable results were found for intracranial meningiomas, as better resectability due to softening and reduction of intraoperative hemorrhage was reported for resections conducted seven to nine days after embolization [59]. Despite this, extreme caution is necessary and scrupulous neurological monitoring must be performed after embolization when dealing with hypervascular skull base neoplasms, especially edematous lesions associated with mid-line shift, because in these cases increased tumor swelling, intratumoral necrosis and hemorrhage may lead to clinical deterioration requiring steroid therapy and, not uncommonly, emergency surgical decompression [56, 62].

Applications

Meningiomas

Meningiomas originate from arachnoid cap cells and develop, maintaining a dural attachment or pedicle at all stages. They are benign, slow-growing neoplasms, accounting for 13% - 18% of intracranial tumors [62]. Treatment is based mostly on complete surgical removal. Meningiomas tend to recur and the risk of recurrence depends mainly on the quality of the resection; the recurrence rate is 9-11% if the dural attachment is excised, 19% - 22% if it is not removed and around 40% in cases of subtotal resection [63-66]. Complete resection is influenced by a series of factors including the patient's clinical conditions dictating surgery tolerability, and features of the meningioma such as its location, volume, density and accessibility of its vascularization to mention the most relevant. In this regard pre-surgical embolization may be beneficial by reducing intraoperative blood loss [18, 67-70], as well as softening and possibly shrinking tumor tissues resulting in much easier, more tolerable, shorter subsequent surgical resection. Furthermore a reduction of intraoperative tumor hemorrhage results in superior outcomes in terms of completeness of resection and preservation of normal structures. Pre-surgical embolization acquires a much more pivotal role when dealing with complex meningiomas associated with vascular anomalies such as aneurysms [62, 71-73].

Vascularization

Intracranial meningiomas receive a vascular supply originating from the ECA with a variable arterial contribution from the ICA [68, 74]. For certain specifically located meningiomas, such as diaphragmatic or tuberculum sellae lesions, the arterial supply is solely from the ICA. Arterial feeders at the dural attachment or pedicle arise from branches of the ECA, such as the MMA, AMA, neuromeningeal branch of the ascending pharyngeal artery or the stylomastoid branch of the occipital artery. From the pedicle the main arterial feeders branch out radially producing the classic angiographic finding known as the "sunburst" sign with the apex of the sunburst corresponding to the point of the dural attachment. Pial or cortical arterial branches supply the capsule of the meningioma. The ICA may contribute to the meningioma dural supply with ethmoidal, cavernous, clival or tentorial branches, depending on the tumor's location. Although angiography is essential to determine the vascularization of the meningioma, the vascular settings and arterial branches, which most likely supply the tumor, can be presumed in advance on the basis of the tumor's location (Table **1**).

Table 1.   Common pattern of arterial supply based on tumor location.

Location	Arterial Supply
Anterior fossa:	
High convexity Parasagittal	Ipsilateral ± contralateral middle meningeal a. A. of the falx cerebri
Frontal convexity Frontal falcine	Meningeal branches of the ethmoidal a. Anterior falcine a.
Olfactory groove meningiomas	Anterior and posterior ethmoidal arteries MMA and distal IMA
Middle fossa:	
Sphenoid wing meningiomas	Recurrent meningeal a. (ophthalmic a.) MMA branches
Paraseller meningiomas	Petrous, cavernous, supraclinoid ICA branches, a. foramen rotondum, a. of the foramen ovale., neuromeningeal trunk of the ascending pharyngeal a.
Posterior fossa:	Posterior meningeal a., MMA, AMA (arterial supply usually shared with lower cranial nerves)
Tentorial	Tentorial branch of the MHT ILT, MMA, AMA *(arterial supply may be shared with cranial nerves III, IV, V and VI)*
Petroclival	Petrosal, petrosquamosal, occipital branches of the MMA Transmastoid branches of the occipital and posterior auricular a. Subarcuate branch of the anterior inferior cerebellar a. Neuromeningeal branches of the ascending pharyngeal a.
Foramen magnum	Posterior meningeal a. (VA); Branches of the ascending pharyngeal a.
Pineal	Meningeal branches of the ECA (i.e. tentorial a.); Medial and posterior choroidal branches; Posterior pericallosal a.; Small branches of the posterior cerebral a.; Branches of the superior vermian and superior cerebellar a.. ± Meningeal branches from the VA and posterior inferior cerebellar a.

Indication and Contraindications

The indications for pre-surgical embolization in the management of intracranial meningiomas are still quite controversial [75] and vary greatly between different institutions and neurosurgical teams. Meningiomas which would most likely benefit from such an approach are hypervascular and deep-seated lesions such as skull base meningiomas, as they usually receive an arterial supply that is not readily accessible during surgery (*e.g.*, the meningohypophyseal trunk, MHT) and, therefore, at the origin of poorly controllable intraoperative hemorrhages [17, 18, 58, 76]. T2 magnetic resonance imaging sequences predicting both hyper-vascularity and the consistency of meningiomas may contribute to the decision-making process [77]. Engelhard summarized the indications for meningioma embolization in his institution as being hypervascular meningiomas supplied predominantly by meningeal arteries (ECA circulation) or by arterial feeders not reachable in the early stages of the surgical approach [50, 57]. Tumors supplied predominantly by ECA branches are better suited to pre-surgical embolization: nonetheless, a contribution from the ICA should always be evaluated. Yoon suggested that once tumors fed by both ICA and ECA branches have been deprived of their ECA contribution, there is a massive increase in blood from the remaining ICA feeders, leading to swelling of the tumor tissue and an increased mass effect [68], justifying extension of the embolization also to these branches [35, 78, 79]. According to Yoon, ICA branches should be embolized when the arterial supply of the tumor originates mostly from the ICA, when angiography rules out any staining of adjacent normal brain tissue during superselective catheterization of these branches, when any doubt concerning an eventual contribution to eloquent and/or speech areas has been resolved by negative provocative tests and, lastly, when it is considered possible to advance a microcatheter just proximal to the tumor [36]. Patients who are not eligible for surgery may gain benefit from palliative embolization as a stand-alone therapeutic approach or as an adjuvant therapy after radiosurgery [27].

Embolization for meningiomas supplied by ICA branches (i.e. branches of the ILT or MHT) is generally considered hazardous and contraindicated. Nevertheless, although the procedure is risky, it is feasible when certain requirements such as equipment availability and expertise are met. Hirohata *et al.* reported on a series of seven patients with petroclival meningiomas who underwent pre-surgical embolization with 150 to 250 μm particles after successful catheterization of branches of both the MHT and the ILT (lateral clival, posterior branch, tentorial branch) [80]. They reported <500 mL blood loss during subsequent surgical resections. They did not use any provocative tests to identify cranial nerve feeders, considering that intra-arterial injection of lidocaine was an unacceptable additional risk for the patients, as already stated by other authors [81, 82]. Robinson described catheterization of the aforementioned ICA branches in five patients with skull base meningiomas. He reported no complications and in 80-100% of cases control angiograms showed no blush images.

Embolization of pial or cortical vessels is strongly contraindicated because of the fragility of these vessels and the consequent risk of hemorrhagic stroke. Nonetheless, Kaji *et al.* [78] embolized distal ICA cortical branches and suggested that such a procedure should be performed for lesions located in non-eloquent areas with a negative amytal test, receiving their arterial supply exclusively from the ICA and using particles rather than acrylic glue.

Although pre-surgical embolization is not canonical management for meningiomas drawing their arterial supply from the ophthalmic artery, given the high risk of visual loss as a result of embolization of the central retinal artery [35, 83], there are case reports of the use of this strategy [35, 79].

The exceptional reports on the feasibility of pre-surgical embolization for skull base meningiomas supplied by the ICA or vertebrobasilar branches (i.e. petrous/cavernous/pial internal carotid branches) are undeniably the prelude to a promising future; however, most authors still consider it dangerous to attempt such procedures and limit pre-surgical embolization to giant convexity meningiomas with multidirectional blood supply which would be the cause of catastrophic blood loss if approached surgically [62]. Embolization of ECA branches supplying a meningioma should be reconsidered if interruption of the branches could be easily achieved early during surgery and if angiography shows the presence of an anastomosis with the intracranial circulation; in this particular case, however, embolization is still feasible provided that smaller particles are avoided since these have a higher penetration potential and, consequently, a higher possibility of entering the intracranial circulation [28]. Large meningiomas associated with peritumoral edema and a shift of midline cerebral structures must be dealt with cautiously, especially when planning a closed-skull procedure such as embolization, as any further increase in tumor volumes (for instance, if post-embolization intratumor infarction occurs) would produce either new neurological deficits or a catastrophic clinical deterioration.

Embolic Materials

The most commonly used embolic material is PVA in different sizes (150 to 350 μm particles are preferable) depending on the tumor's vascular setting, presence of ECA-ICA anastomoses, and positivity of provocative tests identifying an arterial contribution to cranial nerves [12, 24, 27, 84-87] which justify the use of bigger particles ranging from 350 to 500 μm [25, 88, 89]. While smaller particles provide better devascularization results, they carry a higher risk of dissemination or unwanted embolization. Valid alternatives to PVA include trisacryl gelatin microspheres [13, 45, 75], calibrated microspheres [90], cellulose porous beads [13, 42], Gelfoam cut into strips of 1-2 mm x 2-3 mm [24, 69, 84-86, 88], and Onyx for exceptionally hypervascular lesions [88]. Accordingly to Bendszus [45] trisacryl gelatin microspheres provide better results than PVA in terms of reduction of intraoperative blood loss, most likely because of superior penetration potential of the microspheres. Calibrated 400-μm microspheres were found to be safer than smaller PVA particles (45-150 μm) and give results comparable to those achieved with larger PVA particles (150-250 μm) when analyzing the risk of hemorrhagic complications [90]. Komatsu described the use of estrogen because meningiomas may express estrogen/progesterone receptors. The embolic mechanism of action of this hormone is unclear although estrogen tends to cause damage to the vascular endothelium and alter vascular permeability [91].

Outcomes and Complications

Pre-surgical embolization for intracranial meningiomas undoubtedly carries an additional risk of complications although few authors have ever tried to compare outcomes in patients who had pre-surgical embolization and in those treated with surgical resection alone. Among those few, Macpherson *et al.* in 1991, selected 52 patients harboring intracranial meningiomas and subdivided them into two groups: one group comprised patients treated with embolization and surgery, whereas the other consisted of patients treated with surgery alone. The intraoperative blood loss and blood or plasma requirements were less in the embolization group than in the group undergoing surgery alone. A selection bias was later pointed out [75] as patients were assigned to the surgery group if embolization was not feasible or inappropriate, for instance in case of meningiomas with a prevalent ICA supply which, in turn, were extremely challenging when managed surgically [69]. In 2000, Bendszus *et al.* published the results of a two-center prospective study including 60 consecutive meningioma patients of whom 30 were treated with surgery alone and the other 30 were treated in a different center with pre-surgical embolization and subsequent resection. A preliminary study was conducted to ensure that surgical outcomes (intraoperative blood loss, procedure time weighted as a function of the neurosurgeons' experience, size of skin incision and bone flap) when dealing with intracranial meningioma were comparable between the two centers. The results did not reveal any clear advantage from using preoperative embolization with the only exception of operative blood loss, which was less in embolized patients when embolization was subtotal or complete (>90%) [75]. Unfortunately patients were assigned to each therapeutic protocol only on the basis of the center which took care of them in the first place producing, once again, a selection bias that could have compromised the value of the study.

Complication rates for presurgical embolization of meningiomas vary widely in the literature from 0 to 21% [13, 26, 70, 75, 83, 92]. A review by Shah *et al.* [62], published in 2013, included 36 studies on meningiomas treated with presurgical embolization between 1990 and 2011 and showed that 4.6% patients (21 of a total of 459) developed complications. Of the 21 complications, one (4.8%) was considered a major complication and two (9.5%) led to death as a direct result of embolization. These percentages corroborate data collected on the same topic by other authors [12, 13, 28]. Conclusions must be drawn cautiously as the cases were mostly convexity meningiomas (convexity meningiomas = 40.2%; parasagittal meningiomas = 8.4%) which influenced results producing an underestimation of embolization risks. Convexity lesions should rarely be managed with embolization, as their dural arterial feeders are easily manageable in the early stages of the surgical resection, unlike the deep inaccessible arterial feeders supplying skull base meningiomas whose superselective catheterization is nonetheless riskier than that of ECA branches. In 2002 Rosen *et al.* found that the complication rate of pre-surgical embolization for skull base meningiomas was 21% (transient deterioration of neurological examinations in 12.6% cases and a permanent neurological deficit or morbidity in 9%) in a series of 167 lesions. Detailing the complication rates as a function of the specific arterial feeders embolized, he reported that the chances of permanent neurological morbidity were 13%, 11.8% and 10.5% when dealing with the ascending pharyngeal artery, MHT and AMA, respectively. Transient neurological deficits (*e.g.* facial numbness) were more likely when embolizing the ECA or clinoid ICA branches and sphenopalatine artery [83]. In contrast, in a series of 262 meningiomas, of which 119 were classified as skull base meningiomas, Waldron *et al.* [28] reported an outstanding 2.5% rate of complications directly related to embolization and justified the variability in complication rates reported in the literature, in the first place, by the unreasonable aggressiveness of some neuroendovascular surgeons who focus too strongly on "complete devascularization" rather than on "complication avoidance strategies" and in the second place by the lack of numerically adequate case series and well-designed studies concerning, in particular, the management of skull base meningiomas with pre-surgical embolization [35, 36, 79, 80, 82, 92].

The specific complications following meningioma embolization are mainly hemorrhages. Hemorrhages may be classified as subarachnoid, peritumoral or intratumoral [10, 93-96]. The abrupt occlusion of vessels of the ECA in meningiomas fed also by ICA branches may lead to a reactive increase in the blood demand of the latter resulting in either a catastrophic intratumoral hemorrhage or a massive increase in both the mass effect and tissue swelling [22, 97]. Moreover, atypical meningiomas presenting with pathological vessels (reduced wall/lumen ratio, iron deposits suggesting previous hemorrhages) are probably more likely to bleed after embolization, as are cystic meningiomas and lesions with large necrotic areas [13, 96]. To rule out any suspicion of a casual relationship between intratumoral hemorrhage and embolization we note here that meningiomas bleed spontaneously in 1.3% cases [98] and atypical variants, which account for 10% of meningiomas encountered [99], are more likely to bleed [100]. In 2007, Carli *et al.* analyzed results from a series of 747 meningiomas and found a correlation between the use of smaller embolic particles (45-150 μm) and the risk of hemorrhagic complications, as did other authors [21, 67, 76, 87, 93, 95, 101, 102], despite the better results in terms of devascularization when using such sized particles [76, 103, 104].

Ng *et al.* ruled out any suspicion of a histological over-grading of the meningiomas resulting from pre-surgical embolization. Interestingly, accordingly to Ng and Perry the histological patterns of necrotic anaplastic meningiomas differ from those of the necrosis commonly observed after resection of embolized meningiomas [105, 106].

Paragangliomas

Arising from chromaffin cells of the parasympathetic paraganglia of the skull base and neck, paragangliomas are typically benign, slow-growing neoplasms accounting for less than 0.5% of all head and neck tumors. Catecholamine secretion requiring pretreatment with α- and β-blockade has been observed in 4% cases [107-110]. These tumors may violate the intracranial space or produce neurological deficits due to cranial nerve encasement or disruption.

Classification and Vascularization

A topographic classification distinguishes the paragangliomas into carotid, temporal bone, vagal and spinal cord tumors. The most common paragangliomas are those of the carotid bifurcation (glomus caroticum – paraganglia coating the carotid artery in the neck) which are clinically silent until they present as a painless, slow-growing mass in the lateral neck causing vascular and cranial nerve disruption and, not uncommonly, extending into the intracranial space [111-113]. Temporal bone paragangliomas include the glomus tympanicum, arising in the middle ear along the tympanic plexus and commonly presenting with a pulsatile tinnitus, and the glomus jugulare, arising from the paraganglia embracing the jugular bulb [114, 115]. Vagal paragangliomas (glomus vagale - upper parapharyngeal space, glomus nodosum between the jugular vein and carotid artery) extend into the intracranial space through the jugular foramen or posterior to the mastoid tip in 22% cases [116]. Finally, the paragangliomas of the spinal canal are very rare forms of paragangliomas [117]. The Shamblin classification is commonly used for carotid body tumors (Table **2**) [118].

Table 2:   Shamblin classification for carotid bony tumors.

Shamblin Classification	
Class I	Localized tumors touching the carotid with minimal involvement of its vessels. Surgical resection possible with minimal risk of morbidity
Class II	Tumors surrounding the internal and external carotid arteries. Resection is challenging
Class III	Intimately encase the carotid and its vessels and may involve the cranial nerves. Resection is challenging and risky and requires major vascular reconstruction.

The Fisch classification applies to temporal bone paragangliomas (Table **3**) [119]:

Table 3:   The Fisch classification for temporal bone paragangliomas.

Fisch Classification	
A	Paragangliomas confined to the tympanic cavity arising along the tympanic plexus on the promontory.
B	Paragangliomas limited to the tympanomastoid area; invasion of the hypotympanum; cortical bone over the jugular bulb intact.
C_1	Paragangliomas with erosion of the carotid foramen.
C_2	Paragangliomas with destruction of the vertical carotid canal.
C_3	Paragangliomas involving the horizontal portion of the carotid canal; foramen lacerum is intact.
C_4	Paragangliomas invading the foramen lacerum and cavernous sinus
De $_{1/2}$	Paragangliomas with intracranial extradural extension. Subdivided into De$_1$: <2 cm of dural displacement and De$_2$ >2 cm dural displacement.
Di $_{1/2/3}$	Paragangliomas with intracranial intradural extension. Subdivided according to depth of invasion of the posterior cranial fossa: Di$_1$ <2 cm; Di$_2$ between 2 and 4 cm; Di$_3$ >4 cm.

Paragangliomas are supplied mostly by branches of the ECA, in particular the ascending pharyngeal artery [27]. When extending into the intracranial space, for instance in the case of advanced temporal bone lesions, paragangliomas may recruit ICA branches such as the vidian arteries, clival branches or the MHT. Anastomoses between the ECA-ICA circulations may be present and must be identified early to minimize the risk of distal dissemination of particles during embolization [120]. Glomus jugulare tumors often have a multicompartmentalized arterial supply and each should be dealt with separately during embolization to ensure proper devascularization (Table **4**) [18]. Type Di paragangliomas (intracranial, intradural extension) can be supplied by contributors arising from the VA *via* pial feeders from both the anterior cerebellar artery and postero-inferior cerebellar artery [121].

Table 4:   Schematic description of the multicompartmentalized vascularization of glomus jugulare tumors.

Compartment	Vascularization
Inferomedial compartment	Jugular bulb area and hypotympanum, supply from the ascending pharyngeal artery *via* the inferior tympanic artery and jugular branch [121, 122]
Posterolateral compartment	Posterior tympanic cavity and mastoid bone, supply from the stylomastoid branch of the occipital or posterior auricular artery [121, 122]
Anterior compartment	Pericarotid area, supply from both the IMAs *via* the anterior tympanic artery and the caroticotympanic arteries from the petrous portion of the ICA
Superior compartment	Supply from the MMA *via* the superior tympanic artery

Indications

In order to achieve complete surgical resection, pre-surgical embolization is strongly recommended for larger hypervascular paragangliomas to reduce intraoperative blood loss and to provide better visualization of critical structures whose preservation is of the utmost importance [119, 123-126]. Embolization may not be required in the case of glomus tympanicum tumors as the conventional tympanoplasty technique is usually sufficient to enable tumor resection [27]. In contrast, glomus jugulare lesions, especially when they extend intracranially, require preoperative embolization [127]. For tumors encasing the ICA it is recommended that an ICA balloon occlusion test is performed in order to verify tolerance of an eventual sacrifice of this artery during surgical resection. Cohen *et al.* [128] described how a covered stent could be used to preserve ICA patency after tumor devascularization. Lamuraglia *et al.* [129] reported their experience with pre-surgical embolization of carotid body tumors in 11 patients. The authors suggested embolization for tumors >3 cm and recommended surgical resection a few days after devascularization.

Complications

The main complications are accidental dissemination of embolisates from the ECA into the ICA circulation or cranial nerve palsies due to occlusion of branches supplying the vasa nervorum network. Pandya *et al.* [130] described tonsillary herniation following direct puncture and embolization of a glomus jugulare tumor, suggesting a massive tumor infarction as the cause of the malignant posterior fossa edema. Cases of facial palsy following embolization of glomus jugulare tumors, due to disruption of either the stylomastoid artery, petrosal branches of the MMA or AMA which normally supply the facial nerve (VII), have also been reported [131, 132]. The use of PVA is recommended when the cranial nerves are considered at high risk as the following recanalization would restore the arterial supply of cranial nerves in the case of accidental occlusion, unlike glue-based embolic agents which do not offer such a possibility thus requiring provocative tests to identify arterial feeders for the vasa nervorum of cranial nerves. Following subtotal surgical resection, recurrent paragangliomas may be associated with a profound alteration of the vascular supply of the tumors: in these particular cases embolization must be planned with extreme caution [18].

Hemangioblastomas

Hemangioblastomas account for 1.1% - 2% of all craniospinal tumors [133]. Mostly sporadic, these growths occur more frequently in the posterior cranial fossa, precisely in the cerebellar hemispheres and rarely the vermis or cerebello-pontine angle and the brainstem. Approximately 20% are associated with von Hippel-Landau disease. Their main feature is hypervascularization, which also represents the main obstacle during surgical resection and the main source of morbidity and mortality [134] which used to reach rates of 50% prior to the advent of microsurgical techniques [135].

Pre-surgical embolization is indicated for large lesions (>3 cm) [136, 137] with well-defined arterial feeders considered to be inaccessible during surgery. Embolization is usually dangerous considering that hemangioblastomas are more likely to be fed by pial vessels such as branches of the posterior or anterior inferior cerebellar artery. PVA and NBCA are usually the embolic agents of choice. Surgical resection should be performed within 48 to 72 hours to prevent eventual recanalization. Tampieri *et al.* [138] described a massive reduction of intraoperative blood-loss (<100 mL) during surgery in two patients harboring large hemnagiobalstomas of the spine and the posterior fossa who were both treated with pre-surgical embolization. Considering the frequent involvement of the structures of the posterior fossa, massive tumor infarction and swelling following embolization are both to be feared. Eskridge *et al.* [139], reporting on a series of nine craniospinal hemangioblastomas embolized with PVA, described that one patient developed malignant posterior fossa edema with hydrocephalus after the procedure. Conway *et al.* [137] described four of 40 patients with hemangioblastomas treated with preoperative embolization, of whom one suffered a lateral medullary infarction after embolization. Lee *et al.* [140] described four of 14 patients with spinal cord hemangioblastomas treated with pre-surgical embolization. Surgical resection was successful and the neurosurgeon reported a subjectively judged reduction in intraoperative blood loss.

Juvenile Nasopharyngeal Angiofibromas

Accounting for 0.5% of all head and neck tumors [141], juvenile nasopharyngeal angiofibromas (JNAs) are highly vascular, benign neoplasms originating within the posterior margin of the sphenopalatine foramen. They occur mostly in young male patients (mean age at diagnosis is 14 years old). Nasal obstruction and epistaxis are the main presenting symptoms. Despite being benign entities, aggressive local invasion and a high potential for post-surgical recurrence make JNAs difficult to deal with [142, 143]. The macroscopic aspect, observed during nasopharyngeal examination, is usually that of a pink-blue nodular mass located in the oropharynx. Chandler's classification of JNAs [144] includes a stage I referring to JNAs localized in the nasopharyngeal region; stage II which characterizes JNAs extending into the nasal cavities and/or sphenoid sinus; stage III for JNAs invading the infratemporal fossa, orbit or cheek; and stage IV for JNAs with intracranial extension. JNAs, especially when reaching stage IV, require a diagnostic bilateral carotid angiography because there is, not uncommonly, arterial recruitment from the ophthalmic artery, contralateral maxillary artery and branches of the ICA. Other angiographic features include a tortuous vascular network and dense blush during the capillary phase. Ectasic draining veins may be precociously present. The main arterial feeders are usually branches of the IMA; in one-third of the cases the ascending pharyngeal artery is involved [145]. Embolization prior to surgery may reduce intraoperative blood loss and, more importantly, facilitate the most radical resection possible [34, 146]. Roberson *et al.* [145] described how embolization reduced the blood loss from

2400 to 800 mL during surgery. Siniluoto *et al.* [147] compared embolized *versus* non-embolized patients and found that blood loss, resection quality and recurrence rates were better in the embolization group. The main complications following embolization of JNAs include bradycardia, especially after embolization of the IMA and ascending pharyngeal artery, and distal dissemination of embolisates, usually resulting from accidental dissemination of emboli between the ECA and ICA circulations. Gay *et al.* [148] also described palatal necrosis and an oronasal fistula, the latter occurring after surgical resection by transpalatal resection.

Hemangiopericytomas

These tumors arise from the contractile pericytes of Zimmerman coating capillary walls. They account for less than 1% of all central nervous system tumors [149]. Manifesting preferentially in middle-aged patients, hemangiopericytomas occur with equal frequencies in both genders and are aggressive tumors with a high potential for both recurrence and metastatic dissemination [150]. They are hypervascular to such an extent that hemorrhage is the main source of surgical morbidity and mortality and usually hampers complete resection during surgery. Embolization should be aggressive in these cases: a combined approach consisting of pre-surgical embolization and subsequent intraoperative direct intratumoral injection of embolic agents may be required. Embolization is, however, challenging considering that hemangiopericytomas are usually supplied by cortical vessels and the risk of hemorrhagic complications is, therefore, high [140, 149-152].

INTRA-ARTERIAL CHEMOTHERAPY FOR BRAIN TUMORS

Although thousands of patients have been treated for primary and secondary brain tumors by non-selective intra-arterial cerebral infusion, the only phase III trials on this strategy evaluated the effects of nitrosureas (carmustine and PCNU) [153]. However, in the 1990s the use of nitrosureas was discouraged by reports of severe toxicity-related complications [154-156]. To date, there is no confirmation of the efficacy or proof of safety of other concurrent drugs, such as cisplatin, carboplatin, etoposide, methotrexate, antibodies (bevacizumab) and their associations [157, 158].

Various drug administration techniques have been employed. In most cases the drug is administered by a catheter positioned in the ICA at the level of C2. Nagawaka *et al.* [159] and Dropcho *et al.* [160] reported on selective drug infusion by guiding the tip of the intra-arterial catheter into the proximal segments of the terminal branches of the circle of Willis or a major branch of the middle cerebral or basilar artery. Selective catheterization was associated with a lower risk of visual loss than intracarotid infusion, but cerebral infarction and neurotoxic complications other than loss of vision were not reduced [160].

Super-selective intra-arterial cerebral infusion (SIACI) minimizes the neurotoxicity of chemotherapeutic agents and potentiates their efficacy in cases of blood-brain barrier disruption. In contrast, blood-brain barrier disruption in patients treated with non-selective intra-arterial chemotherapy increases the toxicity of the treatment as it exposes normal brain tissue to the drugs. In SIACI, the super-selective catheterization of the tumor's arterial supply enables blood-brain barrier disruption to be used. In most cases, the infusion of 1.4 M mannitol at a rate of 10 mL per 120 seconds is sufficient to open the blood-brain barrier temporarily. The use of hyperosmotic agents to disrupt the barrier results in only a 25% increase of permeability of tumor microvasculature, in contrast to a 10-fold increase of permeability of the normal brain endothelium [161].

In the first few years of the 21st century, SIACI was practiced with carboplatin for the treatment of primary grade III and IV gliomas and secondary neoplasms [162-164]. Although definitive statements about its efficacy should not be made given the restricted cohorts analyzed so far, the toxicity of carboplatin in SIACI appeared to be similar to that in non-selective cerebral infusion [163-165].

In 2007 the first evaluation of the safety of bevacizumab for the treatment of recurrent glioblastoma was published [166]. On the basis of these data, the Food and Drug Administration approved the use of bevacizumab a few years later. Bevacizumab is a monoclonal antibody which binds to vascular endothelial growth factor, reducing tumor-induced neoangiogenesis and also having an effect on the existing vasculature. It reduces brain edema and stabilizes tumor growth. Nevertheless, complications of the intravenous infusion of bevacizumab include infections, venous thromboembolic events and difficulties in wound healing (which occurred in 9.5%, 2.4% and 3.6% of cases, respectively) [167, 168]. The use of bevacizumab with SIACI was intended to minimize these systemic complications typical of intravenous infusion. To date, 37 patients with recurrent glioblastoma, one patient with multiple malignant ependymoma, 26 patients with glioblastoma, three patients with anaplastic astrocytoma and one patient with oligoastrocytoma have been treated [169-175]. Systemic complications that were observed with intravenous infusion were not present with SIACI. Burkhardt *et al.*

[173] and Boockvar *et al.* [171] reported that the incidence of seizures, which responded well to antiepileptic drug therapy, was 7.1% and 6.6%, respectively.

The most recent data on the overall survival of patients affected by glioblastoma were published in 2009 by Stupp *et al.* [176], who reported a 9.8% overall survival rate at 5 years after surgery followed by radiotherapy with concomitant administration of temozolomide. Efficacy data on SIACI of bevacizumab is not currently comparable with that of standard therapies. On the other hand, the minimization of neurotoxicity offered by SIACI has encouraged physicians to retrace their steps along a path that was discouraged in the 1990s by the high rate of complications and limited efficacy. If the use of SIACI is proven to be safe and effective in larger phase II and III trials, a new way to deliver chemotherapy will be an option, giving rise, as happened with the treatment of brain aneurysms, to a new endovascular era [177].

ACKNOWLEDGMENTS

Declared none.

CONFLICT OF INTEREST

The authors confirm that this chapter contents have no conflict of interest.

REFERENCES

[1]   Dawbarn RH. The Treatment of Certain Malignant Growths by Excision. F. A. Davis Company, publishers. Philadelphia. 1903.
[2]   Dawbarn RH. The starvation operation for malignancy in the external carotid area. JAMA 1904; 17: 792-5.
[3]   Djindjian R. The future for angiography in neuroradiology. Neuroradiology 1972; 3: 175-6.
[4]   Djindjian R, Cophignon J, Theron J. Embolization by superselective arteriography from the femoral route in neuroradiology. Review of 60 cases. Neuroradiology 1973; 6: 20-6.
[5]   Manelfe C, Guiraud B, David J, *et al.* [Embolization by catheterization of intracranial meningiomas.] Rev Neurol (Paris) 1973; 128: 339-51 [In French].
[6]   Hekster RE, Matricali B, Luyendijk W. Presurgical transfemoral catheter embolization to reduce operative blood loss. Technical note. J Neurosurg 1974; 41: 396-8.
[7]   French JD, West PM, Von Ameraugh FK, *et al.* Effects of intracarotid administration of nitrogen mustard on normal brain and brain tumors. J Neurosurg 1952; 9: 378-89.
[8]   Peschillo S, Delfini R. Endovascular neurosurgery in Europe and in Italy: what is in the future? World Neurosurg 2012; 77: 248-51.
[9]   American Society of Interventional and Therapeutic Neuroradiology. Head, neck, and brain tumor embolization. AJNR Am J Neuroradiol 2001; 22: S14-5.
[10]   Hayashi T, Shojima K, Utsunomiya H, *et al.* Subarachnoid hemorrhage after preoperative embolization of a cystic meningioma. Surg Neurol 1987; 27: 295-300.
[11]   Horowitz MB, Carrau R, Crammond D, *et al.* Risks of tumor embolization in the presence of an unrecognized patent foramen ovale: case report. AJNR Am J Neuroradiol 2002; 23: 982-4.

[12]   Carli DF, Sluzewski M, Beute GN, *et al.* Complications of particle embolization of meningiomas: frequency, risk factors, and outcome. AJNR Am J Neuroradiol 2010; 31: 152-4.

[13]   Bendszus M, Monoranu CM, Schutz A, Nölte I, Vince GH, Solymosi L. Neurologic complications after particle embolization of intracranial meningiomas. AJNR Am J Neuroradiol 2005; 26: 1413-9.

[14]   Lasjaunias P, Berenstein A. The transosseous peripheral nervous system arterial supply. In: Lasjaunias P, Berenstein A (eds), Surgical Neuroangiography, part 1, functional anatomy of craniofacial arteries. Wien, New York: Springer, 1987: 221-37.

[15]   Garcia-Monaco R. Transcranial arterial anastomoses. Rivista di Neuroradiologia 1994; 7(Suppl 4): 63-6.

[16]   Lasjaunias P, Berenstein A. Dangerous vessels. In: Lasjaunias P, Berenstein A (eds), Surgical Neuroangiography, part 1, functional anatomy of craniofacial arteries. Wien, New York: Springer, 1987: 239-44.

[17]   Nelson PK, Setton A, Choi IS, *et al.* Current status of interventional neuroradiology in the management of meningiomas. Neurosurg Clin N Am 1994; 5: 235-59.

[18]   Gruber A, Bavinzski G, Killer M, *et al.* Preoperative embolization of hypervascular skull base tumors. Minim Invasive Neurosurg 2000; 43: 62-71.

[19]   Chun JY, McDermott MW, Lamborn KR, *et al.* Delayed surgical resection reduces intraoperative blood loss for embolized meningiomas. Neurosurgery 2002; 50: 1231-5; discussion 1235-7.

[20]   Adler JR, Upton J, Wallman J, *et al.* Management and prevention of necrosis of the scalp after embolization and surgery for meningioma. Surg Neurol 1986; 25: 357-60.

[21]   Halbach VV, Hieshima GB, Higashida RT, *et al.* Endovascular therapy of head and neck tumors. In: Vinuela F, Halbach VV, Dion JE, editors. Interventional Neuroradiology: Endovascular Therapy of the Central Nervous System. New York: Raven Press; 1992; 17-28.

[22]   Gruber A, Killer M, Mazal P, *et al.* Preoperative embolization of intracranial meningiomas: a 17-year single center experience. Minim Invasive Neurosurg 2000; 43: 18-29.

[23]   Chan RC, Thompson GB. Ischemic necrosis of the scalp after preoperative embolization of meningeal tumors. Neurosurgery 1984; 15: 76-81.

[24]   Ahuja A, Gibbons KJ. Endovascular therapy of central nervous system tumors. Neurosurg Clin N Am 1994; 5: 541-54.

[25]   Lapresle J, Lasjaunias P. Cranial nerve ischaemic arterial syndromes. A review. Brain 1986; 109(Pt 1): 207-16.

[26]   Dowd CF, Halbach VV, Higashida RT. Meningiomas: the role of preoperative angiography and embolization. Neurosurg Focus 2003; 15: E10.

[27]   Deshmukh VR, Fiorella DJ, McDougall CG, Spetzler RF, Albuquerque FC. Preoperative embolization of central nervous system tumors. Neurosurg Clin N Am 2005; 16: 411-32, xi.

[28]   Waldron JS, Sughrue ME, Hetts SW, *et al.* Embolization of skull base meningiomas and feeding vessels arising from the internal carotid circulation. Neurosurgery 2011; 68: 162-9.

[29]   Horton JA, Kerber CW. Lidocaine injection into external carotid branches: provocative test to preserve cranial nerve function in therapeutic embolization. AJNR Am J Neuroradiol 1986; 7: 105-8.

[30]   Deveikis JP. Sequential injections of amobarbital sodium and lidocaine for provocative neurologic testing in the external carotid circulation. AJNR Am J Neuroradiol 1996; 17: 1143-7.

[31]   Eskridge JM. Interventional neuroradiology. Radiology 1989; 172: 991-1006.

[32]   Theron J, Cosgrove R, Melanson D, *et al.* Embolization with temporary balloon occlusion of the internal carotid or vertebral arteries. Neuroradiology 1986; 28: 246-53.

[33]   Jungreis CA. Skull-base tumors: ethanol embolization of the cavernous carotid artery. Radiology 1991; 181: 741-3.

[34]   Garcia-Cervigon E, Bien S, Rufenacht D, *et al.* Preoperative embolization of naso-pharyngeal angiofibromas. Report of 58 cases. Neuroradiology 1988; 30: 556-60.

[35]   Lefkowitz M, Giannotta SL, Hieshima G, *et al.* Embolization of neurosurgical lesions involving the ophthalmic artery. Neurosurgery 1998; 43: 1298-303.

[36]   Yoon YS, Ahn JY, Chang JH, *et al.* Preoperative embolisation of internal carotid artery branches and pial vessels in hypervascular brain tumours. Acta Neurochir (Wien). 2008; 150: 447-52.

[37]   Capo H, Kuppersmith MJ, Berenstein A, Choi IS, Diamond GA. The clinical importance of the inferolateral trunk of the internal carotid artery. Neurosurgery 1991; 28: 733-8.

[38]   Herrera M, Rysavy J, Kotula F, *et al*. Ivalon shavings: technical considerations of a new embolic agent. Radiology 1982; 144: 638-40.

[39]   Szwarc IA, Carrasco CH, Wallace S, *et al*. Radiopaque suspension of polyvinyl alcohol foam for embolization. AJR Am J Roentgenol 1986; 146: 591-2.

[40]   Kunstlinger F, Brunelle F, Chaumont P, Doyon D. Vascular occlusive agents. AJR Am J Roentgenol 1981; 136: 151-6.

[41]   Berenstein A, Graeb DA. Convenient preparation of ready-to-use particles in polyvinyl alcohol foam suspension for embolization. Radiology 1982; 145: 846.

[42]   Kai Y, Hamada J-I, Morioka M, *et al*. Clinical evaluation of cellulose porous beads for the therapeutic embolization of meningiomas. AJNR Am J Neuroradiol 2006; 27: 1146-50.

[43]   Richling B. Homologous controlled-viscosity fibrin for endovascular embolization. Part I: experimental development of the medium. Acta Neurochir (Wien) 1982; 62: 159-70.

[44]   Richling B. Homologous controlled-viscosity fibrin for endovascular embolization. Part II: catheterization technique, animal experiments. Acta Neurochir. (Wien). 1982 Jan; 64(1-2): 109–24.

[45]   Bendszus M, Klein R, Burger R, *et al*. Efficacy of trisacryl gelatin microspheres versus polyvinyl alcohol particles in the preoperative embolization of meningiomas AJNR Am J Neuroradiol 2000; 21: 255-61.

[46]   Ellman BA, Green CE, Eigenbrodt E, *et al*. Renal infarction with absolute ethanol. Invest Radiol 1980; 15: 318-22.

[47]   Latshaw RF, Pearlman RL, Schaitkin BM, *et al*. Intraarterial ethanol as a long-term occlusive agent in renal, hepatic, and gastrosplenic arteries of pigs. Cardiovasc Intervent Radiol 1985; 8: 24-30.

[48]   Horowitz M, Whisnant RE, Jungreis C, *et al*. Temporary balloon occlusion and ethanol injection for preoperative embolization of carotid-body tumor. Ear Nose Throat J 2002; 81: 536-8,540,542.

[49]   Lonser RR, Heiss JD, Oldfield EH. Tumor devascularization by intratumoral ethanol injection during surgery. Technical note. J Neurosurg 1998; 88: 923-4.

[50]   Probst EN, Grzyska U, Westphal M, *et al*. Preoperative embolization of intracranial meningiomas with a fibrin glue preparation. AJNR Am J Neuroradiol 1999; 20: 1695-702.

[51]   Kumar AJ, Kaufman SL, Patt J, *et al*. Preoperative embolization of hypervascular head and neck neoplasms using microfibrillar collagen. AJNR Am J Neuroradiol 1982; 3: 163-8.

[52]   Kasuya H, Shimizu T, Sasahara A, *et al*. Phenytoin as a liquid material for embolisation of tumours. Neuroradiology 1999; 41: 320-3.

[53]   Kubo M, Kuwayama N, Hirashima Y, Takaku A, Ogawa T, Endo S. Hydroxyapatite ceramics as a particulate embolic material: report of the physical properties of the hydroxyapatite particles and the animal study. AJNR Am J Neuroradiol 2003; 24: 1540-4.

[54]   Kubo M, Kuwayama N, Hirashima Y, *et al*. Hydroxyapatite ceramics as a particulate embolic material: report of the clinical experience. AJNR Am J Neuroradiol 2003; 24: 1545-7.

[55]   Rodesch G, Lasjaunias P. Embolization and meningiomas. In: Al-Mefty O, editor. Meningiomas. New York: Raven Press; 1991: 285-97.

[56]   Duffis EJ, Gandhi CD, Prestigiacomo CJ, *et al*. Head, neck, and brain tumor embolization guidelines. J Neurointerv Surg 2012; 4: 251-5.

[57]   Engelhard HH. Progress in the diagnosis and treatment of patients with meningiomas. Part I: diagnostic imaging, preoperative embolization. Surg Neurol 2001; 55: 89-101.

[58]   Desai R, Bruce J. Meningiomas of the cranial base. J Neurooncol 1994; 20: 255-79.

[59]   Kai Y, Hamada J, Morioka M, *et al*. Appropriate interval between embolization and surgery in patients with meningioma. AJNR Am J Neuroradiol 2002; 23: 139-42.

[60]   Ahuja A, Gibbons KJ, Hopkins LN. Endovascular techniques to treat brain tumors. In: Youmans JR, ed. Neurological Surgery. Philadelphia: W.B. Saunders Co. 1996: 2826-40.

[61]   Pauw BK, Makek MS, Fisch U, *et al*. Preoperative embolization of paragangliomas (glomus tumors) of the head and neck: histopathologic and clinical features. Skull Base Surg 1993; 3: 37-44

[62]   Shah AH, Patel N, Raper DM, *et al*. The role of preoperative embolization for intracranial meningiomas. J. Neurosurg 2013; 119: 364-72.

[63]   Adegbite AB, Khan MI, Paine KW, *et al*. The recurrence of intracranial meningiomas after surgical treatment. J Neurosurg 1983; 58: 51-6.

[64]   Chan RC, Thompson GB. Morbidity, mortality, and quality of life following surgery for intracranial meningiomas. A retrospective study in 257 cases. J Neurosurg 1984; 60: 52-60.

[65]   Jaaskelainen J. Seemingly complete removal of histologically benign intracranial meningioma: late recurrence rate and factors predicting recurrence in 657 patients. A multivariate analysis. Surg Neurol 1986; 26: 461-9.

[66]   Simpson D. The recurrence of intracranial menin giomas after surgical treatment. J Neurochem 1957; 20: 22-39.

[67]   Richter HP, Schachenmayr W. Preoperative embolization of intracranial meningiomas. Neurosurgery 1983; 13: 261-8.

[68]   Manelfe C, Lasjaunias P, Ruscalleda J. Preoperative embolization of intracranial meningiomas. AJNR Am J Neuroradiol 1986; 7: 963-72.

[69]   Macpherson P. The value of preoperative embolization of meningioma estimated subjectively and objectively. Neuroradiology 1991; 33: 334-7.

[70]   Dean BL, Flom RA, Wallace RC, *et al.* Efficacy of endovascular treatment of meningiomas: evaluation with matched samples. AJNR Am J Neuroradiol 1994; 15: 1675-80.

[71]   Javadpour M, Khan AD, Jenkinson MD, Foy PM, Nahser HC. Cerebral aneurysm associated with an intracranial tumour: staged endovascular and surgical treatment in two cases. Br J Neurosurg 2004; 18: 280-4.

[72]   Maekawa H, Tanaka M, Hadeishi H. Middle meningeal artery aneurysm associated with meningioma. Acta Neurochir (Wien) 2009; 151: 1167-8.

[73]   O'Neill OR, Barnwell SL, Silver DJ. Middle meningeal artery aneurysm associated with meningioma: case report. Neurosurgery 1995; 36: 396-8.

[74]   Lasjaunias P, Berenstein A. Dural and bony tumours. In: Lasjaunias P, Berenstein A (eds), Surgical Neuroangiography, part 2, endovascular treatment of craniofacial lesions. Wien, NewYork: Springer, 1987: 57-99.

[75]   Bendszus M, Rao G, Burger R, *et al.* Is there a benefit of preoperative meningioma embolization? Neurosurgery 2000; 47: 1306-11; discussion 1311-2.

[76]   Latchaw RE. Preoperative intracranial meningioma embolization: technical considerations affecting the risk-to-benefit ratio. AJNR Am J Neuroradiol 1993; 14: 583-6.

[77]   Yamaguchi N, Kawase T, Sagoh M, Ohira T, Shiga H, Toya S. Prediction of consistency of meningiomas with preoperative magnetic resonance imaging. Surg Neurol 1997; 48: 579-83.

[78]   Kaji T, Hama Y, Iwasaki Y, *et al.* Preoperative embolization of meningiomas with pial supply: successful treatment of two cases. Surg Neurol 1999; 52: 270-3.

[79]   Terada T, Kinoshita Y, Yokote H, *et al.* Preoperative embolization of meningiomas fed by ophthalmic branch arteries. Surg Neurol 1996; 45: 161-6.

[80]   Hirohata M, Abe T, Morimitsu H, *et al.* Preoperative selective internal carotid artery dural branch embolisation for petroclival meningiomas. Neuroradiology 2003; 45: 656-60.

[81]   Halbach VV, Higashida RT, Hieshima GB, *et al.* Embolization of branches arising from the cavernous portion of the internal carotid artery. AJNR Am J Neuroradiol 1989; 10: 143-50.

[82]   Robinson DH, Song JK, Eskridge JM. Embolization of meningohypophyseal and inferolateral branches of the cavernous internal carotid artery. AJNR Am J Neuroradiol 1999; 20: 1061-7.

[83]   Rosen CL, Ammerman JM, Sekhar LN, Bank WO. Outcome analysis of preoperative embolization in cranial base surgery. Acta Neurochir (Wien) 2002; 144: 1157-64.

[84]   Accreditation Council on Graduate Medical Education. Carotid artery balloon test occlusion. AJNR Am J Neuroradiol 2001; 22(Suppl): S8-9.

[85]   Berdick TR, Hoffer EK, Kooy T, *et al.* Which arteries are expendable? The practice and pitfalls of embolization throughout the body. Semin Intervent Radiol 2008; 25: 191-203.

[86]   Qureshi AI. Endovascular treatment of cerebrovascular diseases and intracranial neoplasms. Lancet 2004; 363: 804-13.

[87]   Kallmes DF, Evans AJ, Kaptain GJ, *et al.* Hemorrhagic complications in embolization of a meningioma: case report and review of the literature. Neuroradiology 1997; 39: 877-80.

[88]   Sekhar LN, Biswas A, Hallam D, *et al.* Neuroendovascular management of tumors and vascular malformations of the head and neck. Neurosurg Clin North Am 2009; 20: 453-85.

[89]   Lasjaunias P, Doyon D. The ascending pharyngeal artery and the blood supply of the lower cranial nerves. J Neuroradiol 1978; 5: 287-301.

[90]   Sluzewski M, van Rooij WJ, Lohle PN, Beute GN, Peluso JP. Embolization of meningiomas: comparison of safety between calibrated microspheres and polyvinyl-alcohol particles as embolic agents. AJNR Am J Neuroradiol 2013; 34: 727-9.

[91]   Suzuki J, Komatsu S. New embolization method using estrogen for dural arteriovenous malformation and meningioma. Surg Neurol 1981; 16: 438-42.

[92]   Oka H, Kurata A, Kawano N, *et al.* Preoperative superselective embolization of skullbase meningiomas: indications and limitations. J Neurooncol 1998; 40: 67-71.

[93]   Suyama T, Tamaki N, Fijiwara K, *et al.* Peritumoral and intratumoral hemorrhage after gelatin sponge embolization of malignant meningioma: case report. Neurosurgery 1987; 21: 944-6.

[94]   Motozaki T, Otsuka S, Sato S, *et al.* Preoperative embolization with gelfoam powder for intracranial meningioma caused an unusual peritumoral hemorrhage. No Shinkei Geka 1987; 15: 95-101.

[95]   Watanabe K, Matsumura K, Matsuda M, *et al.* Meningioma with intratumoral and subdural hemorrhage as an immediate complication of therapeutic embolization. Neurol Med Chir 1986; 26: 904-7.

[96]   Yu SC, Boet R, Wong GK, *et al.* Postembolization hemorrhage of a large and necrotic meningioma. AJNR Am J Neuroradiol 2004; 25: 506-8.

[97]   Teasdale E, Patterson J, McLellan D, *et al.* Subselective preoperative embolization for meningiomas. A radiological and pathological assessment. J Neurosurg 1984; 60: 506-11.

[98]   Modesti LM, Binet EF, Collins GH. Meningiomas causing spontaneous intracranial hematomas. Neurosurgery 1976; 45: 437-41.

[99]   Buccoliero AM, Caldarella A, Taddei A, *et al.* Atypical, aplastic, and unusual meningiomas: morphology and incidence in 300 consecutive cases. Pathologica 2003; 95: 83-7.

[100]   Helle TL, Conley FK. Hemorrhage associated with meningioma: a case report and review of the literature. J Neurol Neurosurg Psychiatry 1980; 43: 725-9.

[101]   Beretta L, Dell'acqua A, Giogi E, *et al.* Complications during preoperative embolization in intracranial meningioma. Minerva Anestesiol 1992; 58(Suppl 4): 111-4.

[102]   Hieshima GB, Everhart FR, Mehringer CM, *et al.* Preoperative embolization of meningiomas. Surg Neurol 1980; 14: 119-27.

[103]   Wakhloo AK, Juengling FD, Van Velthoven V, *et al.* Extended preoperative polyvinyl alcohol microembolization of intracranial meningiomas: assessment of two embolization techniques. AJNR Am J Neuroradiol 1993; 14: 571-82.

[104]   Broaddus WC, Grady MS, Delashaw JB, Ferguson RD, Jane JA. Preoperative superselective arteriolar embolization: a new approach to enhance resectability of spinal tumors. Neurosurgery 1990; 17: 755-9.

[105]   Ng HK, Poon WS, Goh K, *et al.* Histopathology of post-embolized meningiomas. Am J Surg Pathol 1996; 20: 1224-30.

[106]   Perry A, Chicoine MR, Filiput E, *et al.* Clinicopathologic assessment and grading of embolized meningiomas: a correlative study of 64 patients. Cancer 2001; 92: 701-11.

[107]   Azzarelli B, Felten S, Muller J, *et al.* Dopamine in paragangliomas of the glomus jugulare. Laryngoscope 1988; 98: 573-8.

[108]   Blumenfeld JD, Cohen N, Laragh JH, *et al.* Hypertension and catecholamine biosynthesis associated with a glomus jugulare tumor. N Engl J Med 1992; 327: 894-5.

[109]   Farrior J. Surgical management of glomus tumors: endocrine-active tumors of the skull base. South Med J 1988; 81: 1121-6.

[110]   Nelson MD, Kendall BE. Intracranial catecholamine secreting paragangliomas. Neuroradiology 1987; 29: 277-82.

[111]   Lack EE, Cubilla AL, Woodruff JM, *et al.* Paragangliomas of the head and neck region: a clinical study of 69 patients. Cancer 1977; 39: 397-409.

[112]   Meyer FB, Sundt TM Jr, Pearson BW. Carotid body tumors: a subject review and suggested surgical approach. J Neurosurg 1986; 64: 377-85.

[113]   Hodge KM, Byers RM, Peters LJ. Paragangliomas of the head and neck. Arch Otolaryngol Head Neck Surg 1988; 114: 872-7.

[114]   Jackson CG. Glomus tympanicum and glomus jugulare tumors. Otolaryngol Clin North Am 2001; 34: 941-70.

[115]   Rosenwasser H. Glomus jugulare tumors. I. Historical background. Arch Otolaryngol 1968; 88: 1-40.

[116]   Miller RB, Boon MS, Atkins JP, Lowry LD. Vagal paraganglioma: the Jefferson experience. Otolaryngol Head Neck Surg 2000; 122: 482-7.

[117]   Solymosi L, Ferbert A. A case of spinal paraganglioma. Neuroradiology 1985; 27: 217-9.

[118]   Shamblin WR, ReMine WH, Sheps SG, Harrison EG Jr. Carotid body tumor (chemodectoma). Clinicopathologic analysis of ninety cases. Am J Surg 1971; 122: 732-9,

[119]   Offergeld C, Brase C, Yaremchuk S, *et al.* Head and neck paragangliomas: clinical and molecular genetic classification. Clinics 2012; 67(S1): 19-28.

[120]   Djindjian R. Super-selective arteriography of branches of the external carotid artery. Surg Neurol 1976; 5: 133-42.

[121]   Valavanis A. Preoperative embolization of the head and neck: indications, patient selection, goals, and precautions. AJNR Am J Neuroradiol 1986; 7: 943-52.

[122]   Moret J, Delvert JC, Bretonneau CH, Lasjaunias P. Vascularization of the ear: normal – variations – glomus tumors. J Neuroradiol 1982; 9: 209-36.

[123]   Hilal SK, Michelsen JW. Therapeutic percutaneous embolization for extra-axial vascular lesions of the head, neck, and spine. J Neurosurg 1975; 43: 275-87.

[124]   Murphy TP, Brackmann DE. Effects of preoperative embolization on glomus jugulare tumors. Laryngoscope 1989; 99: 1244-7.

[125]   Tikkakoski T, Luotonen J, Leinonen S, *et al.* Preoperative embolization in the management of neck paragangliomas. Laryngoscope 1997; 107: 821-6.

[126]   Young NM, Wiet RJ, Russell EJ, *et al.* Superselective embolization of glomus jugulare tumors. Ann Otol Rhinol Laryngol 1988; 97: 613-20.

[127]   George B. Jugulare foramen paragangliomas. Acta Neurochir (Wien) 1992; 118: 20–6.

[128]   Cohen JE, Ferrario A, Ceratto R, *et al.* Covered stent as an innovative tool for tumor devasculariza-tion and endovascular arterial reconstruction. Neurol Res 2003; 25: 169-72.

[129]   LaMuraglia GM, Fabian RL, Brewster DC, *et al.* The current surgical management of carotid body paragangliomas. J Vasc Surg 1992; 15: 1038-44.

[130]   Pandya SK, Nagpal RD, Desai AP, *et al.* Death following external carotid artery embolization for a functioning glomus jugulare chemodectoma. Case report. J Neurosurg 1978; 48: 1030-4.

[131]   Marangos N, Schumacher M. Facial palsy after glomus jugulare tumour embolization. J Laryngol Otol 1999; 113: 268-70.

[132]   Herdman RC, Gillespie JE, Ramsden RT. Facial palsy after glomus tumour embolization. J Laryngol Otol 1993; 107: 963-6.

[133]   Russell DS, Rubinstein LJ. Tumours and hamartomas of the blood-vessels. In: Pathology of Tumors of the Nervous System. 4th edition. Baltimore: Williams & Wilkins; 1977; 127-45.

[134]   Djindjian M. Successful removal of a brainstem hemangioblastoma. Surg Neurol 1986; 25: 97-100.

[135]   Sanford RA, Smith RA. Hemangioblastoma of the cervicomedullary junction. Report of three cases. J Neurosurg 1986; 64: 317-21.

[136]   Wang C, Zhang J, Liu A, *et al.* Surgical management of medullary hemangioblastoma. Report of 47 cases. Surg Neurol 2001; 56: 218-26.

[137]   Conway JE, Chou D, Clatterbuck RE, *et al.* Hemangioblastomas of the central nervous system in von Hippel-Lindau syndrome and sporadic disease. Neurosurgery 2001; 48: 55-62.

[138]   Tampieri D, Leblanc R, TerBrugge K. Preoperative embolization of brain and spinal hemangioblastomas. Neurosurgery 1993; 33: 502-5.

[139]   Eskridge JM, McAuliffe W, Harris B, *et al.* Preoperative endovascular embolization of craniospinal hemangioblastomas. AJNR Am J Neuroradiol 1996; 17: 525-31.

[140]   Lee DK, Choe WJ, Chung CK, *et al.* Spinal cord hemangioblastoma: surgical strategy and clinical outcome. J Neurooncol 2003; 61: 27-34.

[141]   Magit AE. Tumors of the nose, paranasal sinuses, and nasopharynx. In: Bluestone CD, Stool SE, Kenna MA, editors. Pediatric Otolaryngology. 3rd edition. Philadelphia: WB Saunders; 2004; 893-904.

[142]   Bryan RN, Sessions RB, Horowitz BL. Radiographic management of juvenile angiofibromas. AJNR Am J Neuroradiol 1981; 2: 157-66.

[143]   McCombe A, Lund VJ, Howard DJ. Recurrence in juvenile angiofibroma. Rhinology 1990; 28: 97-102.

[144] Chandler JR, Goulding R, Moskowitz L. Nasopharyngeal angiofibromas: staging and management. Ann Otol Rhinol Laryngol 1984; 93: 322-9.

[145] Roberson GH, Price AC, Davis JM, *et al.* Therapeutic embolization of juvenile angiofibroma. AJR Am J Roentgenol 1979; 133: 657-63.

[146] Pletcher JD, Newton TH, DedoHH, *et al.* Preoperative embolization of juvenile angiofibromas of the nasopharynx. Ann Otol Rhinol Laryngol 1975; 84: 740-6.

[147] Siniluoto TM, Luotonen JP, Tikkakoski TA, *et al.* Value of preoperative embolization in surgery for nasopharyngeal angiofibroma. J Laryngol Otol 1993; 107: 514-21.

[148] Gay I, Elidan J, Gordon R. Oronasal fistula - a possible complication of preoperative embolization in the management of juvenile nasopharyngeal angiofibroma. J Laryngol Otol 1983; 97: 651-6.

[149] Guthrie BL, Ebersold MJ, Scheithauer BW, *et al.* Meningeal hemangiopericytoma: histopathological features, treatment, and long-term follow-up of 44 cases. Neurosurgery 1989; 25: 514-22.

[150] Pandey M, Kothari KC, PatelDD. Haemangiopericytoma: current status, diagnosis and management. Eur J Surg Oncol 1997; 23: 282-5.

[151] Jaaskelainen J, Servo A, Haltia M, *et al.* Intracranial hemangiopericytoma: radiology, surgery, radiotherapy, and outcome in 21 patients. Surg Neurol 1985; 23: 227-36.

[152] Muraszko KM, Antunes JL, Hilal SK, *et al.* Hemangiopericytomas of the spine. Neurosurgery 1982; 10: 473-9.

[153] Newton HB. Intra-arterial chemotherapy of primary brain tumors. Curr Treat Options Oncol 2005; 6: 519-30.

[154] Feun LG, Lee YY, Yung WK, *et al.* Phase II trial of intracarotid BCNU and cisplatin in primary malignant brain tumors. Cancer Drug Deliv 1986; 3: 147-56.

[155] Tonn JC, Roosen K, Schachenmayr W. Brain necroses after intraarterial chemotherapy and irradiation of malignant gliomas - a complication of both ACNU and BCNU? J Neurooncol 1991; 11: 241-2.

[156] Shapiro WR, Green SB, Burger PC, *et al.* A randomized comparison of intra-arterial versus intravenous BCNU, with or without intravenous 5-fluorouracil, for newly diagnosed patients with malignant glioma. J Neurosurg 1992; 76: 772-81.

[157] Stewart DJ. Intraarterial chemotherapy of primary and metastatic brain tumors. In Neurological Complications of Cancer Treatment. Edited by Rottenberg DA. Boston, MA: Butterworth-Heinimann; 1991: 143-70.

[158] Basso U, Londardi S, Brandes AA. Is intra-arterial chemotherapy useful in high-grade gliomas? Expert Rev Anticancer Ther 2002, 2: 507-19.

[159] Nakagawa H, Fujita T, Kubo S, Tsuruzono K, Yamada M. Selective intra-arterial chemotherapy with a combination of etoposide and cisplatin for malignant gliomas: preliminary report. Surg Neurol 1994; 41: 19-27.

[160] Dropcho EJ, Rosenfeld SS, Vitek J, Guthrie BL, Morawetz RB. Phase II study of intracarotid or selective intracerebral infusion of cisplatin for treatment of recurrent anaplastic gliomas. J Neurooncol 1998; 36: 191-8.

[161] Misra A, Ganesh S, Shahiwala A, Shah SP. Drug delivery to the central nervous system: a review. J Pharm Pharm Sci 2003; 6: 252-73.

[162] Chow KL, Gobin YP, Cloughesy T, *et al.* Prognostic factors in recurrent glioblastoma multiforme and anaplastic astrocytoma treated with selective intra-arterial chemotherapy. AJNR Am J Neuroradiol 2000; 21: 471-8.

[163] Gobin YP, Cloughesy TF, Chow KL, *et al.* Intraarterial chemotherapy for brain tumors by using a spatial dose fractionation algorithm and pulsatile delivery. Radiology 2001; 218: 724-32.

[164] Qureshi AI, Suri MF, Khan J, *et al.* Superselective intra-arterial carboplatin for treatment of intracranial neoplasms: experience in 100 procedures. J Neurooncol 2001; 51: 151-8.

[165] Newton HB, Slivka MA, Stevens CL, *et al.* Intra-arterial carboplatin and intravenous etopodise for the treatment of recurrent and progressive non-GBM gliomas. J Neurooncol 2002; 56: 79-86.

[166] Vredenburgh JJ, Desjardins A, Herndon JE, *et al.* Phase II trial of bevacizumab and irinotecan in recurrent malignant glioma. Clin Cancer Res 2007; 13: 1253-9.

[167] Lai A, Filka E, McGibbon B, *et al.* Phase II pilot study of bevacizumab in combination with temozolamide and regional radiation therapy for up-front treatment of patients with newly diagnosed glioblastoma multiforme: interim analysis of safety and tolerability. Int J Radiat Oncol Biol Phys 2008; 71: 1372-80.

[168]   Pope WB, Lai A, Nghiemphu P, *et al*. MRI in patients with high-grade gliomas treated with bevacizumab and chemotherapy. Neurology 2006; 66: 1258-60.

[169]   Riina HA, Fraser JF, Fralin S, *et al*. Superselective intraarterial cerebral infusion of bevacizumab: a revival of interventional neuro-oncology for malignant glioma. J Exp Ther Oncol 2009; 8: 145-50.

[170]   Riina HA, Knopman J, Greenfield JP, *et al*. Balloon-assisted superselective intra-arterial cerebral infusion of bevacizumab for malignant brainstem glioma. A technical note. Interv Neuroradiol 2010; 16: 71-6.

[171]   Boockvar JA, Tsiouris AJ, Hofstetter CP, *et al*. Safety and maximum tolerated dose of superselective intraarterial cerebral infusion of bevacizumab after osmotic blood brain barrier disruption for recurrent malignant glioma. J Neurosurg 2011; 114: 624-32.

[172]   Rajappa P, Krass J, Riina HA, *et al*. Super-selective basilar artery infusion of bevacizumab and cetuximab for multiply recurrent pediatric ependymoma. Interv Neuroradiol 2011; 17: 459-65.

[173]   Burkhardt JK, Riina H, Shin BJ, *et al*. Intra-arterial delivery of bevacizumab after blood-brain barrier disruption for the treatment of recurrent glioblastoma: progression-free survival and overall survival. World Neurosurg 2012; 77: 130-4.

[174]   Jeon JY, Kovanlikaya I, Boockvar JA, *et al*. Metabolic response of glioblastoma to superselective intra-arterial cerebral infusion of bevacizumab: a proton MR spectroscopic imaging study. AJNR Am J Neuroradiol 2012; 33: 2095-102.

[175]   Shin BJ, Burkhardt JK, Riina HA, *et al*. Superselective intra-arterial cerebral infusion of novel agents after blood-brain disruption for the treatment of recurrent glioblastoma multiforme: a technical case series. Neurosurg Clin N Am 2012; 23: 323-9.

[176]   Stupp R, Hegi ME, Mason WP. Effects of radiotherapy with concomitant and adjuvant temozolomide versus radiotherapy alone on survival in glioblastoma in a randomised phase III study: 5-year analysis of the EORTC-NCIC trial. Lancet Oncol 2009; 10: 459-66.

[177]   Peschillo S, Miscusi M, Missori P. Endovascular superselective treatment of brain tumors: a new endovascular era? A quick review. J Neurointerv Surg 2014 Feb 7 [Epub ahead of print].

CHAPTER 9

Dual Antiplatelet Therapy in Neuroendovascular Procedures

Flavia Temperilli[1], Giorgio Re[2] and Fabio M. Pulcinelli[1,*]

[1]Department of Experimental Medicine, "Sapienza" University, Rome, Italy; [2]Department of Cardiovascular, Respiratory, Nephrologic, Anesthesiology and Geriatric Sciences, "Sapienza" University, Rome, Italy

Abstract: Dual antiplatelet therapy is currently used in clinical practice to prevent thrombotic events during and after neuroendovascular procedures.

Despite antiplatelet therapy, a significant number of patients show insufficient platelet inhibition, as measured by laboratory tests. These patients are at greater risk of developing thrombotic events than are patients sensitive to the treatment. This phenomenon is known as "antiplatelet drug resistance". The mechanisms that influence the individual response to antiplatelet therapy are not completely understood and are likely to be multifactorial.

Several platelet function tests have been developed to monitor antiplatelet therapy and may assist in adjusting it to improve outcomes in patients with antiplatelet drug resistance. Nevertheless, the optimal management for these patients has not yet been established. This chapter summarizes information on the available antiplatelet drugs currently used in neuroendovascular procedures, the commonly used tools for platelet function testing and the potential mechanisms underlying suboptimal platelet inhibition by aspirin and clopidogrel.

Keywords: Antiplatelet therapy, aspirin, neuroendovascular procedure, platelet function test, P2Y12 receptor antagonists.

INTRODUCTION

Dual antiplatelet therapy (aspirin plus a P2Y12 receptor antagonist) is at now the main treatment for prevention of coronary stent thrombosis. Clinical trials showed that dual therapy is more effective than aspirin alone for reducing the incidence of major cardiovascular events in high-risk patients [1]. The use of dual antiplatelet therapy is also considered essential in the setting of neurovascular stents and flow

*Corresponding author Fabio M. Pulcinelli: Department of Experimental Medicine, "Sapienza" University, viale Regina Elena 324, 00161, Rome, Italy; Tel: +39 0649973002; Fax: +39 064454820; E-mail: fabio.pulcinelli@uniroma1.it

Simone Peschillo (Ed.)

diverter treatment [2]. Standard practices regarding antiplatelet therapy for stenting are better defined in the cardiac literature [2].

The 2011 ACCF/AHA/SCAI guidelines for Percutaneous Coronary Interventions describe recommendations for dual antiplatelet therapy in patients undergoing coronary stenting. Aspirin in addition to a $P2Y_{12}$ receptor inhibitor, such as clopidogrel, prasugrel or ticagrelor, should be given for at least 12 months. The use of aspirin should be continued indefinitely after implantation of a stent [3].

Minimal literature exists regarding antiplatelet therapy in neurovascular stenting and most protocols are derived from the cardiac setting. Consequently, in neurovascular stenting there is a great heterogeneity of medication protocols, including drugs, doses, timing and platelet reactivity testing [2]. Cardiological guidelines must be applied with caution to the neurovascular setting, since placing a cerebrovascular stent may be inherently different from placing a coronary stent due to the different exposed surface areas of the stents, the different vascular anatomies and the different bleeding rates [2].

The rates of ischemic events associated with stent-assisted coil embolization are reported in the neurovascular literature to be between 2% and 21%, and increase when dual antiplatelet therapy is started incorrectly or stopped prematurely [2].

Conversely, inappropriate use of antiplatelet therapy may also contribute to hemorrhagic complications. Bleeding rates during the administration of dual antiplatelet therapy, after placement of neurovascular stents, have been reported to be between 1% and 4% for carotid artery stenting and approximately 6% for intracranial aneurysms undergoing stent-assisted coil embolization [2]. Thus, adequate dual antiplatelet therapy is necessary prior to the placement of a neurovascular stent.

The World Federation of Interventional and Therapeutic Neuroradiology (WFITN) guidelines recommend a protocol for the management of anticoagulation and antiaggregation in neurointerventional procedures (Table **1**) to avoid embolic complications and to minimize the bleeding risk.

ANTIPLATELET DRUGS

Antiplatelet drugs interfere with platelet function, reducing the risk of ischemic events, but they are associated with an increased risk of bleeding complication [4] (Table **2**).

Table 1.   **WFITN guidelines for anticoagulation and antiaggregation in neurointerventional procedures.**

1. Parameters routinely determined before and after the interventions
• Medical history and current medication
• Pre-procedural INR
• Pre-procedural aPTT
• Pre-procedural blood count
• Pre-/intra-/post-procedural ACT
2. Small neck aneurysm coiling
• Only during the procedure
• Heparin bolus of 5000 U, then 1000 U/L continuously during the procedure, with control of ACT (~200)
• No antiaggregation therapy
3. Wide neck aneurysm coiling
• No pre-treatment
• Intra-procedural: heparin bolus of 5000 U, then 1000 U/L continuously, with control of ACT (~200)
• Post-treatment: aspirin 100 mg, to be continued indefinitely thereafter
4. Aneurysm stenting
• Pre-treatment: 3 days before procedure, aspirin 100 mg and clopidogrel 75 mg
• Intra-procedural: heparin bolus 5000 U, then 1000 U/L continuously, with control of ACT (~200)
• Post-treatment: dual-therapy depending on stent-model, with aspirin to be continued thereafter
5. Aneurysm stenting + coiling
• Pre-treatment: 3 days before procedure, aspirin 100 mg and clopidogrel 75 mg
• Intra-procedural: heparin bolus 5000 U, then 1000 U/L continuously, with control of ACT (~200)
• Post-treatment: dual-therapy depending on stent-model, with aspirin to be continued indefinitely thereafter
6. Aneurysm balloon-remodeling
• Only during the procedure
• Heparin bolus of 5000 U, then 1000 U/L continuously during the procedure, with control of ACT (~200)
• No antiaggregation therapy
7. Drug-eluting stent
• Pre-treatment: 3 days before procedure, aspirin 100 mg and clopidogrel 75 mg
• Intra-procedural: heparin bolus 5000 U, then 1000 U/L continuously, with control of ACT (~200)
• Post-treatment: dual-therapy for one year, with aspirin to be continued indefinitely thereafter
8. Acute stroke intervention
• Because of heterogeneity of duration and dosage, no general recommendation
• The combination of glycoprotein IIb/IIIa inhibitors with recombinant tissue plasminogen activator significantly reduced infarct size and improved neurological outcome in a rat model of embolic stroke
9. Embolization of arteriovenous malformations, dural arteriovenous fistulas and tumors
• Only during the procedure
• Heparin bolus of 5000 U, then 1000 U/L continuously during the procedure, with control of ACT (~200)
INR: International Normalized Ratio
aPTT: activated partial thromboplastin time
ACT: activated clotting time

Table 2.   Comparison of antiplatelet drugs.

Drug	ASA	Clopidogrel (Plavix®)	Prasugrel (Effient®)	Ticagrelor (Brilinta®)
Class	Non-steroidal anti-inflammatory drug (Drug)	Second generation thienopyridine (Prodrug)	Third-generation thienopyridine (Prodrug)	Cyto-pentyl-triazolo-pyrimidine (Drug)
Mechanism of platelet inhibition	Irreversible inhibitor of COX-1.	Irreversible inhibitor of P2Y12 (ADP receptor)	Irreversible inhibitor of P2Y12 (ADP receptor)	Reversible binding of P2Y12 (ADP receptor)
Half-life (active metabolite)	15-20 min	8 hrs	4 hrs	6-9 hrs
Metabolic activation by liver	No	Yes	Yes	No
Recovery of platelet function after discontinuation (days)	7-10	5-10	7-10	5
Frequency of administration	Daily	Daily	Daily	Twice daily

Platelets are anucleated blood cells derived from the cytoplasm of bone marrow megakaryocytes. The life span of circulating platelets is 10 days. Platelets show no interactions with the surface of normal vessels but adhere immediately where endothelial cells are altered or subendothelial extracellular matrix is exposed. This is a critical initial step in both normal hemostasis and pathological thrombosis, and also in inflammatory and immunopathogenic responses [5].

Platelets adhere to exposed subendothelial proteins (collagen and von Willebrand factor), in damaged blood vessels, through interactions with platelet membrane glycoprotein receptors. These interactions produce intracellular signaling cascades that activate platelets [6]. Activated platelets can rapidly recruit additional platelets to the growing hemostatic plug by several feedback amplification loops: they release platelet agonists (such as ADP, ATP and serotonin stored in the delta-granules) and synthesize *de novo* thromboxane A2 (TXA2) [7], which is a potent platelet aggregating agonist and vasoconstrictor.

The local accumulation of these agonists converts integrin receptor glycoprotein IIb/IIIa (GPIIb/IIa) into an active form with a high affinity for fibrinogen and other adhesion molecules, promoting the formation of stable contacts between platelets mediated by bridges of fibrinogen and von Willebrand factor. Generation of fibrin from fibrinogen, due to activation of the coagulation cascade, also contributes to the formation and consolidation of the hemostatic plug [7].

Antiplatelet drugs may have an impact on these processes by inhibiting different steps of platelet function [4]. Three groups of antiplatelet drugs are effective in a clinical setting [8]: (i) cyclooxygenase-1 (COX-1) inhibitors (such as aspirin); (ii) P2Y12 (ADP receptor) antagonists, which may have an irreversible (clopidogrel, prasugrel) or reversible (ticagrelor) mechanism of action; and (iii) glycoprotein IIb/IIIa antagonists (eptifibatide, tirofiban, abciximab) (Fig. **1**).

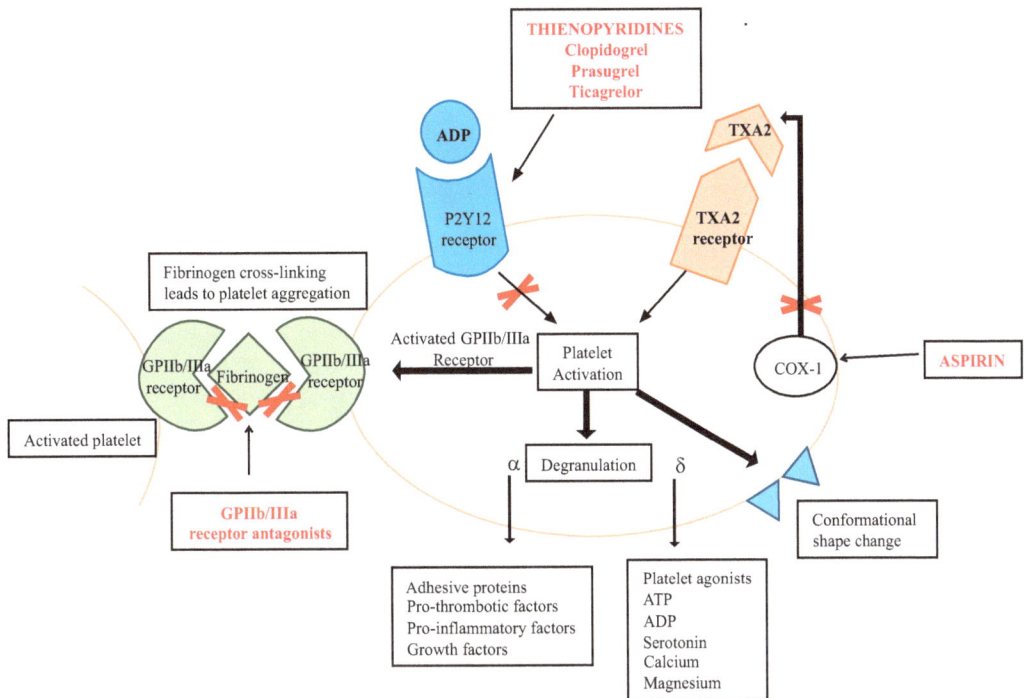

Figure 1: Mechanism of action of antiplatelet drugs. Antiplatelet treatments target different platelet receptors to inhibit platelet function. Abbreviations: GP, glycoprotein; TXA2, thromboxane A2; ADP, adenosine diphosphate; COX-1, cyclooxygenase-1 enzyme; α, alpha granules; δ, delta granules.

Aspirin

The mechanism of action of aspirin depends on its capacity to irreversibly inhibit the enzyme cyclooxygenase (COX). COX is a key enzyme in prostanoid synthesis, existing as two isoforms, COX-1 and COX-2, with a high degree of similarity in their amino acid sequences [9]. COX-1 is an isoform constitutively expressed in nearly all cells and tissues, including platelets. It is responsible for the production of homeostatic prostaglandins, which are involved in diverse normal cellular functions, such as maintenance of renal blood flow, platelet activation and aggregation and gastric mucosal protection. The isoform COX-2 is not present in physiological conditions, but is inducible by proinflammatory cytokines and growth factors and is responsible for the generation of the hyperalgesic and pro-inflammatory prostaglandins [9].

Aspirin irreversibly acetylates platelet COX-1 at the side chain of the Ser529 residue [10], blocking the generation of TXA2, a potent vasoconstrictor and platelet activator [11]. Low doses of aspirin (75-150 mg) administered once daily are sufficient to completely inhibit platelet COX-1 [4]. As platelets are anucleate and cannot regenerate COX-1 once inhibited, new TXA2 biosynthesis depends on new platelet formation. Considering the platelet lifespan of 10 days, only 10% of the platelet pool is recovered daily.

The profound inhibitory effect of low doses of aspirin is, therefore, explained by the irreversible enzyme deactivation and the slow recovery of platelet COX-1 [12]. Conversely, higher doses of aspirin (>300 mg) and a shorter dosing interval are necessary to inhibit COX-2, because nucleated cells can rapidly resynthesize this isoform of the enzyme [4]. Therefore, low doses of aspirin have a selective action on platelets, providing an antithrombotic effect, while high doses provide analgesia and reduction in inflammation.

After oral administration, aspirin is rapidly absorbed both in the stomach and the small intestine [13]. Aspirin reaches peak concentrations in the plasma 30 to 40 minutes after ingestion and the inhibitory effect on platelet function occurs within 1 hour [4]. Aspirin bioavailability is about 50% of administered dose, because it is rapidly biotransformed into its metabolite salicylic acid by endothelial and plasma esterases prior to reaching the systemic circulation. Aspirin has a plasma half-life of approximately 15-20 minutes [13].

Aspirin reaches bone-marrow and inhibits megakaryocyte COX-1, thus blocking thromboxane production in newly formed platelets as well [4].

Aspirin doses of 40-160 mg daily are able to inhibit platelet function [14]. With doses of 75-150 mg daily, a favorable benefit-risk balance is reached [15].

The main side effects of aspirin are gastrointestinal, including ulcers and bleeding.

The gastrointestinal side effects are dose-dependent so an aspirin dose of 300 mg daily is associated with a higher risk of side effects than a dose of 100 mg daily [17].

The effectiveness of aspirin for primary prevention is not proven [15]. In secondary prevention, the European guidelines recommend an initial loading dose of aspirin of 160-325 mg and then a maintenance dose of 75-100 mg daily in patients with acute coronary syndrome (ACS), unless contraindicated [16].

P2Y12 Receptor Antagonists

Thienopyridines specifically inhibit the platelet P2Y12 purinergic receptor (ADP receptor), resulting in inhibition of ADP-induced platelet activation and aggregation [18]. The use of ticlopidine, a first-generation thienopyridine, is associated with bone marrow toxicity; for this reason this drug was replaced by clopidogrel, a second-generation thienopyridine. Currently, clopidogrel in combination with aspirin is the standard therapy in patients with ACS and in patients undergoing percutaneous coronary intervention (PCI) [4].

Prasugrel, a third-generation thienopyridine, has a faster onset of action and a greater inhibitory effect on platelet aggregation compared to clopidogrel, without the interindividual variability of this latter [19]. Prasugrel is associated with a lower incidence of ischemic events with an increased risk of major bleeding complications in patients with ACS undergoing PCI [20]. Clopidogrel and prasugrel are irreversible inhibitors of the P2Y12 receptor, and are prodrugs that need metabolic activation by the hepatic CYP450 enzyme to form their active metabolites.

Ticagrelor belongs to a new class of antiplatelet agents called cyclopentyl-triazolo pyrimidines [21]; it is the first reversible antagonist of P2Y12 receptors, which non-competitively blocks ADP-induced platelet activation. Ticagrelor, unlike clopidogrel and prasugrel, is not a prodrug and does not require metabolic activation by the liver. Like clopidogrel, it is associated with a decreased risk of ischemic events, without increasing the rate of overall major bleeding [21].

Clopidogrel

Clopidogrel is an inactive prodrug rapidly absorbed in the intestine [22] and metabolized in the liver by the CYP450 system (predominantly CYP2C19 and CYP3A4) through two oxidative processes to generate the active metabolite [4]. It binds irreversibly to the platelet P2Y12 receptor, blocking ADP-binding and receptor activation, leading to inhibition of platelet aggregation [4]. The main metabolite of clopidogrel has a half-life of about 8 hours. Effects are obtained within 48 hours with doses of 50 to 100 mg daily and a steady state (about 50%-60% receptor inhibition) is reached after 4 to 7 days of treatment [4].

The recommended dose of clopidogrel is 75 mg for all indications. In the treatment of ACS/PCI patients clopidogrel should be initiated with a single 300/600 mg loading dose, which produces a more rapid and potent antiplatelet effect and should then be continued at 75 mg daily (associated with aspirin 75 mg daily). The recommended duration of treatment is 12 months [3].

It was observed that between 5% and 30% of patients have insufficient responses to clopidogrel [23]. If the initial response is insufficient, an increased dose of clopidogrel may be considered, *e.g.*, an additional loading dose of 600 mg or a doubling of the daily doses for 4-7 days. Several studies have shown a long-term benefit from doubling the daily doses from 75 to 150 mg [24].

In the CAPRIE trial the safety profile of clopidogrel (75 mg daily) was, overall, similar to that of aspirin (325 mg daily) [25].

Prasugrel

Prasugrel is a third-generation thienopyridine administered when clopidogrel is ineffective despite dose optimization. The parent molecule, prasugrel, is rapidly hydrolyzed by esterases, such as those present in the intestine and blood. The intermediate metabolite undergoes subsequent activation by CYP450 (predominantly CYP3A and CYP2B6) through a single step to form the active metabolite that binds irreversibly to the P2Y12 receptor, inhibiting platelet activation and aggregation [26]. The active metabolite of prasugrel reaches peak concentrations in the plasma after about 30 minutes. The plasma half-life of the active metabolite is approximately 4 hours and stable efficacy is attained in 2–4 days [4]. Excretion is mainly urinary [4]. In ACS/PCI patients, prasugrel, in addition to aspirin, is recommended at a single 60 mg loading dose followed by a maintenance dose of 10 mg daily [3].

Consistently with the more potent antiplatelet effects observed with prasugrel than clopidogrel, in the TRITON TIMI study it was found that the third-generation thienopyridines are associated with an increased risk of bleeding, including fatal bleeding [20]. The Food and Drug Administration emanated a warning about the risk of significant or fatal bleeding and provided contraindications to the use of prasugrel in patients with a prior stroke or transient ischemic attack [26].

Ticagrelor

Ticagrelor is the first orally available, reversible antagonist of the P2Y12 receptor. It is not a prodrug and does not need metabolic activation to inhibit the P2Y12 receptor. Ticagrelor is converted in the liver, by CYP3A, into an active metabolite, which is as potent as the parent drug [27].

The plasma peak occurs 2 hours after administration, and with a dose of 90 mg twice daily efficacy stabilizes in 2 to 4 days. The plasma half-lives of ticagrelor and its active metabolite are approximately 6-9 hours and 8-12 hours, respectively. After discontinuation of ticagrelor, the recovery of platelet function occurs after 5 days, which is earlier than after clopidogrel (5-10 days) or prasugrel (7-10 days) discontinuation, but longer than expected, considering its pharmacokinetic half-life. One-third of ticagrelor metabolites are excreted in the urine, and two-thirds in the feces [28].

The PLATO study showed the superiority of ticagrelor compared to clopidogrel in the prevention of ischemic events in patients with ACS, without increasing the rate of overall major bleeding [29].

The recommended dosing is a 180 mg loading dose and then 90 mg twice daily. The adverse effects of ticagrelor include dyspnea, increased frequency of mostly asymptomatic ventricular pauses and asymptomatic increases in uric acid [30].

LOW RESPONSIVENESS TO DUAL ANTIPLATELET THERAPY

Despite the clinical benefit achieved with dual antiplatelet therapy with aspirin and clopidogrel in the setting of ACS and/or PCI, many patients continue to experience cardiovascular events [31].

Multiple and complex factor can cause variations in antiplatelet efficacy response. Standardized methods of platelet function testing may assist in adjusting antiplatelet therapy to reduce cardiovascular complications in patients under antiplatelet treatment. Nevertheless, the optimal management for tailoring antiplatelet treatment has not yet been established. Antiplatelet drug resistance is a heterogeneous phenomenon. Some patients may have low responsiveness either to aspirin or to clopidogrel, or to both agents.

Aspirin Low-Responsiveness

It is estimated that between 5% and 60% of patients taking aspirin for secondary prevention do not respond sufficiently to this drug: the phenomenon is known as 'aspirin resistance' [13]. Although there is no consensual definition of aspirin resistance, the condition can be considered from clinical and laboratory perspectives.

Clinical resistance describes the inability of aspirin to prevent thrombotic events while laboratory resistance denotes the inability of aspirin to inhibit platelet TXA2 production. Laboratory resistance is generally assessed by measuring TXA2 metabolites (serum thromboxane B2 [TXB2] and urinary 11-dehydro-thromboxane B2 [11-dehydro-TXB2]) or by platelet function tests [13].

The question of whether platelet function assays predict clinical outcome is of paramount importance [32]. Recent meta-analyses on the action of aspirin suggest that there is an association between insufficient platelet function inhibition by aspirin and worse clinical outcome [33, 34].

The mechanisms of aspirin resistance are not completely understood. Potential causes of aspirin resistance include:

1. Poor adherence to therapy. A significant proportion of patients do not comply with the recommended aspirin treatment [32]. Poor compliance with aspirin treatment is a frequent problem and likely the main cause of aspirin resistance [35].

2. Long-term aspirin therapy. It has been demonstrated that patients with previously documented sensitivity to aspirin treatment can develop a progressive decrease in platelet sensitivity to the inhibitory effect of aspirin [36].

3. Presence of interacting drugs. (i) *Non-steroidal anti-inflammatory drugs*. Non-steroidal anti-inflammatory drugs such as naproxen, ibuprofen and indomethacin, but not meloxicam, rofecoxib, celecoxib, diclofenac and acetaminophen, interfere with the anti-platelet effect of aspirin. These drugs reversibly bind platelet COX-1, limiting the access of aspirin to the binding site [32]. (ii) *Proton pump inhibitors*. Aspirin is associated with gastrointestinal side effects; for this reason proton pump inhibitors are routinely co-prescribed to patients at high risk of bleeding. The resulting increase in gastric pH leads to

a decrease in the bioavailability of aspirin. The consequences of concurrent aspirin and proton pump inhibitor therapy are not clear, as studies designed to investigate this issue have yielded conflicting results [13].

4. Genetics factors. Although it is possible that modifications in genes encoding for platelet receptors and enzymes alter platelet responses to aspirin in certain individuals, the global contribution of genetic factors to variability in platelet responses to aspirin appears to be minor [32].

5. Plasma factors. Aspirin is rapidly hydrolyzed by esterases in plasma to its inactive metabolite, salicylic acid. Indirect evidence suggests that plasma esterases are involved in the regulation of platelet responses to aspirin [32].

6. Transporters. Multidrug resistance proteins are membrane proteins which form unidirectional channels, capable of pumping a wide range of drugs out of cells. These proteins are involved in cases of drug resistance [13]. One of them, multidrug resistance protein 4 (MRP4), is expressed in human platelet membranes and in membranes of platelet delta-granules. It has been demonstrated in patients undergoing coronary artery bypass graft surgery that insufficient platelet inhibition by aspirin [37] is dependent on overexpression of platelet MRP4. Overexpression of MRP4 increases active transport of aspirin out of the platelet cytosol, reducing its activity on COX-1 and thus affecting the pharmacokinetics of aspirin [38].

7. Diabetes mellitus. Diabetic patients have a higher risk of developing major ischemic events compared to non-diabetic subjects [32]. In diabetic patients, platelets display hypersensitivity to platelet agonists, which seems to be associated with metabolic alterations, oxidative stress and endothelial dysfunction [32, 39]. Furthermore, diabetic patients, with high glucose levels, more frequently display reduced platelet sensitivity to aspirin in comparison to non-diabetics [40]. It has not yet been demonstrated whether greater glycemic control and intensification of aspirin therapy can improve clinical outcomes [32].

8. Persistent TXA2 production. (i) *Regeneration of platelet COX- 1: platelet turnover*. The plasma half-life of aspirin is approximately 20 minutes; however, as platelets cannot generate new COX-1, the effects of aspirin persist for the entire life of platelet (10 days) [9]. As a consequence, the duration of the effect of aspirin depends on the rate of platelet turnover. For this reason, increased platelet turnover can contribute to residual thromboxane production

from new platelet COX-1 or COX-2 activity. High platelet turnover can have numerous causes, which can be divided into primary enhanced turnover of platelets (*e.g.* polycythemia vera) and secondary enhanced turnover (*e.g.* ACS, coronary artery bypass grafting and other surgical treatment) or enhanced platelet-vessel wall interactions (*e.g.* diabetes) [8]; in these clinical conditions, increased platelet turnover has been associated with insufficient platelet inhibition by aspirin [32]. (ii) *TXA2 production independent of COX-1: platelet COX-2*. The origin of residual TXA2 remains unknown. Since TXA2 is derived from both COX-1 and COX-2, persistent TXA2 production, under aspirin treatment, may depend on COX-2 enzymatic activity which is insensitive to the action of aspirin [8]. However, in 2008, Riondino *et al.* demonstrated that residual TXA2 production during aspirin treatment depends on insufficient inhibition of platelet COX-1 and that the level of COX-2-dependent TXA2 was minimal even if platelets overexpress COX-2 [41].

As shown above, several mechanisms may be involved in the phenomenon of aspirin resistance, but poor compliance, concurrent non-steroidal anti-inflammatory drug use and high platelet turnover are likely the most common [13].

Clopidogrel Low-Responsiveness

Among the thienopyridines, clopidogrel has been the most studied. It has been found that between 4% and 30% of patients exhibit "clopidogrel resistance" [42], with the risk of ischemic events enhanced from 1.5 to 5-fold. The mechanisms responsible for variability in clopidogrel responsiveness are not entirely understood and, as for aspirin, are probably multifactorial [1]. The most important mechanisms involved in the resistance to clopidogrel include:

1. Functional variability in CYP450 isoenzyme activity. The conversion of clopidogrel to its active metabolite requires oxidation by the hepatic cytochrome P450-system [4]. Among several polymorphisms of CYP2C19, the two most frequent variants associated with loss-of-function are CYP2C19*2 and CYP2C19*3 [31]. Patients who are carriers of a loss-of-function allele have decreased conversion of clopidogrel to its active metabolite, with higher residual platelet reactivity and with an increased risk of adverse outcomes, such as death, myocardial infarction and stent thrombosis compared with non-carriers [31]. However, despite the significant role of these polymorphisms in clopidogrel responsiveness, only 18% of the variability is explained by genetic

mutations, suggesting that multiple, complex factors are involved in the response to clopidogrel [31].

2. Presence of interacting drugs. A reduced laboratory response to clopidogrel has been observed during co-administration of CYP3A4-metabolized statins (atorvastatin and simvastatin) [43] and CYP2C19-metabolized proton pump inhibitors (especially omeprazole) [44], but whether these pharmacodynamic interactions have clinical relevance is unknown [4].

3. Transporters. The absorption of clopidogrel is modulated by the expression of the intestinal efflux transporter P-glycoprotein. When P-glycoprotein is upregulated as a result of the 3435T/T genetic variant, the oral bioavailability of clopidogrel is limited [45] and there is an associated increase in cardiovascular mortality [13].

4. Clinical factors. The effects of clopidogrel may be reduced in patients with higher pre-treatment platelet reactivity. Increased baseline platelet reactivity has been observed mostly in patients with ACS, increased body mass index, and diabetes mellitus, in particular in insulin-dependent diabetes mellitus. There are other clinical factors that may have a role in clopidogrel responsiveness such as lack of compliance with therapy and underdosing [1].

PLATELET FUNCTION TESTING

A variety of laboratory methods are currently available to monitor the effects of antiplatelet agents in cardiovascular diseases. It is of paramount importance to determine the optimal dose of antiplatelet therapy in these diseases in order to prevent or treat thrombosis while minimizing hemorrhagic side effects. Despite the increased evidence that monitoring the effects of antiplatelet drugs may result in the identification of patients with a higher risk of developing ischemic events, current clinical guidelines do not recommend routine platelet function testing in patients under antiplatelet therapy. This is both because there is no consensus on the platelet function assay to be used and because of the lack of clinical trials proving the impact of treatment modification on clinical outcomes in patients resistant to antiplatelet agents. Moreover, the traditional platelet function assays are expensive, not widely available and need a high degree of technical expertise. It is, therefore, still difficult to reach a rapid and accurate diagnosis of responsiveness to antiplatelet agents [1].

Traditional Tests of Platelet Function

TXB2 assays together with light transmission aggregometry are currently the most accurate tests for identifying aspirin treatment failure. Both tests are specific for the action of aspirin on COX-1.

Serum Thromboxane B2 and Urinary 11-dehydro-thromboxane B2 Measurement

Serum TXB2 and urinary 11-dehydro-TXB2 tests are specific measures of the effects of aspirin on COX enzyme. Arachidonic acid is converted into TXA2 by COX activation in platelets, aspirin inhibits COX-1 and subsequently reduces the production of TXA2. TXA2 has a very short half-life in plasma (30-60 seconds) so it cannot be easily measured in biological samples [32]. Hence, serum/plasma TXB2, the stable metabolites of TXA2, or urinary 11-dehydro-TXB2 is measured, either by immunoassay or mass spectrometry [32].

Serum TXB2 formation requires treatment of whole blood at 37 °C for 1 hour immediately after collection; this results in generation of thrombin, platelet activation, and *in vitro* release of TXA2, followed by clot formation.

In 2009, Frelinger *et al.* in a study of aspirin-treated patients, showed that residual COX-1 function defined by a serum TXB2 level >3.1 pg/ml correlated with subsequent major adverse cardiovascular events [46]. With regards to the urinary 11-dehydro-TXB2 assay, subjects with high levels of 11-dehydro-TXB2 (≥ 67.9 ng/mmol creatinine) were considered aspirin-resistant [32].

Turbidimetric Light Transmission Aggregometry

Light transmission aggregometry is the most common laboratory method used for the detection of aspirin and clopidogrel responsiveness and is considered the gold standard [42]. In this test, platelet aggregation in response to an agonist (arachidonic acid, ADP, epinephrine or collagen) is measured in platelet-rich plasma with a turbidimetric method [10, 47]. The formation of platelet aggregates modifies the optical density of the samples: the optical density is measured and expressed as a percentage of aggregation [47].

Several studies have shown that platelet aggregometry results can predict major adverse cardiovascular events [48].

Although this method is considered the "gold standard" test of platelet function, it has many limitations, such as its low reproducibility, the fact that it is time-consuming, requires a large volume of plasma for sample preparation, needs a skilled technician, and is expensive [10]. It is, therefore, important to follow correct analytical procedures, as reported in Table **3**, and aggregometry guidelines.

Table 3.   **Correct analytical procedure before performing turbidimetric light transmission aggregometry.**

General information on the patient
•   Personal data.
•   Check that the patient has not eaten.
•   Report drugs taken in the preceding two weeks and indicate posology.
•   Past clinical history (with particular reference to coagulation disorders, previous cardiovascular events and recent infections).
Information on the blood sample
•   Report time of collection.
•   Collection carried out avoiding venous stasis and with a 21-gauge needle.
•   Collect blood into 3.8% sodium citrate or ACD formula-A.
•   Samples must not show hemolysis.
Processing
•   Maintain samples at 20/25 °C and prepare platelet-rich plasma (PRP) within one hour of collection of blood.
•   Prepare PRP by centrifuging the sample at 180-200 g for 10 minutes.
•   Prepare platelet-poor plasma by centrifuging the sample at 2000 g for 10 minutes.
•   Check that platelet concentration in PRP is in the instrument's range.
•   If not, dilute PRP with proper buffer.
•   Periodically carry out a control aggregation with PRP from a healthy volunteer.
Instrument for the diagnostic test
•   Check that the instrument is set according to the manufacturer's instructions.
•   Use only cuvettes made of siliconized glass or plastic and check that there are no alterations.
•   Reconstitute reagents according to the indications for the kit and maintain work solutions on ice.
•   Prewarm samples according to the manufacturer's indications.

According to aggregometry guidelines (Platelet Function Testing Aggregometry; Proposed Guideline Clinical and Laboratory Standards Institute *Vol 27 N.19*), each laboratory should establish its own reference intervals by performing platelet aggregation on samples from a minimum of 20 healthy volunteers who have not taken any medication in the 15 days prior to performing the analysis.

Our unpublished data, drawn from 240 patients under dual antiplatelet therapy, demonstrated that insufficient inhibition to collagen- and arachidonic acid-induced platelet aggregation suggests low responsiveness to aspirin, while insufficient inhibition to ADP-induced platelet aggregation suggests low responsiveness to clopidogrel. Thus, this method can differentiate aspirin and clopidogrel resistance (Fig. **2**).

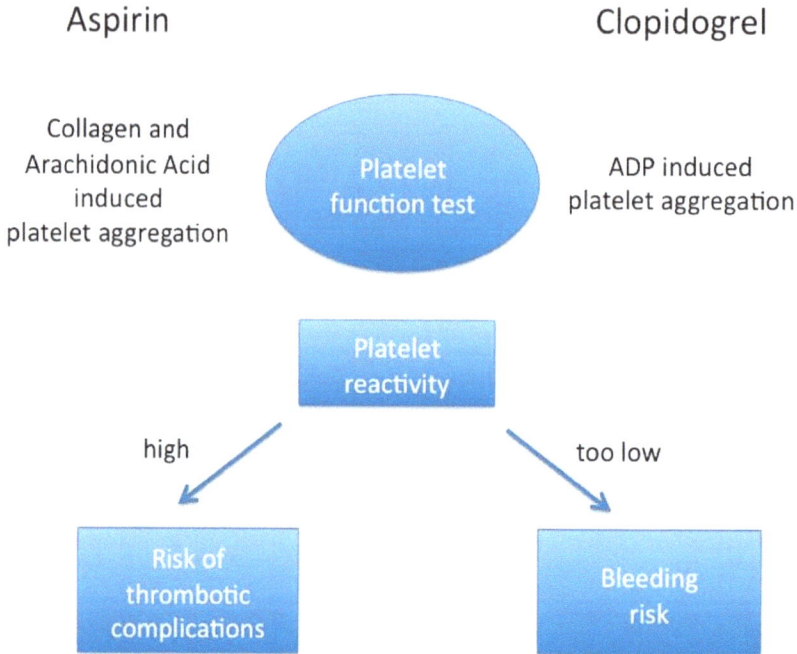

Figure 2: Antiplatelet treatment evaluation in neuroendovascular procedures. Assessment of platelet inhibition with platelet function tests may assist the therapeutic management in neuroendovascular procedures, helping to decrease thrombotic events and to minimize bleeding risk.

Newer Options for Platelet Function Testing

Newer platelet function tests are point-of-care tests that can be used at the patient's bedside without requiring technical expertise. The new tests include VerifyNow (Accumetrics, San Diego, CA, USA) and the Platelet Function Analyzer 100 (PFA-100®; Dade Behring, Newark, DE, USA). These tests have been used for a decade, but their utility in clinical practice remains unclear [49].

VerifyNow and PFA-100® are limited by high variability in platelet count, platelet response, and platelet-receptor concentration [50].

Others tests, such as Impact Cone-and Plate(let) assay (IMPACT-R, DANED SA, Beersel, Belgium), Plateletworks (Helena Laboratories, Beaumont, TX, USA), Thromboelastography platelet mapping system, and Vasodilator-stimulated phosphoprotein (VASP) are limited by poor sensitivity, the fact that they are time-consuming and require expertise to perform and evaluate; they are, therefore, more useful for research than point-of-care use [49].

VerifyNow

The VerifyNow Aspirin is a point-of-care system that measures platelet aggregation in whole blood by an optical turbidimetry method [32]. Whole blood is transferred into standard cartridges containing human fibrinogen-coated beads and arachidonic acid. When platelets aggregate around the fibrinogen-coated beads, light transmission increases and the system converts the change in light transmittance into Aspirin Reaction Units (ARU).

If aspirin has produced the expected antiplatelet effect, inhibiting COX, platelets will show minimal aggregation around beads. The cutoff is set as 550 ARU. A value <550 ARU indicates a platelet dysfunction, consistent with the effect of aspirin in aspirin-sensitive patients. In contrast, a value ≥550 ARU indicates no platelet dysfunction [50] despite aspirin treatment, in aspirin-resistant subjects. This cutoff value was previously associated with an increased risk of adverse ischemic events [32].

In addition to the VerifyNow Aspirin assay (determining sensitivity to aspirin), a VerifyNow P2Y12 assay (sensitive to thienopyridines) and a VerifyNow IIb/IIIa assay (sensitive to glycoprotein IIb/IIIa antagonists) are also available [10].

The VerifyNow P2Y12 assay uses ADP in addition to prostaglandin E1 as the agonist. ADP activates platelets by binding to the P2Y1 and P2Y12 platelet receptors. Prostaglandin E1 suppresses the ADP-induced P2Y1-mediated platelet activation, making this assay more specific and sensitive for the effects of ADP on the P2Y12 receptor. The amount of ADP-induced platelet aggregation is indicated as P2Y12 Reaction Units (PRU). Moreover, the device calculates the percentage of platelet P2Y12 receptor blockade. A low PRU (or high percentage inhibition) reflects high P2Y12-receptor inhibition and a good response to clopidogrel or prasugrel [50]. Clopidogrel resistance is detected when the PRU is ≥ 240 and receptor inhibition is <20% [24].

Platelet Function Analyzer

PFA-100® is a point-of-care instrument developed to simulate, *in vitro*, primary hemostasis in a blood vessel. In disposable test cartridges, citrated whole blood is aspirated through a capillary and an aperture (150 µm-diameter) in a membrane coated with collagen and epinephrine (CEPI) or collagen and ADP (CADP) [10]. Platelets adhere to the membrane and occlude the aperture causing cessation of blood flow. The time taken for a clot to occlude the aperture is referred to as the closure time (CT). Subjects with a closure time in the normal range (CT <193 seconds) despite aspirin treatment are considered aspirin-resistant [51]. This assay is less specific for aspirin resistance than the other assays, which are directly dependent on COX-1 activity [10].

The PFA-100® with CEPI is sensitive to functional alterations of von Willebrand factor [52]. The PFA-100® has also been used to monitor therapy with glycoprotein IIb/IIIa antagonists [10].

Because of the lack of sensitivity of the PFA-100®system for monitoring platelet response to clopidogrel, a new test, INNOVANCE® PFA P2Y*, coated with ADP and prostaglandin E1, was designed to assess the efficacy of clopidogrel treatment [53]. Subjects are considered clopidogrel-resistant if their closure time is <160 seconds, as described in the medical literature [24].

CONCLUSION

Dual antiplatelet therapy is important in maintaining the revascularization benefit in the setting of neuroendovascular procedures. Given the variability in the response to antiplatelet drugs, assessment of platelet inhibition with platelet function tests may improve therapeutic strategies to decrease thrombotic events associated with neuroendovascular procedures.

Although new options for platelet function testing have been developed to monitor the effects of antiplatelet drugs, the gold standard test remains light transmission aggregometry. This method can differentiate aspirin and clopidogrel resistance. Insufficient inhibition of collagen- and arachidonic acid-induced platelet aggregation suggests low responsiveness to aspirin, while insufficient inhibition of ADP-induced platelet aggregation suggests low responsiveness to clopidogrel.

ACKNOWLEDGEMENTS

The authors would like to thank Dr. Anna Lisa Montemari for her advice.

CONFLICT OF INTEREST

The authors confirm that this chapter contents have no conflict of interest.

REFERENCES

[1]   Angiolillo DJ, Fernandez-Ortiz A, Bernardo E, *et al*. Variability in individual responsiveness to clopidogrel: clinical implications, management, and future perspectives. J Am Coll Cardiol 2007; 49: 1505-16.

[2]   Faught RW, Satti SR, Hurst RW, Pukenas BA, Smith MJ. Heterogeneous practice patterns regarding antiplatelet medications for neuroendovascular stenting in the USA: a multicenter survey. J Neurointerv Surg 2014. Jan 3 [Epub ahead of print]

[3]   Levine GN, Bates ER, Blankenship JC, *et al*. 2011 ACCF/AHA/SCAI Guideline for Percutaneous Coronary Intervention: executive summary: a report of the American College of Cardiology Foundation/American Heart Association Task Force on Practice Guidelines and the Society for Cardiovascular Angiography and Interventions. Circulation 2011; 124: 2574-609.

[4]   Eikelboom JW, Hirsh J, Spencer FA, Baglin TP, Weitz JI. Antiplatelet drugs: Antithrombotic Therapy and Prevention of Thrombosis, 9th ed: American College of Chest Physicians Evidence-Based Clinical Practice Guidelines. Chest 2012; 141: e89S-119S.

[5]   Ruggeri ZM, Mendolicchio GL. Adhesion mechanisms in platelet function. Circ Res 2007; 100: 1673-85.

[6]   Fitzgerald DJ. Vascular biology of thrombosis: the role of platelet-vessel wall adhesion. Neurology 2001; 57: S1-4.

[7]   Jennings LK. Mechanisms of platelet activation: need for new strategies to protect against platelet-mediated atherothrombosis. Thromb Haemost 2009; 102: 248-57.

[8]   Kuzniatsova N, Shantsila E, Blann A, Lip GY. A contemporary viewpoint on 'aspirin resistance'. Ann Med 2012; 44: 773-83.

[9]   Awtry EH, Loscalzo J. Aspirin. Circulation 2000; 101: 1206-18.

[10]   Michelson AD, Frelinger AL 3rd, Furman MI. Current options in platelet function testing. Am J Cardiol 2006; 98: 4N-10N.

[11]   Grinstein J, Cannon CP. Aspirin resistance: current status and role of tailored therapy. Clin Cardiol 2012; 35: 673-81.

[12]   Maree AO, Curtin RJ, Dooley M, *et al*. Platelet response to low-dose enteric-coated aspirin in patients with stable cardiovascular disease. J Am Coll Cardiol 2005; 46: 1258-63.

[13]   Floyd CN, Ferro A. Mechanisms of aspirin resistance. Pharmacol Ther 2014; 141: 69-78.

[14]   Bochner F, Lloyd JV. Aspirin for myocardial infarction. Clinical pharmacokinetic considerations. Clin Pharmacokinet 1995; 28: 433-8.

[15]   Antithrombotic Trialists Collaboration, Baigent C, Blackwell L, Collins R, *et al*. Aspirin in the primary and secondary prevention of vascular disease: collaborative meta-analysis of individual participant data from randomised trials. Lancet 2009; 373: 1849-60.

[16]   Task Force for Diagnosis and Treatment of Non ST-Segment Elevated Acute Coronary Syndromes of European Society of Caridiology, Bassand JP, Hamm CW, Ardissino D, *et al*. Guidelines for the

diagnosis and treatment of non-ST-segment elevation acute coronary syndromes. Eur Heart J 2007; 28: 1598-660.

[17] Farrell B, Godwin J, Richards S, Warlow C. The United Kingdom transient ischaemic attack (UK-TIA) aspirin trial: final results. J Neurol Neurosurg Psychiatry 1991; 54: 1044-54.

[18] Herbert JM, Savi P. P2Y12, a new platelet ADP receptor, target of clopidogrel. Semin Vasc Med 2003; 3: 113-22.

[19] Janssen PW, ten Berg JM. Platelet function testing and tailored antiplatelet therapy. J Cardiovasc Transl Res 2013; 6: 316-28.

[20] Wiviott SD, Braunwald E, McCabe CH, *et al.* Prasugrel versus clopidogrel in patients with acute coronary syndromes. N Engl J Med 2007; 357: 2001-15.

[21] Cannon CP, Harrington RA, James S, *et al.* Comparison of ticagrelor with clopidogrel in patients with a planned invasive strategy for acute coronary syndromes (PLATO): a randomised double-blind study. Lancet 2010; 375: 283-93.

[22] Lins R, Broekhuysen J, Necciari J, Deroubaix X. Pharmacokinetic profile of 14C-labeled clopidogrel. Semin Thromb Hemost 1999; 25(Suppl 2): 29-33.

[23] Gurbel PA, Bliden KP, Hiatt BL, O'Connor CM. Clopidogrel for coronary stenting: response variability, drug resistance, and the effect of pretreatment platelet reactivity. Circulation 2003; 107: 2908-13.

[24] Patti G, Barczi G, Orlic D, *et al.* Outcome comparison of 600- and 300-mg loading doses of clopidogrel in patients undergoing primary percutaneous coronary intervention for ST-segment elevation myocardial infarction: results from the ARMYDA-6 MI (Antiplatelet therapy for Reduction of MYocardial Damage during Angioplasty-Myocardial Infarction) randomized study. J Am Coll Cardiol 2011; 58: 1592-9.

[25] CAPRIE Steering Committee. A randomised, blinded, trial of clopidogrel versus aspirin in patients at risk of ischaemic events (CAPRIE). CAPRIE Steering Committee. Lancet 1996; 348: 1329-39.

[26] Wiviott SD, Antman EM, Braunwald E. Prasugrel. Circulation 2010; 122: 394-403.

[27] Husted S, Emanuelsson H, Heptinstall S, Sandset PM, Wickens M, Peters G. Pharmacodynamics, pharmacokinetics, and safety of the oral reversible P2Y12 antagonist AZD6140 with aspirin in patients with atherosclerosis: a double-blind comparison to clopidogrel with aspirin. Eur Heart J 2006; 27: 1038-47.

[28] Siller-Matula JM, Trenk D, Krahenbuhl S, Michelson AD, Delle-Karth G. Clinical implications of drug-drug interactions with P2Y12 receptor inhibitors. J Thromb Haemost 2014; 12: 2-13.

[29] Wallentin L, Becker RC, Budaj A, *et al.* Ticagrelor versus clopidogrel in patients with acute coronary syndromes. N Engl J Med 2009; 361: 1045-57.

[30] Abergel E, Nikolsky E. Ticagrelor: an investigational oral antiplatelet treatment for reduction of major adverse cardiac events in patients with acute coronary syndrome. Vasc Health Risk Manag 2010; 6: 963-77.

[31] Garabedian T, Alam S. High residual platelet reactivity on clopidogrel: its significance and therapeutic challenges overcoming clopidogrel resistance. Cardiovasc Diagn Ther 2013; 3: 23-37.

[32] Lordkipanidze M. Advances in monitoring of aspirin therapy. Platelets 2012; 23: 526-36.

[33] Krasopoulos G, Brister SJ, Beattie WS, Buchanan MR. Aspirin "resistance" and risk of cardiovascular morbidity: systematic review and meta-analysis. BMJ 2008; 336: 195-8.

[34] Snoep JD, Hovens MM, Eikenboom JC, van der Bom JG, Huisman MV. Association of laboratory-defined aspirin resistance with a higher risk of recurrent cardiovascular events: a systematic review and meta-analysis. Arch Intern Med 2007; 167: 1593-9.

[35] Shantsila E, Lip GY. 'Aspirin resistance' or treatment non-compliance: which is to blame for cardiovascular complications? J Transl Med 2008; 6: 47.

[36] Pulcinelli FM, Pignatelli P, Celestini A, Riondino S, Gazzaniga PP, Violi F. Inhibition of platelet aggregation by aspirin progressively decreases in long-term treated patients. J Am Coll Cardiol 2004; 43: 979-84.

[37] Zimmermann N, Wenk A, Kim U, Kienzle P, Weber AA, Gams E, *et al.* Functional and biochemical evaluation of platelet aspirin resistance after coronary artery bypass surgery. Circulation 2003; 108: 542-7.

[38]   Mattiello T, Guerriero R, Lotti LV, *et al*. Aspirin extrusion from human platelets through multidrug resistance protein-4-mediated transport: evidence of a reduced drug action in patients after coronary artery bypass grafting. J Am Coll Cardiol 2011; 58: 752-61.

[39]   Angiolillo DJ. Antiplatelet therapy in type 2 diabetes mellitus. Curr Opin Endocrinol Diabetes Obes 2007; 14: 124-31.

[40]   Pulcinelli FM, Biasucci LM, Riondino S, *et al*. COX-1 sensitivity and thromboxane A2 production in type 1 and type 2 diabetic patients under chronic aspirin treatment. Eur Heart J 2009; 30: 1279-86.

[41]   Riondino S, Trifiro E, Principessa L, *et al*. Lack of biological relevance of platelet cyclooxygenase-2 dependent thromboxane A2 production. Thromb Res 2008; 122: 359-65.

[42]   Gorog DA, Sweeny JM, Fuster V. Antiplatelet drug 'resistance'. Part 2: laboratory resistance to antiplatelet drugs-fact or artifact? Nat Rev Cardiol 2009; 6: 365-73.

[43]   Zahno A, Brecht K, Bodmer M, Bur D, Tsakiris DA, Krahenbuhl S. Effects of drug interactions on biotransformation and antiplatelet effect of clopidogrel *in vitro*. Br J Pharmacol 2010; 161: 393-404.

[44]   Angiolillo DJ, Gibson CM, Cheng S, *et al*. Differential effects of omeprazole and pantoprazole on the pharmacodynamics and pharmacokinetics of clopidogrel in healthy subjects: randomized, placebo-controlled, crossover comparison studies. Clin Pharmacol Ther 2011; 89: 65-74.

[45]   Taubert D, von Beckerath N, Grimberg G, *et al*. Impact of P-glycoprotein on clopidogrel absorption. Clin Pharmacol Ther 2006; 80: 486-501.

[46]   Frelinger AL 3rd, Li Y, Linden MD, *et al*. Association of cyclooxygenase-1-dependent and -independent platelet function assays with adverse clinical outcomes in aspirin-treated patients presenting for cardiac catheterization. Circulation 2009; 120: 2586-96.

[47]   Born GV. Aggregation of blood platelets by adenosine diphosphate and its reversal. Nature 1962; 194: 927-9.

[48]   Gum PA, Kottke-Marchant K, Welsh PA, White J, Topol EJ. A prospective, blinded determination of the natural history of aspirin resistance among stable patients with cardiovascular disease. J Am Coll Cardiol 2003; 41: 961-5.

[49]   Gorog DA, Fuster V. Platelet function tests in clinical cardiology: unfulfilled expectations. J Am Coll Cardiol 2013; 61: 2115-29.

[50]   Hussein HM, Emiru T, Georgiadis AL, Qureshi AI. Assessment of platelet inhibition by point-of-care testing in neuroendovascular procedures. AJNR Am J Neuroradiol 2013; 34: 700-6.

[51]   Lordkipanidze M, Pharand C, Schampaert E, Turgeon J, Palisaitis DA, Diodati JG. A comparison of six major platelet function tests to determine the prevalence of aspirin resistance in patients with stable coronary artery disease. Eur Heart J 2007; 28: 1702-8.

[52]   Madsen EH, Schmidt EB, Maurer-Spurej E, Kristensen SR. Effects of aspirin and clopidogrel in healthy men measured by platelet aggregation and PFA-100. Platelets 2008; 19: 335-41.

[53]   Linnemann B, Schwonberg J, Rechner AR, Mani H, Lindhoff-Last E. Assessment of clopidogrel non-response by the PFA-100 system using the new test cartridge INNOVANCE PFA P2Y. Ann Hematol 2010; 89: 597-605.

Frontiers in Neurosurgery, Vol. 1, 2015, 232-252

CHAPTER 10

Anesthesia Options for Endovascular Neurosurgery

Italia La Rosa[*], Filippo Pecorari and Giovanni Rosa

Department of Cardiovascular, Respiratory, Nephrologic, Anesthesiology and Geriatric Sciences, "Sapienza" University, Rome, Italy

Abstract: Many intracranial vascular pathologies are now being successfully managed by interventional neuroradiology techniques. The procedures have become increasingly complex, requiring planning and coordination. Key roles are played by the anesthesiologist and close collaboration with neuroradiologist is crucial for successful results. The optimal conduct of anesthesia in a neuroradiology suite requires careful planning of each procedure and detailed evaluation of the individual patient. The basic principles of neuroanesthesia cannot be avoided: optimization of cerebral blood flow, perfusion pressure, control of intracranial pressure and close monitoring of hemodynamic values, respiratory patterns, fluid status and body temperature are all necessary. Rapid awakening must be ensured so that the patient's neurological status can be assessed quickly. The provision of anesthesia outside the operating room has its own inherent risks. This chapter will focus on perioperative anesthesiologic care and strategies to avoid or deal with complications if they do occur.

Keywords: Anesthesiologist, endovascular neurosurgeon, neuroanesthetist, neurointerventionalist.

INTRODUCTION

Interventional neuroradiology procedures have become increasingly complex in the past decades and have come to have an established role in the management of many neurological and neurosurgical conditions. As the field of interventional neuroradiology expands, the neuroanesthetist will become increasingly involved in the management of patients undergoing neuroradiology procedures. In fact, the role of the anesthesiologist is of paramount importance and close collaboration with the neuroradiologist is crucial for successful results.

In spite of the relatively non-invasive nature of interventional neuroradiology procedures, serious, even fatal, complications may occur. The perioperative care

---

*Corresponding author Italia La Rosa: Department of Cardiovascular, Respiratory, Nephrologic, Anesthesiology and Geriatric Sciences, "Sapienza" University, viale del Policlinico 155, Rome, Italy; Tel: +39064997119; E-mail: italia.larosa@uniroma1.it

Simone Peschillo (Ed.)

of patients with complex intracranial pathologies must therefore be based on cooperation between specialists in this field, operating room staff and intensive care unit personnel. Planning the anesthetic and postoperative management is essential to avoid complications.

For optimal anesthetic management, the anesthesiologist should be familiar with specific radiological procedures and their potential complications. Conditions and procedures in which interventional neuroradiology can play a role include (I) cerebral angiography; (II) embolization procedures for intracranial aneurysms, arteriovenous malformations, or fistulas in the brain or spine, preoperative embolization of tumors; (III) temporary or permanent occlusion procedures for intracranial or extracranial arteries; (IV) stenting and intracranial angioplasty for cerebral atherosclerosis; and (V) acute ischemic stroke.

Interventional neuroradiology procedures require carefully planning by an experienced anesthetist and all staff of the radiology suite should be familiar with emergency protocols. Further difficulties are raised by performing procedures outside the operating room and the increasingly aging population of patients with medical comorbidities.

EVALUATION OF PATIENTS AND PREOPERATIVE PLANNING

An early neurological examination is essential to determine a patient's psychological status, focusing on his or her ability to cooperate. Level of consciousness, focal neurological deficits, reactivity and pupil size should be recorded and classified according to the Glasgow Coma Scale and American Society of Anesthesiologists (ASA) Physical Status levels (Table **1**) to tailor the anesthetic approach prior to the neuroradiology procedures.

Table 1.   Definitions of American society of anesthesiology's physical status (ASA PS) class levels.

ASA PS	Definition
I	A normal healthy patient
II	A patient with mild systemic disease
III	A patient with severe systemic disease
IV	A patient with severe systemic disease that is a constant threat to life
V	A moribund patient who is not expected to survive without the operation
VI	A declared brain-dead patient whose organs are being removed for donor purposes

Airway evaluation includes the routine evaluation of potential difficulty with laryngoscopy. The term "difficult airways" spans different clinical situations, from difficulty in providing mask ventilation or inability to intubate the patient. The combination of difficult ventilation with the inability to intubate is the worst event with a high risk of brain damage.

The general examination should include respiratory assessment, auscultation of the chest and blood-gas analysis, if needed.

Cardiovascular status and arterial pressure should be studied before the procedure.

In order to determine the best balance between cardiac risks and risks of delaying a procedure, the cardiac risk associated with the particular operation and anesthesia must be assessed. A cardiological review and specific tests of cardiac function (echocardiography) and ischemic potential (coronary angiography) can be useful. The critical points are to decide whether the patient will be in a better state if the procedure is postponed and to determine how long it will take to obtain clinical reports.

Subarachnoid hemorrhage may lead to significant electrocardiographic changes, left ventricular systolic dysfunction and dysrhythmias due to hyperactivity of the sympathetic system and release of catecholamines. These changes do not affect the procedure but require adequate management and monitoring of cardiac function in all cases.

Diagnostic and laboratory studies should be directed towards concomitant illnesses and according to clinical need.

There is no indication in the Italian Society of Anesthesia Analgesia Resuscitation and Intensive Care (SIAARTI) Guidelines for routine electrocardiography, chest X-ray or blood chemistry analyses in ASA 1 or 2 patients to be subjected to sedation alone [1]. Nevertheless if cranial nerve deficits or compromised protective reflexes or hemodynamic changes are present, chest X-ray and electrocardiography studies are recommended; the results should be annotated in the patient's records.

Laboratory investigations include studies of liver and kidney function, protein electrophoresis, glycemia, hemoglobin and electrolyte changes. Hyperglycemia is common in the elderly as is the use of steroid medications. Persistent and severe high levels of glucose in the blood are well known to be associated with medical and neurological complications. Maintaining blood glucose levels between 130-140 mg/dL and infusing insulin when needed is reasonable to avoid poor outcomes. Electrolyte disturbances are common both before and after neurological procedures. Changes in brain volume is related with changes in serum sodium. Using diuretics and steroids in often associated with potassium loss. These disturbances and abnormalities should be corrected when they are present.

As anticoagulation is employed in most procedures, coagulation should be assessed and recorded in the clinical charts.

Nephropathy induced by contrast is a complication of interventional procedures and is associated with long hospital stay and adverse clinical outcomes, particularly in patients with pre-existing chronic kidney disease [2, 3]. "Radiological procedures utilizing intravascular injections of iodinated contrast media are being widely applied for both diagnostic and therapeutic purposes" [4].

"An absolute (≥ 0.5 mg/dL) or relative ($\geq 25\%$) increase in serum creatinine at 48-72 hours after exposure to a contrast agent, compared to baseline serum creatinine values is definied as a contrast-induced nephropathy".

Patients with pre-existing cardiovascular or renal disease are far more exposed to renal function impairment following radiological procedures (up to 20% risk) than patients with no such comorbidities (risk ranging from 0.6% to 2.3%).

Elderly diabetic patients who are given large doses of high osmolar contrast are especially at risk. According to Weisbord *et al.* [5], effective strategies to prevent contrast-induced nephropathy should focus on: "(i) administration of less nephrotoxic contrast agents; (ii) provision of pre-emptive hemofiltration and hemodialysis to remove contrast from the circulation; (iii) utilization of pharmacological agents to counteract the nephrotoxic effects of contrast media; and (iv) expansion of the intravascular space and enhanced diuresis with intravenous fluids".

Antioxidants and drugs inhibiting renal vasoconstriction, alone or combined, are considered to be useful in the prophylaxis of contrast-induced nephropathy however no pharmacological agents have been approved for the prevention of this condition yet. Furosemide, dopamine, fenoldopam, calcium channel blockers, and mannitol have failed to demonstrate any significant benefit. Moreover the role of

N-acetylcysteine, ascorbic acid (vitamin C), and statins, object of discussion of systemic reviews and meta-analysis, remains unclear [2, 3].

In the past it was noted that in patients with multiple myeloma, especially the forms secreting Bence-Jones protein, the administration of contrast material could lead to precipitation of proteins in the renal tubules. This phenomenon could be caused by dehydration, and perhaps partly also by a direct effect of the contrast agent on the polypeptide chains. The low incidence of nephropathy with low osmotic contrast media has led to the current view that, in patients with normal renal function and adequate hydration, multiple myeloma does not represent a contraindication to the administration of contrast material and, therefore, the search for urinary Bence-Jones protein is not necessary prior to giving the contrast medium. A review of seven series of patients with myeloma (476 patients) showed that contrast media are not a risk factor for the development of contrast-induced nephropathy in these patients [6]. Nevertheless, it is common for clinical pathology laboratories to perform/report urgent serum electrophoresis studies or the search for Bence-Jones proteinuria.

Intravenous contrast medium is used for many different diagnostic procedures in neuroradiology to enhance the visibility of the blood vessels.

From when it is used a new low osmolar non-ionic contrast media it is shown a generalized reduction of contrast reaction. The reactions usually happen after 5-30 minutes from exposure to the contrast. They occur with generalized skin reactions, angioedema or cardiovascular failure and difficult breathing. When dealing with patients considered at high-risk, such as those with a history of serious reactions, all the precautions available should be taken. Iodine and shellfish allergies are particularly relevant. The prophylactic use of corticosteroids is recommended in these patients [5, 7]. "Antihistamines (H1 and H2) and ephedrine have also been advocated for high-risk patients, often in combination with corticosteroids": in patients considered to be at elevated risk appropriate doses are 50 mg oral prednisone or 32 mg methylprednisolone 12 hours before the procedure plus 50 mg diphenhydramine 2 hours before the procedure. The use of antihistamine H1 and H2 receptor antagonists and ephedrine to reduce the risk of adverse reactions to contrast media has not become yet part of the common clinical practice. "Life-threatening reactions or even death may still occur in patients who receive pre-medication and low osmolar contrast media" [2]. Protamine can cause anaphylaxis and acute pulmonary hypertension. First-line assistance for serious contrast reactions should be promptly available and include adequate control of airways, oxygen supplementation, intravascular fluid and close monitoring of vital signs. Adrenaline increase pressure, reverses vasodilatation and bronchoconstriction, produces inotropic and chronotropic cardiac effects; it may be given *via* intramuscular injection (0.5 mL of 1:1000 preparation) or intravenously if necessary.

Fever is common in intensive care neurology patients, especially those with subarachnoid hemorrhage, and is often due to a local inflammatory response and dysregulation of the hypothalamic temperature control center. A body temperature >38.5 °C can be associated with an increased risk of vasospasm and poor outcome [8]. Post-treatment shivering and a correlated reduction in tissue oxygenation should be avoided. Thus a close control of body temperature seems appropriate. Finally, given the possibility of significant exposure to radiation, the possibility of pregnancy in females should be explored.

EQUIPMENT AND MONITORING

The variety and complexity of conditions treated in interventional neuroradiology suites require different and specific techniques and these procedures are often conducted in a location remote from other services. Nevertheless, monitoring and equipment standards should be equal to those adopted in any operating room and are mandatory to conduct anesthesia and mild/deep sedation safely. The SIAARTI Study Group for Safety in Anesthesia and Intensive Care therefore drafted a guideline document for anesthesiologists carrying out anesthesia in locations other than an operating room, in accordance with other international scientific societies [1].

Before undertaking any action, a preliminary evaluation should be made to check that there is sufficient space in the room, adequate illumination, a reliable source of oxygen and compressed air, as well as an adequate system for suction and scavenging waste anesthetic gases.

Standard monitoring should be applied, regardless of the anesthetic technique, and includes an ECG pulse oximetry probe, and non-invasive blood pressure measurements.

For intravenous sedation, capnography sampling *via* a nasal cannula is useful. More invasive cardiac monitoring should be guided by the patient's ASA. In mechanically ventilated patients, additional control of end tidal CO_2 and ventilator function is recommended using expiratory spirometry and analysis of volatile gases.

Invasive blood pressure monitoring *via* an arterial cannula is essential in hypertensive patients and when the blood pressure will be manipulated. This allows mean pressures to be assessed easily and may be used to monitor the induction of either hypertension or hypotension. The cannula can be used to take samples for blood-gas analyses and assays of blood glucose or activated clotting time.

A urinary catheter is useful in long procedures when large volumes of intravenous heparinized flush solutions and radiographic contrast are required. Furthermore, it may be necessary to administer diuretics such as mannitol and furosemide. A nasogastric tube is inserted to administer antiplatelet drugs enterally in stent procedures. A warming device is essential to maintain normothermia in the very cold radiologic suite and a temperature probe is especially useful.

Intraoperative neurophysiological monitoring is performed using a variety of neurophysiological techniques, including electroencephalography, somatosensory evoked potentials, electromyography, and transcranial motor evoked potentials, which are then interpreted by physicians to assess the integrity of neural pathways and contribute to the patient's safety. Near-infrared spectroscopy may be of additional value in these patients. In the neuroradiological setting, cerebral oximetry using near-infrared spectroscopy offers advantages over other techniques in terms of simplicity. However, the evidence defining clear cut-off points for cerebral ischemia or identification of patients at high risk is limited. A large prospective study is needed to assess the role and relative advantages of the various monitoring modalities [9-11].

ANESTHETIC TECHNIQUE

The complexity and duration of interventional neurological procedures require detailed attention by the anesthesiologist and knowledge of the technical aspects is necessary to ensure the quality of the anesthetic care and to maintain the patient's safety.

General Anesthesia

The anesthetic technique varies among centers and depending on the degree of neurological impairment. Most centers routinely use general anesthesia for complex or prolonged procedures. Patients may be aphasic, paretic, or unable to remain motionless and the experience may cause significant distress. General anesthesia minimizes movement artifacts, thereby improving the quality of images and facilitating navigation of endovascular catheters. Patient movements might produce a modification of intracranial arteries position in relation to a previously acquired "vascular map" resulting in increased technical difficulties and, more importantly, a higher risk of complications. General anesthesia may improve the patient's comfort and many people carrying out these neurological procedures and anesthetists prefer to use general anesthesia because of better cardio-respiratory control.

A reduction in mean arterial pressure decreases cerebral perfusion pressure and hence cerebral blood flow; raised intracranial pressure might further reduce cerebral perfusion. In a healthy brain with intact autoregulation, the mean arterial pressure of the cerebral blood flow ranges from 50 to 150 mmHg. Injuries of various natures to the brain might impair the autoregulation mechanism. Hence, in clinical practice, the mean arterial pressure should be manipulated to keep the cerebral perfusion pressure near 70 mmHg.

It's important to maintain a stable pressure during the crucial stages for the anesthesiologist, such as induction and intubation, avoiding hypotensive or hypertensive episodes.

All patients undergoing general anesthesia need airway management *via* endotracheal intubation or through the use of a laryngeal mask to ensure airway protection and prevent pulmonary aspiration in patients at risk. Adequate neuromuscular paralysis is induced prior to intubation.

The $PaCO_2$ of intubated, ventilated patients should be maintained in the range of normocapnia or mild hypocapnia (4.0-4.5 kPa; 30-35 mmHg), consistent with the safe delivery of positive pressure ventilation. "If a patient increased intracranial pressure, prophylactic mild hypocapnia may be indicated during induction and maintenance of general anesthesia" [9, 10, 12].

There is no evidence that one anesthetic technique is superior to another.

A target-controlled infusion (TCI) of propofol/remifentanil for induction and maintenance of total intravenous anesthesia (TIVA) allows cardiovascular stability and rapid emergence [13]. The relatively short context-sensitive half-life of remifentanil, a potent opioid analgesic drug, allows obtaining both quick induction and recovery as the desired blood plasma level may be rapidly achieved. Sevoflurane is the volatile agent of choice, with coupling of the cerebral blood flow and cerebral metabolic rate of oxygen ($CMRO_2$) maintained up to 1-1.2 the minimum alveolar concentration. Nitrous oxide may expand microair emboli and increase intracranial pressure and should, therefore, be avoided in endovascular procedures [9, 10].

Monitored Anesthesia Care

According to the ASA, "monitored anesthesia care is a planned procedure during which the patient undergoes local anesthesia together with sedation and analgesia" [14]. Understanding the various depths of sedation is essential to provide safe and effective procedural sedation and analgesia. The ASA has defined the various depths of sedation (Table **2**) [15].

Table 2:   **American society of anesthesiologists classification of levels of sedation.**

Minimal sedation (anxiolysis):
- Response to verbal stimulation is normal.
- Cognitive function and coordination may be impaired.
- Ventilatory and cardiovascular functions are unaffected

Moderate sedation/analgesia (formerly called conscious sedation)
- Depression of consciousness is drug-induced.
- Patient responds purposefully to verbal commands.
- Airway is patent, and spontaneous ventilation is adequate.
- Cardiovascular function is usually unaffected.

Deep sedation/analgesia
- Depression of consciousness is drug-induced.
- Patient is not easily aroused but responds purposefully following repeated or painful stimulation.
- Independent maintenance of ventilatory function may be impaired.
- Patient may require assistance in maintaining a patent airway.
- Spontaneous ventilation may be inadequate.
- Cardiovascular function is usually maintained

Various drugs are available to provide procedural sedation. A short-acting benzodiazepine (e.g., midazolam), either alone or in combination with an opioid analgesic (e.g., fentanyl, morphine, remifentanyl), is commonly selected for monitored anesthesia care. Combining a benzodiazepine and an opiate may be preferable for longer procedures but does increase the risk of oxygen desaturation and cardiorespiratory complications. Specific reversal agents for opiates (naloxone) and benzodiazepines (flumazenil) must be readily available during the procedure.

Dexmedetomidine is utilized for procedural sedation in pediatric and adult patients [16, 17]. It is an α_2-adrenergic agonist that provides sedation, anxiolysis, hypnosis, analgesia, and sympatholysis. Dexmedetomidine has several characteristics that make its use for procedural sedation very appealing. First, it provides little to no respiratory depression. Also, patients are able to follow commands and respond to verbal and tactile stimuli but fall quickly asleep when not stimulated. Although it does provide some pain relief, the use of other analgesics is necessary for the more painful procedures. Minimal cardiovascular effects are seen and include mild bradycardia and a decrease in systemic vascular resistance [18]. The acceptance and use of this agent in many settings is growing rapidly and its role in monitored anesthesia care is expected to expand as more studies review its reliability.

Clonidine, another α_2 agonist, has several beneficial actions during the peri-procedural period, such as improving hemodynamic stability in response to stress, reducing opioid requirement and causing sedation, anxiolysis and analgesia. Thus far the Food and Drug Administration has only approved its use for short-term mechanically ventilated adults in the intensive care unit, but it is currently being used off-label in many settings outside the intensive care unit [16, 18, 19].

Finally, many interventional neuroradiology procedures can easily be performed with sedation techniques by repeated bolus injections or continuous infusion.

COAGULATION MANAGEMENT

Heparin is required and routinely administered to prevent thromboembolic complications during microcatheter manipulation and stent placement. The activated clotting time should be measured and maintained at two to three times the baseline value by intravenous administration of heparin (70 IU/kg of body weight). Additional boluses must be given every hour on the basis of the activated clotting time. Infusion of heparine should be continued after the procedure to protect the endothelium from trauma and, at the same time, to protect against the inherently thrombogenic nature of the material implanted, which can be a cause of retrograde thrombosis in embolized vessels. Switching from bovine to porcine heparin or vice versa can be useful in the rare patients refractory to this anticoagulant. A suspicion of antithrombin III deficiency should prompt an even more careful management of coagulation; fresh-frozen plasma may be necessary to achieve the desired anticoagulant effect.

Antiplatelet agents *via* a nasogastric tube may also be required in cases of thromboembolic vascular occlusion. Although still controversial in the acute setting [16], "antiplatelet agents (aspirin, the glycoprotein IIb/IIIa receptor antagonists, and the thienopyridine derivatives) are increasingly being used for cerebrovascular disease management. Abciximab has been used to treat thromboembolic complications" as a rescue treatment in cases of acute intrastent thrombosis [20].

Thrombin inhibitors and antiplatelet agents do not have a known specific antidote, moreover platelet transfusion is considered non-specific when reversal of the effects of these drugs is necessary. The half-life of the individual drugs is, therefore, a major selection criterion.

Heparin may be reversed with protamine sulfate in the case of intraprocedural complications, such as vessel rupture during manipulation. The dose is 1.0-1.5 mg, given intravenously, for every 100 IU of active heparin; the total should not exceed 50 mg. Adverse reactions, especially in patients with allergy to fish, may include hypotension and bronchoconstriction resulting from massive release of histamine. In order to counter unwanted side effects it is strongly recommended to proceed with a slow infusion.

In brief, the anesthetist plays a key role in the meticulous control and management of coagulation during neuroradiological procedures.

CEREBRAL PROTECTION

The role of neuroprotective strategies during periods of neuronal vulnerability has been studied in recent years. Despite decades of basic and clinical research and some successes, these strategies have not been planned carefully. Collectively, neuroprotective measures to avoid and/or minimize brain damage improving neurological outcomes can be classified into non-pharmacological and pharmacological [21]. The anesthesiologist can easily manipulate some important physiological variables, such as body temperature, cerebral perfusion pressure, blood glucose level and hemoglobin concentration. Furthermore brain oxygen tension and arterial CO_2 partial pressure can be modified and brain size may be controlled by osmotic drugs.

Many pharmacological strategies for neuroprotection have been tested in the laboratory with the aim of inhibiting or reversing of the pathways that lead to ischemic cell death, but few have reached clinical use. Agents targeting specific molecular sites, such as NMDA antagonists, calcium-channel agonists and sodium-channel antagonists, free radical-trapping drugs, citicoline and erythropoietin, were among the strategies that did not show favorable results [21-23].

Magnesium sulfate infusion was found to have a neuroprotective effect in experimental models and in pilot clinical trials. However a systemic review and a recent multicenter trial did not confirm a benefit in terms of neurological outcome [22, 23].

Since pharmacological neuroprotective agents do not currently exist, the anesthesiologist is compelled to use the non-pharmacological strategies that seem to work: (i) liberal normoglycemia (7.8-10 mmol/L or 140-180 mg/dL), taking care to avoid hypoglycemia; (ii) maintenance of mean arterial pressure ≥ 80 mmHg or induced hypertension (~20%) in special situations; and (iii) ensuring a hemoglobin concentration ≥9 g/dL to promote sufficient oxygen delivery to the brain.

MANAGEMENT OF SPECIFIC NEUROLOGICAL PROCEDURES

Cerebral Angiography

Most patients requiring diagnostic cerebral angiography are awake. It is essential that patients remain immobile during the procedure to facilitate imaging. Patients should be warned about a hot sensation in face and in the head, impaired vision during the injection and headache due to traction during vessel manipulation.

The interventional neuroradiology team should identify those patients requiring only an anxiolytic (e.g. intravenous midazolam at a dose of 0.035 mg/kg) and those who must be given a general anesthesia because their neurological status does not enable cooperation. Local anesthesia in the groin area is generally performed by the proceduralist.

Endovascular Treatment of Cerebral Aneurysms

"Coil embolization of intracranial aneurysms has become the routine first-choice therapy for many lesions" and can be performed under conscious sedation (intravenous midazolam and fentanyl 0.7-1.4 µg/kg or remifentanil hydrochloride 0.025-0.1 µg/kg/min). The drug administration rate must be adjusted to the age of the patient, severity of the disorder and invasiveness of the procedure [10, 24].

Coils combined with balloons or stent-assisted coils are used for the treatment to prevent extension into proximal arteries and fill the aneurysm more easily. Antiplatelet drug administration may be planned in advance when a stent is contemplated or in the case of unruptured aneurysms. The procedure implies an ever-present risk of vascular rupture and thromboembolism accidents leading to vessel occlusion.

A recent review reported a "technical success rate of 93%, significant hemorrhagic complications in 8% of cases and significant thromboembolic events in 6% with a mortality rate of 19%" [25], compared with endovascular coiling without stents.

Complications during the treatment of aneurysms can be rapid and catastrophic. There should, therefore, be equally rapid and good communication between the neuroradiologist and anesthetist in order to manage any events that do occur as quickly as possible.

Many proceduralists and anesthetists prefer general anesthesia especially in the care of patients with subarachnoid hemorrhage because of better radiological images and cardio-respiratory management as well as greater comfort for the patients. Patients with subarachnoid hemorrhage often have increased intracranial pressure and secondary damage to the brain from hydrocephalus or ischemia. Patients with hydrocephalus need ventricular drainage in the operating room prior to the procedure.

Careful management of general anesthesia is necessary to maintain cardiovascular stability, optimal cerebral perfusion and intracranial pressure. Blood pressure manipulation is essential and should be closely controlled beat-to-beat by invasive arterial pressure monitoring.

Critical elevation of blood pressure up to 160 mmHg may lead to rupture of the aneurysm and must be controlled by antihypertensive drugs. The choice of appropriate agents should be based on experience, clinical findings, and potential side effects. Labetalol and esmolol exert minimal effects on cerebral circulation and intracranial pressure. Vasodilators can increase intracranial pressure and cerebral blood volume and must be used carefully.

At the same time hypotension must be avoided in order to maintain the cerebral perfusion. Adequate fluid replacement and rapid control of the depth of anesthesia can help to minimize hemodynamic changes. Phenylephrine or metaraminol infusion may be used to maintain a specific blood pressure target.

In patients in whom general anesthesia has been induced, a Cushing response (bradycardia and hypertension) or the proceduralist's diagnosis of extravasation of contrast may be the only clue to a rupture. In this event reversal with protamine should be agreed with colleagues.

Relative normocapnia or mild hypocapnia is generally desired in neuroanesthesia and becomes important in the prevention of increased intracranial pressure and post-rupture events. Mannitol (0.25-0.5 g/kg) or furosemide may be given to reduce cerebral edema.

In the event of an occlusive complication normocapnia is beneficial and the arterial pressure should be raised to increase blood flow. Antiplatelet agents, administered by the intravenous or intra-arterial route, may be used with care.

Cerebral vasospasm has been reported to occur in 30-70% of subarachnoid hemorrhages [10] and may be a complication of interventional neuroradiology procedures, as well. Calcium antagonists (nimodipine, nicardipine and verapamil) are effective in reversing this complication, but repeated endovascular treatment is frequently required. The hemodynamic effect of vasodilatation may persist beyond the acute period and could worsen cerebral perfusion pressure so that vasopressors (phenylephrine or noradrenaline) are often required. Tight control of arterial pressure is needed.

The complications of the endovascular treatment of aneurysms include vascular access complications such as groin hematoma and retroperitoneal bleeding, particularly in anticoagulated patients, and should be promptly investigated and treated.

Embolization of Cerebral Arteriovenous Malformations

Cerebral arteriovenous malformations consist in a nidus fed by one or more pial arteries draining into one or more veins without interposition of a capillary bed resulting in an arteriovenous shunt. These vascular lesions are often associated with intracranial aneurysms. The flow in the arteriovenous shunt can be high and patients may present with spontaneous hemorrhage, seizures, focal neurological signs, or headaches. The current treatment options include, individually or in combination, surgical resection, embolization alone or to reduce the nidus size before surgery, and radiosurgery. Endovascular treatment may be staged often reaching several interventional neuroradiology sessions. A preliminary endovascular approach may be useful to reduce the risk and difficulty of surgical resection or improve the effectiveness of radiosurgery. The embolic material used is either n-butyl cyanoacrylate, a thrombogenic glue, or Onyx, a non-adhesive and radiolucent compound that precipitates on contact with blood. The injection may be painful and an analgesic bolus should be administered before the injection [26].

General anesthesia is preferred to maintain immobility during the procedure to facilitate imaging. Temporary apnea and the Valsalva maneuver should also improve visualization.

Hypotension can be useful to reduce the flow across an arteriovenous malformation and facilitate the safe deployment of embolic material. It is recommended that normal blood pressure or hypotension is maintained in the perioperative period to reduce the risk of bleeding and cerebral edema as a consequence of neovascularization and hyperemia in the feeding vessel [10].

Complications include cerebral edema and retention of materials in the brain. In addition, in smaller patients, the glue can cause symptomatic pulmonary emboli. Pulmonary edema and acute respiratory distress syndrome may also occur.

"Curative embolization of small cerebral arteriovenous malformations is an efficient and safe alternative to neurosurgical and radiosurgical methods. Careful angiographic assessment of individual arteriovenous malformations can be performed under sedation before treatment".

Dural Arteriovenous Fistulas

"Intracranial dural arteriovenous fistulas (DAVFs) are pathological shunts between dural arteries and dural venous sinuses, meningeal veins, or cortical veins. DAVFs account for 10%-15% of intracranial arteriovenous malformations". Symptoms are related to the location of the lesion and the pattern of venous drainage. A hemorrhagic presentation is more frequent in high-grade lesions. Treatment and management decisions should be made by a multidisciplinary team. The anesthetic considerations are related to the presence of symptoms due to heart failure, a mass effect, and seizures that may occur [10, 27].

Embolization of Spinal Arteriovenous Malformations

Spinal arteriovenous malformations are rare vascular lesions. "DAVFs are the most common spinal vascular malformations and can be a significant cause of myelopathy although they are under-diagnosed". Surgical or embolization treatment of spinal DAVFs has improved significantly in the last decade.

However, a high percentage of patients are still left with severe disability. Recent small studies reported the effective use of Onyx glue for embolization [10, 28].

General anesthesia and adequate analgesia are indicated to improve the precision of images and reduce movement artefacts. Arterial hypotension decreases the flow through the malformation before glue injection; however, stable blood pressures are required for proper records of any neurological monitoring. Neuro-physiological monitoring with somatosensory and motor evoked potentials is useful in this context. Knowledge of the impact of various anesthetic agents on neuro-physiological parameters is essential to reduce and control their repercussions on the reliability of neuro-physiological monitoring.

Inhalational anesthetics and neuromuscular blockade influence transcranical motor evoked potentials (MEP) and they are a cause of significative changes in MEPs. Also hypothermia has an influence in monitoring. Opioids, in contrast, have little influence on motor evoked potentials. Total intravenous anesthesia (TIVA) minimize the change of amplitude and latency of motor evoked potentials. Optimal anaesthetic regimen maintanance of a stable concentration of inhalational or intravenous anesthetics optimizes monitoring *via* transcranial motor evoked potentials [29].

Stenting and Intracranial Angioplasty

"Early results of the Stenting and Aggressive Medical Management for Preventing Recurrent stroke in Intracranial Stenosis (SAMMPRIS) trial provided insufficient data to establish whether stenting offered any longer-term benefit". [30]. Patients may be treated with either aggressive management comprising antiplatelet agents, statins and antihypertensive therapy or medical management plus percutaneous angioplasty and stenting.

Such procedures have been successfully performed under general or local anesthesia. Some proceduralists prefer monitoring the neurological status all the time. Mild sedation with titrated fentanyl and midazolam has been demonstrated to be a feasible alternative to avoid general anesthesia [10, 31]. However conversion from sedation to general anesthesia is required in the case that the patient moves excessively or intraprocedural complications occur, such as vessel perforation or acute thrombosis. Headache is a common symptom and patients do not tolerate a long period of lying supine and motionless.

In certain specific lesions, such as stenosis of the basilar artery, general anesthesia is preferred to ensure better airway control.

The general anesthesia requires very careful planning. An experience neuroanesthetist is needed to manage any cardiovascular disease and severe illnesses present. Systemic blood pressure should be maintained below 140/90 mmHg, or 130/80 mmHg in diabetics, in the perioperative period, although hypotension must be avoided. Careful control of coagulation is essential to avoid hemorrhagic complications.

Rapid recovery from anesthesia at the end of the procedure enables early neurological examination and monitoring.

Acute Ischemic Stroke

Intra-arterial mechanical thrombectomy is a technique available for removing intracranial arterial occlusions in acute ischemic stroke. Anesthetic management during these endovascular procedures includes local anesthesia with a range of conscious sedation and general anesthesia. There is no general agreement on the process of anesthesia during endovascular therapy. However, several recently published retrospective analyses have shown adverse and poorer outcomes in patients in whom general anesthesia is used [32]. Thus, the decision between sedation or general anesthesia requires a careful balance and should be tailored to the individual patient's neurological status and ability to collaborate. Many stroke patients are unable to communicate and cooperate sufficiently with the proceduralist because of their neurological impairment. Such patients may be aphasic, paretic or display unpleasant restlessness.

The navigation of microcatheters and devices is easier and safer in immobile patients. Movements can disrupt the navigation and increase the risk of complications such as distension and perforation and also prolong the procedure. Extraction of the clot is, therefore, often painful and causes discomfort in a significant number of cases.

General anesthesia with endotracheal intubation is an attractive management in endovascular intra-arterial thrombolysis and patients are comfortable, painless and motionless and the airways are protected.

Conscious sedation with analgesia may make the patient more comfortable but may not be adequate for restless patients and patients with higher scores on the

National Institutes of Health Stroke Scale (NIHSS). In any case, the perception of pain during angioplasty and extraction remains unchanged. Dexmedetomidine has been used for sedation and in this setting the patient is awake and cooperative without respiratory depression. Experimental data suggest an associated reduction of infarct volume. Clinical evidence remains elusive [10].

The use of conscious sedation and analgesia was examined in numerous observational and interventional studies [31-34]. The largest study was performed by Abou-Chebl *et al.* a retrospective review of 980 stroke cases [31]. This study did not show differences in hemorrhagic complications between patients managed with either general anesthesia or conscious sedation. However, the patients managed with general anesthesia had higher probabilities of poor neurological outcome and mortality in comparison with the patients manage with conscious sedation. In 2012, Davis *et al.* [35] in 2012 presented 6-year results of his experience with arterial revascularization in patients managed with general anesthesia or conscious sedation. In thise study the patients who received general anesthesia were "sicker" and had higher baseline NIHSS scores, longer preprocedural times or lower levels of consciousness. Davis *et al.* postulated that additional factors may contribute to poor outcomes. The most unwelcome general anesthesia-related effect in acute stroke is hypotension. A reduction in cerebral perfusion pressure may lead to a reduction in collateral perfusion and progressive complete infarction.

Induction of general anesthesia frequently causes a decrease in blood pressure. In addition, high blood pressure (systolic >180 mmHg or diastolic >105 mmHg) is a contraindication to the use of intravenous recombinant tissue plasminogen activator, the first-line treatment for acute stroke. The importance of avoiding hypotension in stroke patients is related to the need to maintain adequate cerebral perfusion, particularly in the penumbral area. In a retrospective series, a systolic blood pressure <140 mmHg was associated with a worse neurological outcome.

Beat-to-beat blood pressure monitoring (through an arterial catheter specifically placed for the purpose of continuous blood pressure monitoring) is useful considering the rapid time constants in this setting for changes in systemic or cerebral hemodynamics. Many stroke patients have preexisting systemic hypertension and associated intravascular volume depletion. Depletion may worsen the vasodilatory effects of induction of general anesthesia and adequate saline infusion is needed to maintain mean arterial pressure. Careful induction and maintenance of general anesthesia could improve the management of acute stroke patients.

At present there is no clinical evidence to support general anesthesia over conscious sedation or the efficacy of neuroprotective strategies in endovascular stroke treatment. Neuroanesthesia care must ensure that hyperthermia, hypotension, hyperglycemia and hypoglycemia are avoided, just as in trauma and neurosurgical patients. Close control and monitoring of vital parameters is necessary.

POSTOPERATIVE CARE

The pivotal features of post-procedure anesthetic care are maintenance of stable cardiovascular parameters and gas-exchange and meticulous control of systemic physiological variables. Most patients can be nursed on the ward, unless their neurological condition dictates admission to an intensive care unit. Close control of hydration is important, as is the prevention and treatment of nausea and vomiting due to the contrast media and anesthetic agents used during the procedure. Continuous neurological observation is essential to identify complications and new neurological deficits. Their quick and aggressive management contributes to improving patients' outcome. An open channel of communication between the neuroradiologist and anesthesiologist is important for routine care but is crucial for successful results.

ACKNOWLEDGEMENTS

Declared none.

CONFLICT OF INTEREST

The authors confirm that this chapter contents have no conflict of interest.

REFERENCES

[1]   SIAARTI Study Group for Safety in Anesthesia and Intensive Care. Recommendations for anesthesia and sedation in nonoperating room locations. Minerva Anestesiol 2005; 71: 20.
[2]   Hung YM, Lin SL, Hung SY, Huang WC, Wang PY. Preventing radiocontrast-induced nephropathy in chronic kidney disease patients undergoing coronary angiography. World J Cardiol 2012; 4: 157-72.
[3]   Pahade JK, LeBedis CA, Raptopoulos VD, *et al.* Incidence of contrast-induced nephropathy in patients with multiple myeloma undergoing contrast-enhanced CT. Am J Roentgenol 2011; 196(5): 1094-101.

[4]   Dickinson MC, Kam PCA Intravascular iodinated contrast media and the anaesthetist. Anaesthesia 2008; 63: 626-34.

[5]   Weisbord SD, Palevsky PM. Review Strategies for the prevention of contrast-induced acute kidney injury. Curr Opin Nephrol Hypertens 2010; 19: 539-49.

[6]   McCarthy CS Becker JA. Multiple myeloma and contrast media. Radiology 1992; 183: 519-21.

[7]   Heinrich MC, Häberle L, Müller V, Bautz W, Uder M. Nephrotoxicity of iso-osmolar iodixanol compared with nonionic low-osmolar contrast media: meta-analysis of randomized controlled trials. Radiology 2009; 250: 68-86.

[8]   Shahlaie K, Keachie K Hutchins IM. Risk factors for posttraumatic vasospasm J.Neurosurg 2011; 115: 602-11.

[9]   Reddy U, Smith M. Anesthetic management of endovascular procedures for cerebrovascular atherosclerosis Curr Opin Anaesthesiol 2012; 25: 486-92.

[10]   Hayman MW, Paleologos MS, Kam PC. Interventional neuroradiological procedures - a review for anaesthetists. Anaesth Intensive Care 2013; 41: 184-201.

[11]   Mazzeo AT, Di Pasquale R, Settineri N. Usefulness and limits of near infrared spectroscopy monitoring during endovascular neuradiologic procedures. Minerva Anestesiol 2012; 78: 34-45.

[12]   Schulenburg E, Matta B. Anaesthesia for interventional neuroradiology. Current Opin Anaesthesiol 2011; 24: 426-32.

[13]   Lee CZ, Young WL. Anesthesia for endovascular neurosurgery and interventional neuroradiology Anesthesiol Clin 2012; 30: 127-47.

[14]   Ghisi D, Faneli A, Tosi M. Monitored anesthesia care. Minerva Anestesiol 2005; 71: 533-8.

[15]   American Society of Anesthesiologists. Continuum of depth of sedation definition of general anesthesia and levels of sedation/analgesia. October 27, 2004.

[16]   Miner JR, Moore JC, Plummer D, Gray RO, Patel S, Ho JD. Randomized clinical trial of the effect of supplemental opioids in procedural sedation with propofol on serum catecholamines. Acad Emerg Med 2013; 20: 330-7.

[17]   Jewett J, Phillips WJ. Dexmedetomidine for procedural sedation in the emergency department. Eur J Emerg Med 2010; 17: 60.

[18]   Panzer O, Moitra V, Sladen RN. Pharmacology of sedative-analgesic agents: dexmedetomidine, remifentanil, ketamine, volatile anesthetics, and the role of peripheral Mu antagonists. Anesthesiol Clin 2011; 29: 587-605.

[19]   Pichot C, Ghignone M, Quintin L. Dexmedetomidine and clonidine: from second-to first line sedative agents in the critical care setting. J Intensive Care 2012; 27: 219-37.

[20]   Pumar JM, Banguero A, Arias-Rivas S. The administration of abciximab as a rescue treatment seems safe in cases involving the formation of acute intrastent thromboses. Rev Neurol 2014; 58: 113-6.

[21]   El Beheiry H. Protecting the brain during neurosurgical procedures: strategies that can work. Curr Opin Anesthesiol 2012; 5: 548-55.

[22]   Venkatasubba Rao CP, Suarez JI. Magnesium and neuroprotection in subarachnoid hemorrhage. Lancet 2012; 380: 9-11.

[23]   Wong GK, Boet R, Poon WS, *et al*. Intravenous magnesium sulphate for aneurysmal subarachnoid hemorrhage: an updated systemic review and meta-analysis. Crit Care 2011; 15: R52.

[24]   Ogilvy CS, Yang X, Jamil OA, *et al*. Neurointerventional procedures for unruptured intracranial aneurysms under procedural sedation and local anestesia: a large-volume, single-center experience. J Neurosurg 2011; 114: 120-8.

[25]   Bodily KD, Cloft HJ, Lanzino G, Fiorella DJ, White PM, Kallmes DF. Stent-assisted coiling in acutely ruptured intracranial aneurysm. A review. AJNR Am J Neuroradiol 2011; 32: 1232-6.

[26]   Szajner M, Roman T, *et al*. Onyx in endovascular treatment of cerebral arteriovenous malformations – a review. Acta Neurochir Suppl 2013; 115: 45-8.

[27]   Gandhi D, Chen J, Pearl M, Huang J, Gemmete JJ, Kathuria S. Intracranial arteriovenous fistulas: classification and treatments. AJNR Am J Neuroradiol 2012; 33: 1007-13.

[28]   Lanzino G, D'Urso PI, Kallmes DF. Onyx embolization of extradural spinal arteriovenous malformations Neurosurgery 2012; 70: 329-33.

[29]   Wang AC, Than KD, Etame AB, La Marca F, Park P. Impact of anesthesia on transcranial electric motor evoked potential monitoring during spine surgery: a review of the literature. Neurosurg Focus 2009; 27: E7.

[30]   Derdeyn CP, Chimowitz MI, Lynn MJ, *et al.* Aggressive medical treatment with or without stenting in high-risk patients with intracranial artery stenosis (SAMMPRIS): the final results of a randomised trial. Lancet 2014; 383: 333-41.

[31]   Abou-Chebl A, Krieger DW, Bajzer CT, Yadav JS. Intracranial angioplasty and stenting in the awake patients. J Neuroimaging 2006; 16: 216-23.

[32]   John N, Mitchell P Dowling R Yan B. Is general anaesthesia preferable to conscious sedation in the treatment of acute ischaemic stroke with intra-arterial mechanical thrombectomy? A review of the literature. Neuroradiology 2013; 55: 93-100.

[33]   Brekenheld C, Zhang F Ruiz-Ares G, *et al.* General is better than local anesthesia during endovascular procedures. Stroke 2010; 41: 2716-27.

[34]   Langner S Khaw AV Fretwurst T, Angermaier A, Hosten N, Kirsch M. [Endovascular treatment of acute ischemic stroke under conscious sedation compared to general anesthesia -safety, feasibility and clinical and radiological outcome.] Rofo 2013; 185: 320-7.

[35]   Davis MJ Menon BK Baghirzarda LB, *et al.* The Calgary Stroke Program. Anesthetic management and outcome in patients during endovascular therapy for acute stroke. Anesthesiology 2012; 116: 396-405.

APPENDIX

Dangerous　Extracranial-Intracranial　Anastomoses　-　Vessels　the Neurointerventionalist Needs to Know

Simone Peschillo[1], Antonio Santodirocco[2] and Alessandro Caporlingua[3]

[1]Department of Neurology and Psychiatry, Endovascular Neurosurgery/Interventional Neuroradiology, "Sapienza" University of Rome, Rome, Italy; [2]Department of Neurology and Psychiatry, Interventional Neuroradiology, "Sapienza" University of Rome, Rome, Italy; [3]Department of Neurology and Psychiatry, Neurosurgery, "Sapienza" University of Rome, Rome, Italy

ABBREVIATIONS

ECA	=	External Carotid Artery
ICA	=	Internal Carotid Artery
OA	=	Ophtalmic Artery
MMA	=	Middle Meninegal Artery
IMA	=	Internal Maxillary Artery
STA	=	Superficial Temporal Artery
FA	=	Facial Artery
MHT	=	Meningohypophiseal Trunk
ILT	=	Infero-Lateral Trunk
AMA	=	Accessory Meningeal Artery
SCA	=	Superior Cerebellar Artery
AICA	=	Anteroinferior Cerebellar Artery

The embryologic and phylogenetic development of the cranial and facial arteries links the **external carotid artery (ECA)** to the **internal carotid artery (ICA)** circulations, creating several anastomotic routes that the neurointerventionist needs to keep in mind while doing any intracranial embolization procedure,

Knowledge of cranial nerves arterial supply is also crucial to avoid post-operative cranial nerve palsies.

Connections between the **ECA - ICA** circulations are concentrated in the following anatomic regions:

- ORBITAL REGION (Table **1**);

- PETROUS-CAVERNOUS REGION (Table **2**, **3** and **4**);

- UPPER CERVICAL REGION (Table **5**).

1) ORBITAL REGION (TABLE 1)

Anastomoses between branches of the **ECA,** and the **Ophtalmic Artery (OA)**, branch of the **ICA**. Embolization procedures involving this territory entails a risk of **central retinal artery** occlusion resulting in blindness.

These anastomoses develop as follows:

INTERNAL MAXILLARY ARTERY (IMA) COLLATERALS

Proximal Collaterals

- **Meningo-ophtalmic artery:** remnant of the embriologic stapedial artery, it may take over the entire supply of the ophtalmic artery, resulting in supply to the OA, including central retinal artery and ciliary arteries exclusively from the middle meningeal artery (MMA) from which the meningo-ophtalmic artery originates.

- **MMA:** connections between MMA and its orbital branches and the superficial recurrent meningeal branch of the lacrimal artery and the anterior falcine artery that arises from distal OA.

Distal Collaterals

- **Anterior deep temporal artery** and **Infraorbital artery:** they have anastomoses with the inferior branch of the lacrimal artery of the OA.

- **Sphenopalatine artery:** through the septal arteries it anastomoses with the anterior and posterior ethmoidal arteries originating from the OA.

Cutaneous Collaterals

- **Superficial temporal artery (STA):** connects with the sopraorbital branch of OA.

- **Facial artery (FA):** anastomoses with the dorsal nasal artery of the OA at the angular termination.

2) CAVERNOUS-PETROUS REGION (TABLES 2, 3 and 4)

In this region 3 major anastomotic territories connecting the ECA with the ICA are described. The **petrous, clival** and **cavernous territories.** ICA branches involved in these anstomotic routes are:

- **Petrous territory:** Mandibular artery and caroticotympanic artery

- **Clival territory:** meningohypophyseal trunk (MHT) and lateral clival artery.

- **Cavernous territory:** infero-lateral trunk (ILT)

Tables **2-4** illustrate further details on these vascular connections.

3) UPPER CERVICAL REGION (TABLE 5)

In this region there are anastomoses between the ECA and Vertebral artery, through the following collaterals:

- Occipital artery and Stylomastoid artery

- Ascending pharyngeal collaterals

There are also two anastomotic routes that connect the subclavian artery to the vertebral artery, through the **ascending cervical artery and the deep cervical artery**. When an aberrant origin of the vertebral artery from the thyrocervical or costocervical truck is detected, knowledge of these anastomoses is key to avoid intra-procedural embolic accidents.

CRANIAL NERVE SUPPLY

- **III: Mesencephalic perforators** (Vertebrobasilar system)

  ILT (ICA)

- **IV: Marginal artery of the tentorium cerebelli** (MHT)

  ILT (ICA)

- **V: superior cerebellar artery (SCA), anteroinferior cerebellar artery (AICA) V$_2$: ILT, IMA V$_3$: ILT, AMA**

  MMA, Ascending Pharyngeal Artery

  ILT

- VII, VIII: AICA

- IX, X: Neuromeningeal Trunk

- XI: Cervical arteries, muscolospinal branch of Ascending pharingeal artery

- XII: Neuromeningeal trunk

Table 1.   Anastomoses of the orbital region. An extreme anatomic variation not displayed in this table is the meningo-ophtalmic artery, remnant of the stapedial artery (embryologic connection between ICA/ECA), which may takes over the entire supply of the ophtalmic artery territory.

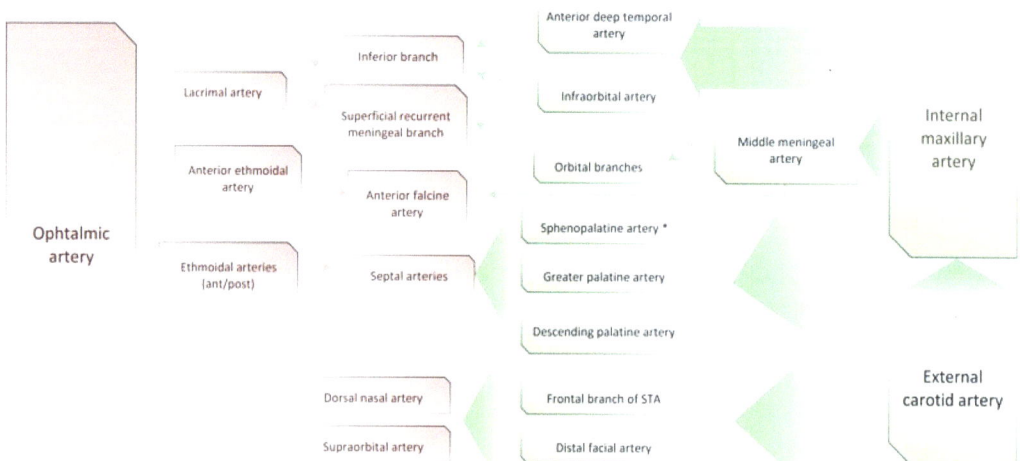

*When embolization of the sphenopalatine artery is required (i.e. epistaxis) particles >80 μm are recommended (septal arteries diameter is <80 μm).

Table 2.   Anastomotic routes in the petrous region.

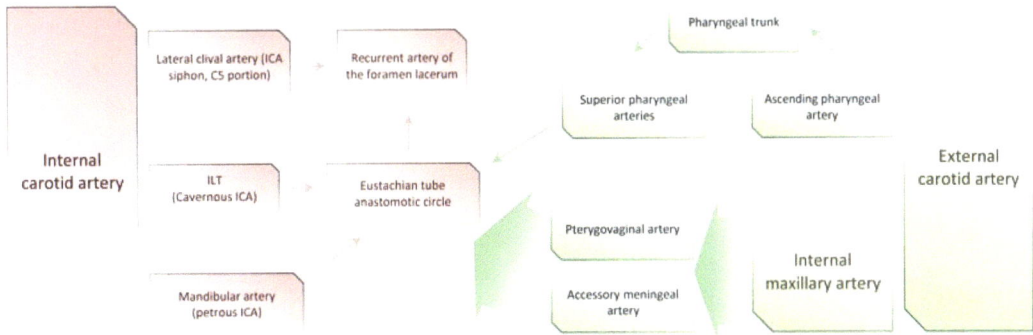

Table 3.   Anastomoses in the clival region.

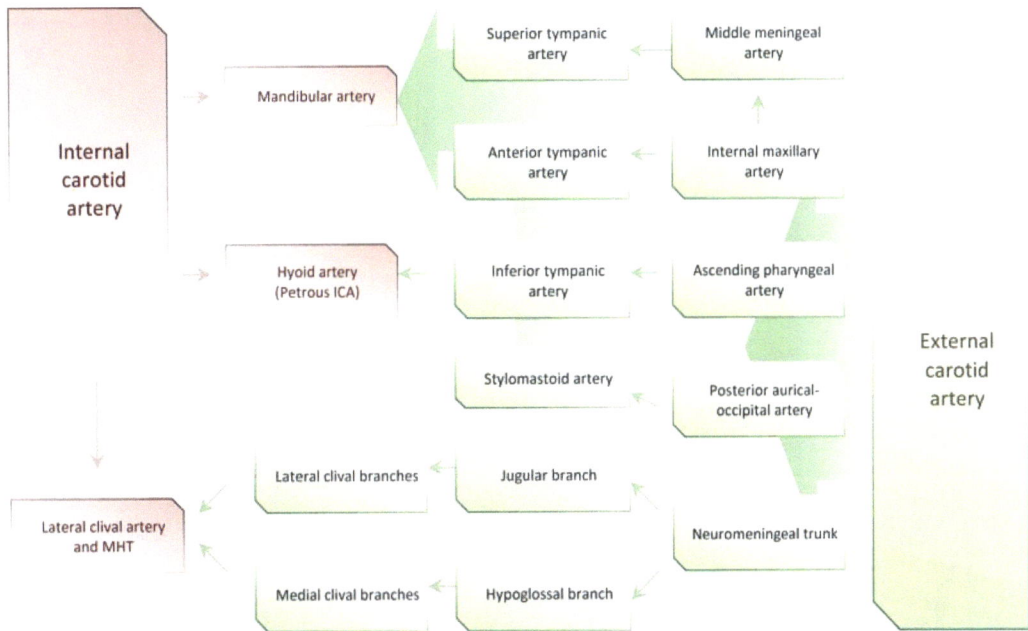

Table 4.   Anastomotic routes in the cavernous region.

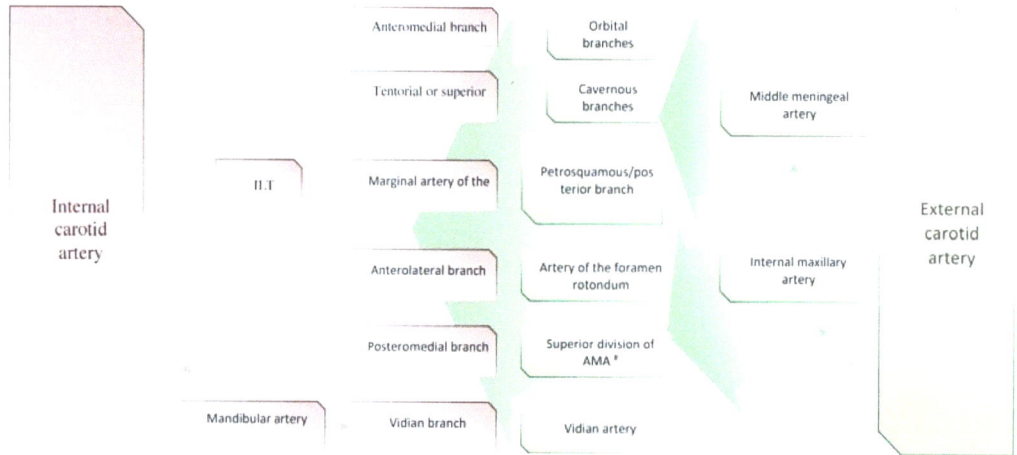

*The marginal artery of the tentorium may originate from the ophtalmic artery or the MHT of the ICA. #In 20% cases the AMA may take over the entire supply of the ILT territory.

Table 5.   Anastomoses in the cervical region.

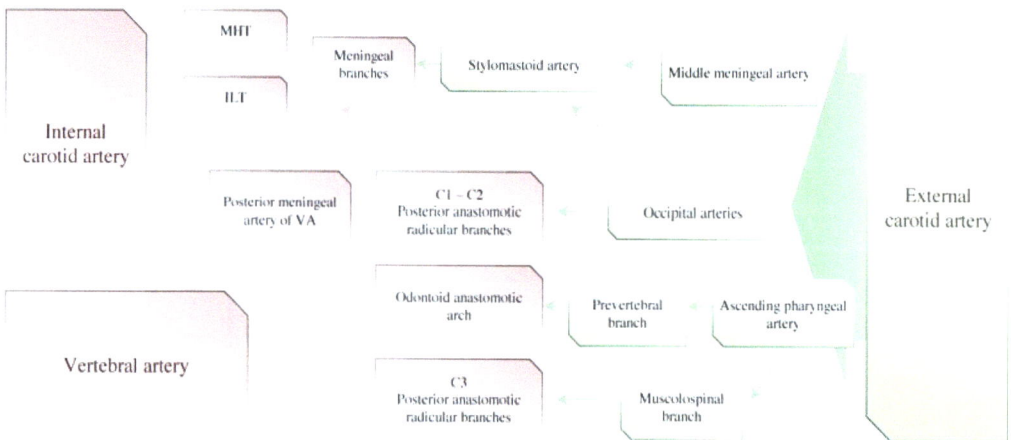

Subject Index

A

Abciximab 145, 215, 242

Accessory meningeal artery (AMA) 46-47, 62, 183, 190-91, 195, 199

ACE catheter 173

Activation, metabolic 214, 217, 219

Acute coronary syndrome (ACS) 217-19, 222-23

Acute ischemic stroke 139-40, 142-43, 145, 154-55, 174, 233, 248

ADP-induced platelet activation 217

ADP-induced platelet aggregation 226-27

ADP receptor 214-15, 217

Agents 113, 219, 241-42, 244
 endogenous lytic 186, 188-89

Alcohol, polyvinyl 159, 184-85

Analgesia 216, 240, 41, 248, 49

Anastomoses 39, 45, 54, 104, 107-9, 112, 124, 184, 188, 193, 198

Anesthesia 88, 232, 234, 237, 244, 248

Anesthesiologist 113, 232-33, 237-39, 242-43, 250

Anesthetic technique 237-39

Anesthetists 233, 239, 242, 244

Aneurysmal sac 7, 12-14, 24, 94, 101-4, 111

Aneurysm balloon-remodeling 213

Aneurysm cavity 169

Aneurysm coiling 154, 159, 161, 170

Aneurysm neck 25-26, 101, 113, 115, 154, 161-62, 164-69

Aneurysm occlusion 25, 163
 efficient 162

Aneurysms 4-8, 13-14, 17, 20, 26, 54, 58, 70, 74-75, 78, 94-96, 101-3, 109, 112-17, 121, 127, 154, 159, 161-64, 190, 243-44
 anterior cerebral artery 13
 basilar artery 15
 berry 13, 15, 17
 bleeding berry 14
 cervical carotid artery 5
 common carotid artery 23
 communicating artery 8
 endovascular treatment of 245
 false symptomatic popliteal 5
 intracavernous 41, 58
 intranidal 70, 125
 large-necked 24
 large ophthalmic artery 116
 management of 5, 7, 94
 midbasilar artery 113
 patient's 6

 small-necked 24
 spinal 133
 terminal-type 25-26
 venous 70
 wide-necked 17, 25

Aneurysm sac 13, 17, 110, 159, 163, 168

Aneurysm stenting 213

Aneurysm treatment 165

Angioarchitecture 33, 126-27, 136

Angiogram 53, 55, 169

Angiography 3, 10-11, 27, 38, 56-58, 77-78, 86-87, 95, 111-13, 115-16, 126, 129, 132, 147, 180, 185, 188, 191-93, 200, 233-34, 243
 green 86-87
 post-treatment 77

Angioplasty 145, 148-51, 170, 249

Annual mortality risk 34, 74-75

Anterior circulation 95, 117, 146

Anterior cranial fossa 36, 51-52, 54-55

Anterior meningeal artery 52, 54

Anterograde 35

Antiaggregation therapy 213

Anticoagulation 43, 212-13, 235

Antiplatelet agents 170, 217, 223, 241-42, 245, 247

Antiplatelet drugs 211-12, 214-15, 228, 238

Antiplatelet therapy 145, 211-12, 223

Antiplatelet treatment 219

Antiplatelet treatment evaluation 226

Antiplatelet treatments target 215

Anxiolysis 240-41

Arachidonic acid 224-25, 227

Arachnoid 121

Area, eloquent cerebral 84

Arterial aneurysms 4, 131
 unrelated 71

Arterial bifurcations 14-15, 19, 114

Arterial branches 18, 36, 191
 perforating 114-15

Arterial feeders 37-38, 40, 60, 68, 74, 129, 135, 190, 192, 195, 199

Arterial grafts 105, 108

Arterial ligation 3, 5, 115

Arterial pressure 122, 234, 239, 243, 245, 249

Arterial steal 125, 131-32

Arterioles 33-34

Arteriovenous fistulas 33, 54, 62
 direct 33, 53, 60
 giant spinal cord dural 125
 intracranial dural 246

www.ingramcontent.com/pod-product-compliance
Lightning Source LLC
Chambersburg PA
CBHW050819220326
41598CB00006B/254